AF147141

Desmopressin in Bleeding Disorders

NATO ASI Series

Advanced Science Institutes Series

A series presenting the results of activities sponsored by the NATO Science Committee, which aims at the dissemination of advanced scientific and technological knowledge, with a view to strengthening links between scientific communities.

The series is published by an international board of publishers in conjunction with the NATO Scientific Affairs Division

A	**Life Sciences**	Plenum Publishing Corporation
B	**Physics**	New York and London
C	**Mathematical and Physical Sciences**	Kluwer Academic Publishers
D	**Behavioral and Social Sciences**	Dordrecht, Boston, and London
E	**Applied Sciences**	
F	**Computer and Systems Sciences**	Springer-Verlag
G	**Ecological Sciences**	Berlin, Heidelberg, New York, London,
H	**Cell Biology**	Paris, Tokyo, Hong Kong, and Barcelona
I	**Global Environmental Change**	

Recent Volumes in this Series

Volume 239—The Mammalian Cochlear Nuclei: Organization and Function
edited by Miguel A. Merchán, José M. Juiz, Donald A. Godfrey, and Enrico Mugnaini

Volume 240—Regulation of Gene Expression in Animal Viruses
edited by Luis Carrasco, Nahum Sonenberg, and Eckard Wimmer

Volume 241—Iodine Deficiency in Europe: A Continuing Concern
edited by F. Delange, J.T. Dunn, and D. Glinoer

Volume 242—Desmopressin in Bleeding Disorders
edited by G. Mariani, P. M. Mannucci, and M. Cattaneo

Volume 243A—Biological Effects and Physics of Solar and Galactic Radiation, Part A
edited by Charles E. Swenberg, Gerda Horneck, and E. G. Stassinopoulos

Volume 243B—Biological Effects and Physics of Solar and Galactic Radiation, Part B
edited by Charles E. Swenberg, Gerda Horneck, and E. G. Stassinopoulos

Volume 244—Forest Development in Cold Climates
edited by John Alden, J. Louise Mastrantonio, and Søren Ødum

Series A: Life Sciences

Desmopressin in Bleeding Disorders

Edited by

G. Mariani

University of Rome "La Sapienza"
Rome, Italy

P. M. Mannucci and M. Cattaneo

University of Milan
Milan, Italy

Springer Science+Business Media, LLC

Proceedings of a NATO Advanced Research Workshop on
Desmopressin in Bleeding Disorders,
held April 27–30, 1992,
in Il Ciocco, Tuscany, Italy

NATO-PCO-DATA BASE

The electronic index to the NATO ASI Series provides full bibliographical references (with keywords and/or abstracts) to more than 30,000 contributions from international scientists published in all sections of the NATO ASI Series. Access to the NATO-PCO-DATA BASE is possible in two ways:

—via online FILE 128 (NATO-PCO-DATA BASE) hosted by ESRIN, Via Galileo Galilei, I-00044 Frascati, Italy

—via CD-ROM "NATO-PCO-DATA BASE" with user-friendly retrieval software in English, French, and German (©WTV GmbH and DATAWARE Technologies, Inc. 1989)

The CD-ROM can be ordered through any member of the Board of Publishers or through NATO-PCO, Overijse, Belgium.

Library of Congress Cataloging in Publication Data

Desmopressin in bleeding disorders / edited by G. Mariani, P.M. Mannucci, and M. Cattaneo.
p. cm. — (NATO ASI series; Series A. Life sciences; vol. 242)
"Proceedings of a NATO Advanced Research Workshop on Desmopressin in Bleeding Disorders, held April 27–30, 1992, in Il Ciocco, Tuscany, Italy"—T.p. verso.
"Published in cooperation with NATO Scientific Affairs Division."
Includes bibliographical references and index.
ISBN 978-0-306-44414-2
1. Desmopressin—Therapeutic use—Congresses. 2. Hemorrhagic diseases—Chemotherapy—Congresses. I. Mariani, Guglielmo. II. Mannucci, P.M. (Pier Mannuccio) III. Cattaneo, Marco. IV. North Atlantic Treaty Organization. Scientific Affairs Division. V. NATO Advanced Research Workshop on Desmopressin in Bleeding Disorders (1992; Il Ciocco, Italy) VI. Series.
[DNLM: 1. Desmopressin—pharmacology—congresses. 2. Desmopressin—therapeutic use—congresses. 3. Hemostasis—drug effects—congresses. 4. Hemophilia—drug therapy—congresses. 5. Von Willebrand's Disease—drug therapy—congresses. QV 160 D464 1993]
RC633.D47 1993
615'.718—dc20
DNLM/DLC
for Library of Congress 93-13097
CIP

ISBN 978-0-306-44414-2 ISBN 978-1-4615-2922-4 (eBook)
DOI 10.1007/978-1-4615-2922-4

Originally published by Plenum Press, New York 1993

PREFACE

Before the introduction of DDAVP, central diabetes insipidus was treated by the administration of a more or less purified extract from bovine or porcine posterior pituitaries, and the preparations were mostly given in the form of nasal snuff.

In 1956, the structure of vasopressin became known and two forms were found, namely arginine vasopressin (AVP) in humans and most other species, and lysine vasopressin (LVP) which was found in the pig.

In 1967, Zaoral et al. were the first to synthesize 1-desamino-8-D-arginine vasopressin, DDAVP. In comparison with the compounds which were previously available, DDAVP offered increased antidiuretic potency and an equally distinct shift of the antidiuretic to pressor potency ratio.

As a result of the pioneering studies of Cash and Mannucci, numerous publications appeared in the medical literature of the 80's, widening the fields of clinical application of the drug.

A very important aspect of this drug is that it can be used as an alternative treatment for mild factor VIII deficiencies, mild hemophilia A and von Willebrand's disease. These congenital deficiencies are far from rare and have, up to now, been treated with plasma-derived factor VIII concentrates; in the countries in which desmopressin has not been used a consistent proportion of these patients have seroconverted for HIV1 and hepatitis.

This drug is to be considered of great interest in the developing countries. The World Federation of Hemophilia has, in a recent meeting, defined Desmopressin as the "first recommended drug in mild factor VIII deficiencies", which are far more frequent than severe hemophilia A cases. Other indications, such as acquired and congenital platelet defects and some surgical situations, have subsequently emerged.

Though a great deal of progress has been made in the last decade, several questions have remained unanswered. These concern, among other aspects, the drug's mechanisms of action, the efficacy of the different routes of administration, the therapeutic protocols, and its interaction with other drugs.

The aim of this workshop was to collect an ample mass of data from different specialists, to foster discussion among them and to form a consensus on treatment protocols and indications.

G. Mariani

ACKNOWLEDGEMENTS

The workshop was organized under the patronage of the World Federation of Haemophilia to whom the editors would like to extend their thanks.

It was made possible by the financial and organizational support of the Scientific Affairs Division of N.A.T.O.

Alma Derivati S.p.A. and Sclavo S.p.A. should also be thanked for their additional assistance in the organization and in the financing of the workshop.

Finally thanks are due to Mr. David Holmes for his assistance with the preparation of the manuscript of this publication.

CONTENTS

I. HEMOSTASIS AND DESMOPRESSIN

II. PHEMACOLOGY AND PHARMACODYNAMICS OF DESMOPRESSIN

III. DESMOPRESSIN IN RENAL DISEASE

IV. DESMOPRESSIN AND PLATELETS

V. DESMOPRESSIN AND SURGERY

VI. DESMOPRESSIN AND BLOOD DONATION

VII CLINICAL APPLICATIONS OF DESMOPRESSIN IN HEMOPHILIA AND von WILLEBRAND'S DISEASE
(First Part)

REGULATION OF HAEMOSTASIS:

THE ROLE OF ARGININE VASOPRESSIN

P.J. Grant

Academic Unit of Medicine
Martin Wing
The General Infirmary at Leeds
Leeds, LS1 3EX, UK

INTRODUCTION

The posterior pituitary stores the peptide hormone 8-Arginine vasopressin and secretes it in response to osmoregulatory stimulii, changes in blood volume and various physical stresses.

The major physiological action of vasopressin lies in the area of renal water homeostasis. Under certain circumstances, the levels of vasopressin seen in the circulation are much above those for a maximal renal effect. Evidence has accumulated to indicate that at these higher levels vasopressin has additional effects on other systems, notably the coagulation and fibrinolytic pathways and various vascular beds. High physiological concentrations of vasopressin, such as occur in response to surgery, hypotension or nausea, are associated with increases in factor VIII coagulant activity, von Willebrand factor and fibrinolytic activity. Vasopressin seems to have a role in the physiology of haemostasis under certain conditions, particularly associated with physical stress. The significance of these effects in relation to the pathogenesis of vascular disorders is uncertain.

THE PHYSIOLOGY OF VASOPRESSIN SYNTHESIS AND SECRETION

Although the original anatomical description of the hypophysis cerebri was made by Galen[1], there was relatively little advance in knowledge about the pituitary until the advent of light microscopy allowed Rathke to study its anatomical development.[2] The pituitary gland is divided into the anterior lobe, the intermediate lobe and the posterior lobe (posterior pituitary) which is connected to the hypothalamus by the infundibular stalk. The dominant features of the neurohypophysis (hypothalamic - neural stalk - posterior pituitary unit) are the supra-opticohypopyseal and paraventriculohypophyseal nerve tracts. Originating from magnocellular neurons in the paraventricular and supra-optic nucleii within the hypothalamus, these tracts pass through the neural stalk to terminate as dilated endings on capillaries of the hypophyseal portal system within the posterior pituitary.

Desmopressin in Bleeding Disorders, Edited by G. Mariani *et al.*
Plenum Press, New York, 1993

Vasopressin is a nonapeptide ring structure that is produced by the neurons of the supra-optic and paraventricular nucleii in the hypothalamus.[3] The neurosecretory granules migrate down the axons of the tracts at rates of 200 mm per day before storage in the nerve endings. Phasic firing of the nerve bodies stimulates secretion of free vasopressin. Vasopressin in plasma passes freely through peripheral and glomerular capillary membranes and is rapidly distributed in the extracellular space.[4] The half-life of aVP in the plasma is of the order of 5-6 min.[5] In humans, total clearance of aVP, representing metabolic clearance and renal excretion produces a biological half-life of approximately 30 min. Suppression of aVP leads to a change from the antidiuretic state in 30-40 minutes.[4]

Two varieties of peripheral vasopressin receptors have been identified; the 'V_1' receptor on smooth muscle and the 'V_2' receptors in renal epithelia. Only the latter receptors activate adenylate cyclase.[6] V_1 receptor stimulation causes a rise in cytosolic Ca^{++} concentration via an increase in membrane phosphatidylinositol turnover, generally producing contraction in vascular smooth muscle and glycogenolysis in hepatocytes.

PHYSIOLOGICAL CONTROL MECHANISMS FOR VASOPRESSIN SECRETION

Maintenance of blood water concentrations and plasma osmolality is probably the major homeostatic function of the neurohypophysis. Under normal conditions of hydration, the kidney is maximally stimulated to conserve water at plasma aVP concentrations of 1-5 pg/ml.[7] Plasma osmolality is normally set at approximately 282 mOsm/Kg and a rise to 287 mOsm/Kg initiates release of aVP which thereafter increases rapidly with rising osmolality.[8] Water loading suppresses aVP release.

Decrease in blood volume or pressure both produce significant increases in circulating levels of plasma vasopressin.[8] Under normal conditions, osmolality is the prime determinant of aVP release, however during hypotension the osmotic set point is altered so that minor changes in osmolality cause increased secretion of aVP. With severe loss of blood volume the osmotic control is overridden and massive increments in aVP may occur without marked changes in osmolality.[9]

Early experiments on water regulation in dogs indicated that emotional stress might increase aVP secretion. Robertson has shown, however, that this is not the case.[8] Physical stress, however, is commonly associated with increased aVP secretion and this response appears to be independent of osmolality and volume control. Apomorphine-induced nausea causes increments of aVP of up to 500 pg/ml[8] and the area postrema in the wall of the IVth ventricle is thought to mediate this response.[10] Insulin- induced hypoglycaemia produces small increments of aVP, up to 8 pg/ml, although the area in the brain responsible for this response is unknown. Baylis et al concluded that this might be due to the effect of insulin[11] which has been shown to bind to the nucleus tractus solitairius and the area postrema.[12] Major surgical procedures are associated with marked increments in plasma aVP concentrations that closely follow skin incision and bowel traction.[13]This was thought to be mediated by pain rather than through volume receptors, as the response was abolished by cervical cordotomy, but unaffected by vagotomy. There is, however, evidence to suggest that pain does not stimulate aVP release [14] and other work has suggested that the response of aVP during operations is in fact mediated by volume and pressure receptors. [15]

VASOPRESSIN AND HAEMOSTASIS

Coagulation and Fibrinolysis . The coagulation and fibrinolytic systems are two separate, but interlinked enzyme pathways that act to regulate the production and breakdown of fibrin. The coagulation system consists of a series of reactions that have been described as a 'cascade'[16] or 'waterfall'[17] that ultimately terminate in the conversion of fibrinogen to fibrin. The demonstration that blood in the absence of tissue factor was able to generate pro-coagulant activity led to the concept of an intrinsic pathway.[18]

In this model, activated factor XII initiates a sequence of reactions through factors IX, XI and X to convert prothrombin to thrombin. Factor VIII coagulant protein (FVIII:C) has an important role as a cofactor in this process as demonstrated by the bleeding disorder associated with haemophilia. Factor VIII exists in the circulation as a complex of FVIII:C and von Willebrand factor, the latter taking part in platelet- subendothelial binding and acting to protect FVIII:C in the circulation. In contrast the extrinsic pathway is initiated by tissue factor which activates factor VII. Factor VII can act directly on factor X, but an alternative pathway through factor IX and the intrinsic pathway has recently been described.[19]

The fibrinolytic system counteracts the activity of the coagulation cascade in that it is concerned with the regulation of generation of plasmin which acts to breakdown crosslinked fibrin. The conversion of plasminogen to plasmin occurs by the action of two biochemically distinct plasminogen activators (PA's), tissue-type PA (t-PA) and urokinase.[20] The activity of t-PA and u-PA are in turn regulated by circulating inhibitors of which PA inhibitor-1 (PAI-1) is considered to be the most important. A second inhibitor (PAI-2) has been described in relation to pregnancy, but there is little evidence that it has a major role in the regulation of fibrinolysis in other circumstances. Evidence exists to indicate that PAI-1 has an important role in the development of vascular disease. Work from Hamsten et al[21] has described higher levels of PAI-1 in young survivors of myocardial infarction who go on to have further vascular events. PAI- 1 concentrations are elevated in a number of conditions associated with vascular disorders including type 2 diabetes mellitus, obesity and after major surgery.[22,23] The regulation of PAI-1 has been of considerable interest with evidence from population studies [24,25] and in-vitro work[26,27] that insulin may have important effects. This has not yet been supported by studies of the direct effect of insulin in vivo.[28,29] In-vitro studies indicate that many of the growth factors such as platelet derived growth factor and insulin-like growth factor-1 may increase PAI- 1.[30] Similarly cytokines such as tumour necrosis factor and interleukin-1 suppress cell mediated fibrinolysis by induction of PAI-1 synthesis and secretion.[31,32]

Physical stress such as occurs in response to surgery, hypoglycaemia, exercise and hypotension has been known for many years to cause changes in coagulation and fibrinolysis. The original observations linking hormones to these responses were made in the early part of this century and formed the basis of the idea that adrenergic mechanisms are responsible.[33,34] The major changes seen during stress are increases in factor VIII coagulation activity (FVIII:C), von Willebrand factor (vWF) and enhanced fibrinolytic activity. In the circulation the factor VIII molecule exists as a complex of FVIII:C and vWF. FVIII:C acts as a co-factor in the intrinsic coagulation cascade and deficiency of this protein is the primary defect in classical haemophilia. VWF takes part in platelet-subendothelial binding and deficiency of vWF occurs in von WIllebrands disease. The fibrinolytic system consists of activators and inhibitors that regulate the conversion of plasminogen to plasmin which acts to lyse fibrin. The principal activators of plasminogen are tissue plasminogen activator (t-PA) and urokinase (u-PA), whilst the most important inhibitor of t-PA and u-PA is PA inhibitor-1 (PAI-1).

In 1961 Schneck and von Kaulla showed that intravenous pitressin (a mixture of arginine and lysine vasopressin) caused an increase in plasminogen activator activity, and attributed this to the vasoconstrictive actions of aVP.[35] Similar results were obtained with pharmacological doses of aVP[36,37] but it was suggested that the increase in plasminogen activator could be a non-specific response as it appeared to correlate with the severity of side effects, notably abdominal pain. The discovery that the synthetic analogue, DDAVP, produced increases in factor VIII:C, vWF:Ag and plasminogen activator,[38] yet produced no abdominal pain and had a lack of vasoconstrictive effects suggested the existence of specific receptors for vasopressin on vascular endothelial cells. The effects of DDAVP on coagulation and fibrinolysis and its relative lack of side effects led to its clinical use and a rapid decline in interest in the parent molecule. The pharmacological effects of DDAVP have been recently reviewed.[39]

Although it was thought that the levels of aVP required to affect coagulation and fibrinolysis were too high to be of any physiological significance, the development of sensitive radioimmunoassays for this peptide has led to studies that indicate this may not be the case. Infusion of aVP into normal volunteers has shown that increases in fibrinolysis occur at plasma concentrations of about 15-20 pg/ml[40] and in FVIII:C and vWF at 20-25 pg/ml.[40,41] The increase in fibrinolytic activity is due to a rise in t-PA rather than a fall in PAI-1.[42] Although such levels of aVP are not seen under normal circumstances, they are within the range that occur during various forms of physical stress and the results support the idea that in specific conditions, aVP may have a role in the regulation of coagulation and fibrinolysis.

Further studies of the relationship between aVP and changes in haemostasis have been hampered by the lack of availability of a specific aVP receptor blocker for use in man. However, during major abdominal surgery increases in aVP to median values of 51 pg/ml immediately after bowel manipulation were temporally associated with increases in both FVIII:C and fibrinolytic activity.[43] A similar relationship was observed during hip surgery.[44] The study of insulin induced hypoglycaemia[45] and apomorphine induced nausea[46] highlighted some of the problems in presuming that these temporal relationships indicated cause and effect. During hypoglycaemia, similar changes in haemostasis occur, yet the increase in aVP is insufficent to have an effect. Additionally, during both hypoglycaemia and nausea there was a parallel increase in adrenaline concentrations which could have been responsible for the observed changes. In order to tease out the effects of aVP from those of adrenaline, two further studies were carried out in which adrenaline release does not occur. In a study of the effects of modified ECT there were increases in aVP levels associated with enhanced fibrinolytic activity, but no change in either adrenaline or FVIII concentrations.[47] These results suggest that aVP has only a minor role in the regulation of FVIII and that it is more important in fibrinolytic responses. To support this view, similar results were obtained in the study of patients with rare forms of autonomic failure and their responses to postural hypotension.[48] Patients with Shy-Drager syndrome release neither adrenaline nor aVP in response to hypotension, whereas in Progressive Autonomic Failure (PAF), aVP is released normally and there is no adrenaline response. Results from this study, in albeit a small number of patients, showed that postural hypotension in Shy-Drager syndrome led to no change in adrenaline, aVP, FVIII or fibrinolysis whereas in PAF, the rise in aVP was associated with marked increases in fibrinolysis, but no change in adrenaline or FVIII.

The mechanisms by which aVP exerts its effect on haemostasis remain unclear. It was initially considered that aVP caused an effect through its vasoactive properties, although the similar haemostatic effects of DDAVP argue against this view. Cash et al and Prowse et al have studied the structural requirements for the factor VIII and plasminogen activator responses to aVP. By using analogues of aVP they concluded that the whole molecule was required for both FVIII and plasminogen activator release and the putative receptor could be differentiated from that on smooth muscle. On a molar basis aVP was found to be 80 times as potent as adrenaline for its effect on fibrinolytic responses. In addition intra arterial infusion with venous sampling produced significant increases in plasminogen activator with adrenaline but had no effect with aVP.[49,50] Adrenaline releases vWF:Ag fron endothelial cell cultures,[51] but aVP has not been shown to act directly to release either factor VIII:C or vWF:Ag.[52] At present there is no evidence to suggest that the haemostatic effects of vasopressin are mediated by a direct effect on endothelial cells. It has been proposed that vasopressin might act by releasing a second messenger from the hypothalamus which acts directly on endothelial cells to produce changes in haemostasis.[52] Alternatively, vasopressin may act on one or more organs, such as the liver or kidney, distinct from vascular endothelial cells. It is also possible that aVP interacts in some way with catecholamines as there is a complex, partially understood relationship between autonomic function and aVP release. Although aVP does not increase catecholamine concentrations in peripheral blood[53] it is possible that an effect occurs either centrally or that adrenaline and vasopressin act synergistically.

ADRENALINE AND HAEMOSTASIS

The initial observation that catecholamines might have a role in the control of haemostatic function was made by Vosburgh and Richards in 1903 when they noticed acceleration of blood clotting after giving adrenaline to dogs[33]. This observation was confirmed and extensively investigated in a series of classical experiments by WB Cannon and associates at the beginning of the First World War.[34] The effect of adrenaline infusions and splanchnic circulation were investigated under various conditions in anaethetised cats. From these experiments Cannon et al concluded that the effect of adrenaline on blood coagulation was dose-dependent, that adrenaline had to circulate through the abdominal viscera, thus implicating a 'hepatic factor' which was released into the circulation, and that the integrity of the splanchnic nerves were vital in producing the effect on coagulation. These findings produced much of the early knowledge on which later theories regarding the hormonal control of haemostasis were based. Further comprehensive studies on the effect of adrenaline on coagulation were to wait until 1957 when Forwell and Ingram published work confirming the findings of Cannon and also demonstrating that adrenaline infusions in man produced a consistent reduction in the coagulation time.[54] They attributed this finding to an effect of adrenaline on factor V concentrations in the plasma. The observation that adrenaline infusions in man produced increases in the factor VIII complex[55] led to an investigation into the effects of alpha and beta- receptor blockade. Ingram and Vaughan Jones demonstrated that the increase following adrenaline infusion was blocked by propranolol but unaffected by phentolamine.[56] From this they concluded that the effect of adrenaline on the FVIII complex was mediated by beta-receptors. Subsequent reports that the rise in FVIII:C during insulin-induced hypoglycaemia could be blocked by prior treatment with propranolol[57] tended to confirm the view that adrenaline was a major mediator of haemostatic function under conditions of stress.

The role of adrenergic mechanisms in the control of fibrinolysis is, however, less certain. Cash et al investigated the systemic plasminogen activator response to adrenaline infusions in normal subjects, with and without, prior ß-blockade.[58] They reported marked increases in plasminogen activator following adrenaline infusion, a response that was only partially reduced (by 26%) by prior treatment with propranolol, a $ß_2$- receptor blocker, and unaffected by a $ß_1$ blocker. They postulated the existence of two separate adrenergic pathways for plasminogen activator, one of which is unaffected by $ß_2$ blockade. Cohen et al[59] reported, however, that prior $ß_2$-receptor blockade with propranolol had no effect on the plasminogen activator response to exercise and it has been demonstrated that the rise in adrenaline during exercise occurs after the increase in fibrinolysis.[60] Thus, although adrenergic mechanisms seem to have a role in the regulation of fibrinolysis, there is evidence to suggest the existence of other stimulatory pathways, perhaps involving other hormones.

CONCLUSION

The nonapeptide antidiuretic hormone, 8-Arginine vasopressin, acts potently on the kidney to conserve water at low plasma concentrations. Plasma levels above those required for a maximal renal effect are commonly seen during various forms of physical stress and have been shown to modulate a number of physiological systems. Amongst these are changes in coagulation and fibrinolysis with vasoactive effects on the microcirculation.

The significance of the changes in haemostasis remain unclear, although there is reason to believe that the acute increase in factor VIII may produce a tendency to a hypercoaguable state. The increase in systemic fibrinolytic activity may have a role in protecting the intact circulation from developing distant thrombosis in the event of local tissue injury. Further hamostatic regulation would be acheived by the generally vasoconstrictive effects of aVP in the skin microcirculation. The actions of higher levels of aVP may prepare the organism for the classic fight or flight response by redistributing cardiac output and activating the haemostatic systems. In this context, it is possible that whilst at low concentrations aVP acts as the antidiuretic hormone, at higher levels aVP could function as an "antihaemmorrhagic" hormone to maintain vascular integrity in the event of injury.

REFERENCES

1. W.L.H. Duckworth. "Galen on Anatomical Procedures, the Later Books." Translation M.C. Lyons, B. Towerts, eds., Cambridge University Press (1962).

2. M.H. Rathke, Uber die Enstehung der Glandula pituitaria, *Ar. Anat. Phys.* 4:483-485 (1838).

3. H. Sachs, P. Fawcett, Y. Takabatake, R. Portanova, Biosynthesis and release of vasopressin and neurophysin, *Recent Prog. Horm. Res.* 25:447-484 (1969).

4. G. Bauman, J.F. Dingman, Distribution, blood transport, and degradation of antidiuretic hormone in man, *J. Clin. Invest.* 57:1109-1116 (1976).

5. M. Fabian, M.L. Forsling, J.J. Jones, S.S. Pryor, The clearance and antidiuretic potency of neurohypophyseal hormones in man, and their plasma binding and stability, *J. Physiol.* 204:653-668 (1969).

6. W.H. Sawyer, M. Manning, Effective antiagonists of the antidiuretic action of vasopressin in rats, *Ann. N.Y. Acad. Sci.* 394:464-472 (1982).

7. T.H. Thomas, M.R. Lee MR, The specificity of antisera for the radioimmunoassay of arginine vasopressin in himan plasma and urine during water loading, *Clin. Sci. Mol. Med.* 51:525-36 (1976).

8. G.L. Robertson, Functional and morphological aspects of hypothalamic neurons, *Physiol. Rev.* 57:574-658 (1977).

9. F.L. Dunn, T.J. Brennan, A.E. Nelson, G.L. Robertson, The role of blood osmolality and volume in regulating vasopressin secretion in the blood, *J. Clin. Invest.* 52:212- 219 (1973).

10. K.L. Barnes, C.M. Ferrario, Anatomical and physiological characterisation of the sympathofacilitative area postrema pathways in the dog, in: "Central nervous system mechanisms in hypertension", J.P. Buckely, C.M. Ferrario CM eds., Raven Press, New York, (1981).

11. P.H. Baylis, R.L. Zerbe, G.L. Robertson, Arginine vasopressin response to insulin induced hypoglycaemia in man, *J. Clin. Endocrinol. Metab.* 53(5):935-40 (1981).

12. M. Van Houten, B.I. Posner, B.M. Kopriwa, J.R. Brawer, Insulin binding sites in the rat brain: in vivo localisation to the circumventricular organs by quantitative radioautography, *Endocrinology* 105:666-673 (1979).

13. W.H. Moran, B. Zimmerman, Mechanisms of antidiuretic hormone (ADH) control of importance to the surgical patient, *Surgery* 62:639-644 (1967).

14. T.C. Brennan, R.L. Shelton, G.L. Robertson, Effects of stress on plasma vasopressin and corticosterone in rats, *Clin.Res.* 23:234A (1975).

15. J.S.P. Cochrane, M.L. Forsling, N. Menzies Gow, L.P. Le Quesne, Arginine vasopressin release following surgical operations, *Br. J. Surg.* 68:209-213 (1981).

16. R.G. MacFarlane, An enzyme cascade in the blood clotting mechanism, and its function as a biochemical amplifier, *Nature* 202:498-499 (1964).

17. E.W. Davie, O.D. Ratnoff, Waterfall sequence for intrinsic blood clotting, *Science* 145:1310-1312 (1964).

18. R. Biggs, A.S. Douglas, R.G. MacFarlane, The formation of thromboplastin on human blood, *J. Physiol.* 119:89-101 (1953).

19. M. Berrettini, B. Lammle, J.H. Griffin, Initiation of coagulation and relationships between intrinsic and extrinsic coagulation pathways, in: "Thrombosis and Haemostasis", M. Verstraete, J. Vermylen, R. Lijnen, J. Arnout, eds., Leuven University Press (1987).

20. O. Saksela, Plasminogen activation and the regulation of pericellular proteolysis, *Biochim. Biophys. Acta.* 823:35-65 (1985).

21. A. Hamsten, U. De Faire, G. Walldius, G. Dahlén, A. Szamosi, C. Landou et al, Plasminogen activator inhibitor in plasma: risk factor for recurrent myocardial infarction, *Lancet* iv:3-9 (1987).

22. P.J. Grant, M.H. Stickland, N.A. Booth, C.R.M. Prentice, Metformin causes a reduction in basal and post-venous occlusion plasminogen activator inhibitor-1 in type 2 diabetic patients, *Diabetic Med.* 8:361-365 (1991).

23. E.K.O. Kruithof, A. Gudinchet, F. Bachman, Plasminogen activator inhibitor 1 and plasminogen activator inhibitor 2 in various disease states, *Thromb. Haemostas.* 59:7-12 (1988).

24. I. Juhan-Vague, P. Vague, M.C. Alessi, C. Badier, J. Valadier, M.F. Aillaud, Relationships between plasma insulin, triglyceride, body mass index and plasminogen activator inhibitor 1, *Diabete Metabol.* 13:331-336 (1987).

25. P. Vague, I. Juhan-Vague, M.F. Aillaud, C. Badier, R. Viard, M.C. Alessi, et al, Correlation between blood fibrinolytic activity, plasminogen activator inhibitor level, plasma insulin level and relative body weight in normal and obese subjects, *Metabolism* 2:250-253 (1986).

26. T. Kooistra, P.J. Bosma, H.A.M. Tons, A.P. van den Berg, P. Meyer, H.M.G. Princen, Plasminogen activator inhibitor 1: Biosynthesis and mRNA level afe increased by insulin in cultured human hepatocytes, *Thromb. Haemostas.* 62:723-728 (1989).

27. P.J. Grant, M. Rüegg, R.L. Medcalf, Basal expression and insulin-mediated induction of PAI-1 mRNA in Hep G2 cells, *Fibrinolysis* 5:81-86 (1991).

28. P.J. Grant, E.K.O. Kruithof, C.P. Felley, J.B. Felber, F. Bachmann, Short-term infusions of insulin, triacylglycerol and glucose od not cause acute increases in plasminogen activator inhibitor-1 in man, *Clin. Sci.* 79:513-516 (1990).

29. B.J. Potter van Loon, A.C.W. de Bart, J.K. Radder, M. Frölich, C. Kluft, A.E. Meinders, Acute exogenous hyperinsulinaemia does not result in elevation of plasma plasminogen activator inhibitor-1 (PAI-1) in humans, *Fibrinolysis* 4 (suppl 2):93-94 (1990).

30. P.J. Grant, M.H. Stickland, P. Zenobi, J.P. Sebastian, P. Belchetz, The effects of IGF-1 on plasminogen activator inhibitor-1concentrations: results from in vivo and in vitro studies, *Diabetic Med.* abstract, in press (1992).

31. V.W.M. van Hindsbergh, T. Kooistra, E.A. van den Berg, H.M.G. Princen, W. Fiers, J.J. Emeis, Tumour necrosis factor increases the production of plasminogen activator inhibitor in human endothelial cells in vitro and rats in vivo, *Blood* 72:1467-1473 (1988).

32. J.J. Emeis, T. Kooistra, Interleukin 1 and lipopolysaccharide induce an inhibitor of tissue-type plasminogen activator in vivo and in cultured endothelial cells, *J. Exp. Med.* 1643:1260-1266 (1986).

33. C.H. Vosborgh, A.N. Richards, An experimental study of the sugar content and extra vascular coagulaton of the blood after administration of adrenalin, *Am. J. Physiol.* ix:35-51 (1903).

34. W.B. Cannon, H. Gray H Factors affecting the coagulation time of blood II: The hastening or retading of coagulation by adrenalin injections., *Am. J. Physiol.* 24: 232-42 (1914).

35. S.A. Schweck, K.N. von Kaulla, Fibrinolysis and the nervous system, *Neurology* II:959-969 (1961).

36. P.M. Mannucci, G.L. Barbi, Effect of cyclic AMP and related drugs on plasminogen activator, *Eur. J. Clin. Invest.* 3:253 (1973).

37. J.D. Cash, A.M.A. Gader, J. Da Costa, The release of plasminogen activator and factor VII by LVP, AVP, DDAVP, ATIII and OP in man, *Brit. J. Haematol.* 27:363- 364 (1974).

38. P.M. Mannucci, M. Aberg, I.M. Nilsson, B. Robertson, Mechanism of plasminogen activator and factor VIII increase after vasoactive drugs, *Br. J. Haematol.* 30:81 (1975).

39. P.M. Mannucci, Desmopressin: a non transfusional treatment for congenital and acquired bleeding disorders, *Blood* 72:1449-55 (1988).

40. P.J. Grant, J.A. Davies, G.M. Tate, M. Boothby, C.R.M Prentice, Effects of physiological concentrations of vasopressin on haemostatic function in man, *Clin. Sci.* 69: 471-476 (1985).

41. S.S. Nussey, D.H. Bevan, V.T.Y. Ang, J.S. Jenkins, Effects of arginine vasopressin (AVP) infusions on circulating concentrations of platelet AVP, factor VIII:C and von Willebrand factor, *Thromb. Haemostas.* 55(1): 34-36 (1986).

42. H. Hariman, P.J. Grant, J.R. Hughes, J.A. Davies, C.R.M. Prentice, The effects of physiological concentrations of vasopressin on components of the fibrinolytic pathway, *Thromb. Haemostas* . 61:298-300 (1989).

43. P.J. Grant, G.M. Tate, N.S. Williams, J.A. Davies, C.R.M. Prentice, Intra-operative activation of coagulation - a stimulus to thrombosis mediated by vasopressin? *Thromb. Haemostas.* 55(1):104-107 (1986).

44. J. Wilson, P.J. Grant, J.A. Davies, M. Boothby, P.J. Gaffney, C.R.M. Prentice, The relationship between plasma vasopressin and changes in coagulation and fibrinolysis during hip surgery, *Thromb. Res.* 52:439-445 (1988).

45. P.J. Grant, M.H. Stickland, P.G. Wiles J.A Davies, J.K. Wales, C.R.M. Prentice, Hormonal control of haemostasis during hypoglycaemia in diabetes mellitus, *Thromb. Haemostas.* 57:341-344 (1987).

46. P.J. Grant, J.R. Hughes, H.G. Dean, J.A Davies, Prentice, C.R.M., Vasopressin and catecholamine secretion during apomorphine-induced nausea mediate acute changes in haemostatic function in man, *Clin.Sci.* 71:621-624 (1986).

47. K.K. Hampton, P.J. Grant, M. Boothby, H.G. Dean, J.A. Davies, C.R.M. Prentice, The effect of modified electroconvulsive therapy on vasopressin release and haemostasis in man, *Blood Coag. Fib.* 1:293-297 (1990).

48. K.K. Hampton, P.J. Grant, M. Boothby, J.A. Davies, C.R.M. Prentice, Vasopressin and the regulation of fibrinolysis: haemostatic responses to hypotension in the absence of adrenaline. Thromb. Haemost. 58:93- (1987).

49. C.V. Prowse, G. Sas, A.M.A. Gader, J.H. Cort, J.D Cash, Specificity in the factor VIII response to vasopressin infusion in man, *Br. J. Haematol.* 41:437-447 (1979).

50. J.D. Cash, A.M.A. Gader, J.L. Mulder, J.H. Cort, Structure- activity relations of the fibrinolytic response to vasopressin in man, *Clin. Sci. Mol. Med.* 54:403-409 (1978).

51. R.T. Wall, R.B. Counts, L.A. Harker, G.E. Striker, Binding and release of factor VIII/von Willebrand factor by human endothelial cells, *Br. J. Haem.* 46:287-298 (1980).

52. J.H. Cort, A.J. Fishman, W.J. Dodds, J.H. Rand, I.L. Schwartz, New category of vasopressin receptor in the central nervous system, *Int. J. Pept. Protein Res.* 17:14- 22 (1981).

53. P.J. Grant, P.G. Wiles, H.G. Dean, J.A. Davies, C.R.M. Prentice, The physiological effects of vasopressin on haemostasis are not mediated by catecholamine release, *Thromb. Res.* 45:839-843 (1987).

54. G.D. Forwell, G.I.C. Ingram, The effect of adrenaline infusion on human blood coagulation, *J. Physiol.* 135: 371-383 (1957).

55. G.C. Ingram, Increase in anti-haemophilic globulin activity following infusion of adrenaline, *J. Physiol.* 156:217-224 (1961).

56. G.I.C. Ingram, R. Vaughan Jones, The rise in clotting factor VIII induced in man by adrenaline: effect of and ß blockers, *J. Physiol.* 187:447-454 (1966).

57. R.J.M. Gorral, R.G. Webber, B.M. Frier, Increase in coagulation factor VIII activity in man follwing acute hypoglycaemia: Mediation via an adrenergic mechanism, *Br. J. Haem.* 44:301-305 (1980).

58. J.D. Cash, D.G. Woodfield, A.G.E. Allan, Adrenergic mechanisms in the systemic plasminogen activator response to adrenaline in man, *Br. J. Haem.* 18:487-494 (1970).

59. R.J. Cohen, S.E. Epstein, L.S. Cohen, L.H. Dennis , Alterations of fibrinolysis and blood coagulation induced by exercise and the role of beta adrenergic-receptor stimulation, *Lancet* ii:1264-1266 (1968).

60. C.M. Hankey, B.J. Britton, W.G. Wood, M. Peele, M.H. Irving, Changes in blood catecholamine levels and blood coagulation and fibrinolytic activity in response to graded exercise in man, *Br. J. Haem.* 29:377-384 (1975).

DISCUSSION

Vilhardt (Denmark): You used Shy Drager and Progressive Autonomic Failure patients. Of course, they are rare: diabetes insipidus is much more common, with a population prevalence of 1:24,000. Have any studies of coagulation factors and fibrinolytic activity been performed in abdominal surgery in diabetes insipidus patients? They would have no vasopressin to release.
Grant: This is not necessarily true. They would have no osmotic response, but they do respond to stress with vasopressin release.
Vilhardt: Some patients have an absolute block of biosynthesis of vasopressin, so that they would not.
Grant: I know of no such studies.

Kobrinski (United States): We can support the diabetes insipidus hypothesis. Patients with nephrogenic diabetes insipidus have a blunted response of Factor VIII and vWf, but their basal levels are elevated, suggesting an adrenaline response. Also, desmopressin is a vasodilator: it would be interesting to look at how desmopressin infusion would affect VP blood levels. Does it cause secondary release of arginine vasopressin?
Grant: It would have an effect on vasopressin release only if the hypotension was significant enough. Minor hypotension would not affect vasopressin release.

Kobrinski: In anaesthesia, controlled hypotension is a means of reducing blood loss. A fall of mean blood pressure of about 8 mm Hg is needed. Would that have an effect?
Grant: Probably not. You may get a small rise, but you need about 15-20 pg/ml vasopressin concentration before there is an effect on haemostasis.

Vilhardt: Most current AVP antibodies cross-react with DDAVP. In our laboratory we have measured both AVP and DDAVP, and did not find any change in AVP after desmopressin infusion. This suggests that the cardiovascular effects are not large enough.

Bichet (Canada): The process may be more complicated. Receptors on the pituitary with a feedback loop may lead to infusion with DDAVP shutting down AVP secretion. We have used DDAVP levels of 1000 mg/l: there was a very small increase in AVP, but it is impossible to determine whether this was due to cross-reactivity. With cloning of the receptor it may be possible to see if there is a feedback loop.

Brommer (The Netherlands): You showed the effect of DDAVP on enhancement of thrombin generation. How did you measure that?
Grant: The patients were infused with DDAVP. The blood samples were defibrinated, and thrombin generation measured using a chromogenic substrate and recalcification.

Mannucci (Italy): Most of us dealing with DDAVP have not found an increase in fibrinopeptide A. You found a huge increase. Experts say that this level cannot be generated in the circulation, and that levels above 10 nanomols are artefactual. How is this? Are you certain that thrombin was not formed in vitro?
Grant: The method used was circulating FPA generation time. I remained unconvinced about this test. It is true that a rise in FPA cannot be picked up in this tests: it is not sensitive enough. This is a separate issue: FPA generation time uses thrombin generation as part of the test.

VON WILLEBRAND FACTOR AND P-SELECTIN TARGETING TO AND RELEASE FROM ENDOTHELIAL CELL-SPECIFIC STORAGE GRANULES

Tanya N. Mayadas

Center for Hemostasis and Thrombosis Research
Division of Hematology/Oncology
and Department of Medicine
New England Medical Center
Boston, MA 02111

INTRODUCTION

A readily releasable pool of von Willebrand factor (vWf) was first realized after Prentice and colleagues (1972) observed that exercise or the administration of adrenaline caused an increase in circulating vWf. vWf was later reported in the alpha granules of platelets (Zucker et al., 1979; Jeanneau et al., 1984) and the Weibel-Palade bodies of endothelial cells (Weibel and Palade, 1964; Wagner et al.,1982). Recently, a transmembrane protein, P-selectin (PADGEM, GMP140, CD62), was also identified in these two cell-specific storage granules (Stenberg et al., 1985; Berman et al., 1986; Bonfanti et al., 1989; McEver et al., 1989). The release of Weibel-Palade bodies occurs by stimulation of the endothelium with various secretagogues which are effective within minutes in inducing the release of von Willebrand factor (for review, Wagner 1990) and P-selectin (Hattori et al., 1989) which are the only proteins known to be stored in these storage granules. There is substantial evidence that the increased circulating levels of vWf observed in patients treated with 1-desamino-8-d-arginine vasopressin (DDAVP), a pharmacological analogue of the hormone L-arginine vasopressin, originates from a storage pool of vWf present in the endothelium. However, DDAVP *in vitro* does not directly cause Weibel-Palade body release (for review, Mannucci, 1986). vWf is an adhesive multimeric glycoprotein which has at least two functions in hemostasis: it is important in the initial events in hemostasis such as platelet adhesion to the subendothelium, and platelet aggregation and spreading and it complexes with fVIII, the factor deficient in hemophilia A, to

Desmopressin in Bleeding Disorders, Edited by G. Mariani *et al.*
Plenum Press, New York, 1993

protect it from proteolysis. The highest molecular weight multimers are the most biologically effective in adhesion but all multimeric forms are capable of complexing with fVIII (Wagner, 1990). P-selectin is a transmembrane protein present on the surface of activated endothelium and platelets and is effective in the early stages of inflammation and wound healing by recruiting neutrophils and monocytes (Larsen et al., 1989; Hamburger and McEver 1990; Geng et al., 1990) through recognition of Sialyl-Le^{X} antigen (Larsen et al., 1990; Corral et al., 1990; Polley et al., 1991) on these white blood cells.

The following topics will be the focus of this review 1) the targeting of vWf and P-selectin to the secretory granules 2) the formation and replenishment of Weibel-Palade bodies and 3) vWf and P-selectin secretion

VON WILLEBRAND FACTOR AND P-SELECTIN TARGETING TO STORAGE GRANULES

vWf is synthesized by endothelial cells and megakaryocytes as a large precursor which undergoes various processing steps including dimerization and glycosylation in the endoplasmic reticulum, and subsequent carbohydrate processing, multimerization of the dimers and propeptide cleavage in the trans Golgi apparatus. Multimerization of vWf continues in the Weibel-Palade bodies and the prosequence is cleaved most efficiently in these secretory granules. The Weibel-Palade bodies preferentially store the highly multimeric forms of vWf which are stored prior to propolypeptide cleavage, whereas the lower multimeric forms are secreted constitutively. Only 5% of the total vWf synthesized by human umbilical vein endothelial cells is stored (Wagner, 1990).

The large propolypeptide, identical to vWf antigen II (Fay et al., 1986), is required for vWf multimerization (Verweij et al., 1987; Wise et al., 1988; Mayadas and Wagner, 1989). Since it is cleaved after the highest molecular weight multimers are stored (Wagner et al., 1987; Ewenstein et al., 1987), we postulated that, as in the case of prosomatostatin (Sevarino et al., 1987; Stoller and Shields, 1989), the propolypeptide of vWf may also play an important role in targeting vWf to storage granules. To determine the role of the propolypeptide in vWf targeting and to elucidate other criteria for vWf storage, we expressed full-length vWf cDNA and cDNA lacking the propolypeptide in heterologous cell lines that have a regulated pathway of secretion, and cells that only secrete proteins constitutively. vWf-containing granules with a rod-shaped morphology characteristic of Weibel-Palade bodies, formed only in cells that normally store endogenous hormones, such as AtT-20 cells (a mouse pituitary cell line) and RIN 5F cells (a mouse insulinoma cell line), and that were transfected with full-length vWf cDNA (Figure 1). In these two cell types, the expression of vWf cDNA in which the propolypeptide was deleted did not lead to the formation of vWf-containing storage granules. Pro-vWf molecules lacking the C-terminal region involved in interchain disulfide bonding were stored. Furthermore, vWf-containing granules did not codistribute with granules containing the cells' endogenous hormones. Our studies concluded that 1) the signal for storage is universal, since

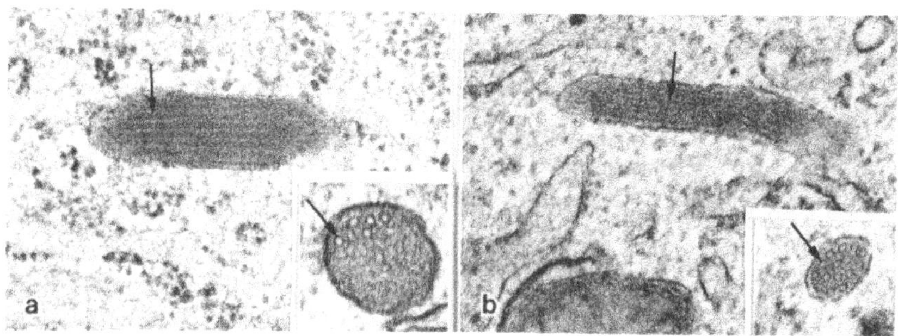

Figure 1. Electron micrographs of Weibel-Palade bodies and of similar organelles formed in transfected RIN 5F cells. (a) section of a human umbilical vein endothelial cell containing a Weibel-Palade body with tubules arranged parallel to its long axis (arrow). Inset: transversal section of a Weibel-Palade body shows a juxtaposition of several tubules (arrow) embedded in a dense matrix. (b) Section of a RIN 5F cell expressing pro-vWf. The micrograph shows an organelle morphologically identical to a Weibel-Palade body. Inset: typical tubular elements are seen on cross-section of the organelle (arrow). Weibel-Palade body-like structures were not seen in sections of mock-transfected RIN 5F cells. Bar=0.1μm. Reproduced with permission from Wagner et al. (1991).

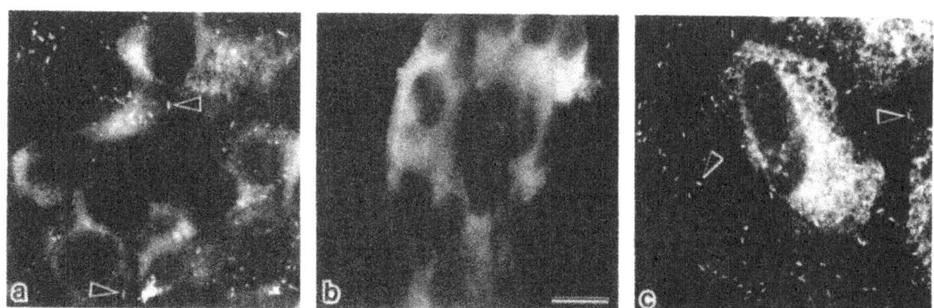

Figure 2. Distribution of vWf in AtT-20 cells transfected with pro-vWf containing a mutation in the propolypeptide that results in the inhibition of vWf multimerization, and a mutant of vWf lacking the propolypeptide. Distribution of vWf in endothelial cells is shown for comparison. vWf in permeabilized cells grown on glass coverslips was visualized by immunofluorescence with a polyclonal antiserum to vWf. (a) AtT-20 cell expressing pro-vWf that is unable to multimerize. (b) AtT-20 cells expressing vWf with the propolypeptide deleted (Wagner et al., 1991). (c) First-passage endothelial cells from human umbilical vein. The perinuclear staining is indicative of vWf present in the endoplasmic reticulum and the Golgi apparatus. Arrowheads point to Weibel-Palade bodies of endothelial cells and vWf-containing Weibel-Palade body-like organelles in AtT-20 cells. AtT-20 cells expressing vWf cDNA with the propolypeptide deleted (b) lack vWf-containing storage granules (Wagner, et al., 1991). (Bar = 10μm). Reproduced with permission from Mayadas T.N. and Wagner, D.D. 1992.

an adhesive protein is stored by a endocrine cell line, 2) vWf is responsible for the formation of rod-shaped granules, and 3) the propolypeptide is responsible for vWf targeting to secretory granules (Wagner et al., 1991). Interestingly, when vWf cDNA engineered with a mutation in the propolypeptide that abolishes vWf multimerization was expressed in AtT-20 cells, the resulting dimers were stored in Weibel-Palade body-like structures (Figure 2) (Mayadas and Wagner, 1992). This demonstrated that the mutation did not affect the capacity of the propolypeptide to direct vWf storage despite the elimination of its ability to promote interchain disulfide bonding, and that covalent multimerization was not a prerequisite for vWf storage. More recently, A. Journet, S. Saffaripour and D.D. Wagner (unpublished observations) have found that prosequence cleavage is a prerequisite for vWf storage. Although the vWf cleavage-mutant formed large multimers, the presence of the propolypeptide may have hindered crystal structure formation which could be a prerequisite for vWf storage. Another possibility is that the dibasic cleavage site is recognized as part of the targeting signal for vWf storage.

P-selectin is a member of the selectin family of molecules whose members include E-selectin (ELAM1) and L-selectin (MEL14 antigen). They share domain and structural homology and they all participate in heterologous cell-cell interactions required for wound healing and the inflammatory response (Springer, 1990; Bevilacqua et al., 1991). P-selectin is composed of a C-type lectin domain, an epidermal growth factor repeat, nine complement binding repeats, a transmembrane domain and a cytoplasmic tail (Johnston et al., 1989). Unlike vWf, where only a small percentage of the total protein is stored, P-selectin is efficiently stored in endothelial cells. The targeting of this transmembrane proteins has been recently elucidated. P-selectin expressed in AtT-20 cells was stored in granules which codistributed with endogenous adrenocorticotrophin hormone (ACTH) containing granules (Figure 3) and was released upon stimulation of these cells with the cAMP analogue, 8-bromo-cAMP (Koedam et al., 1992; Disdier et al., 1992). This suggested that P-selectin contains "targeting signal(s)" that directs it to storage granules. Other studies have reported that the cytoplasmic tail of membrane proteins directed to lysosomes (Williams and Fukuda, 1990; Peters et al., 1990), or retained in the endoplasmic reticulum (Jackson et al., 1990) carry important targeting information. Disdier et al (1992) and Koedam et al (unpublished observations) demonstrated that a deletion of the cytoplasmic tail of P-selectin abolished its storage and resulted in the constitutive secretion of P-selectin to the membrane surface. These studies established an important role for the cytoplasmic tail in the targeting of P-selectin to storage granules. Furthermore, Disdier et al (1992) expressed a fusion protein, composed of the extracellular domains and transmembrane domain of tissue factor, a plasma membrane protein, fused to the cytoplasmic domain of P-selectin in AtT-20 cells. They reported that the fusion protein was diverted to secretory granules, indicating that the cytoplasmic tail is sufficient for targeting of heterologous proteins to secretory granules.

Although P-selectin and vWf are the only known proteins in Weibel-Palade bodies there appears to be no intracellular sorting relationship between them since AtT-20 or RIN 5F cells expressing pro-vWf store vWf in the absence of P-selectin (Wagner et al., 1991), and P-

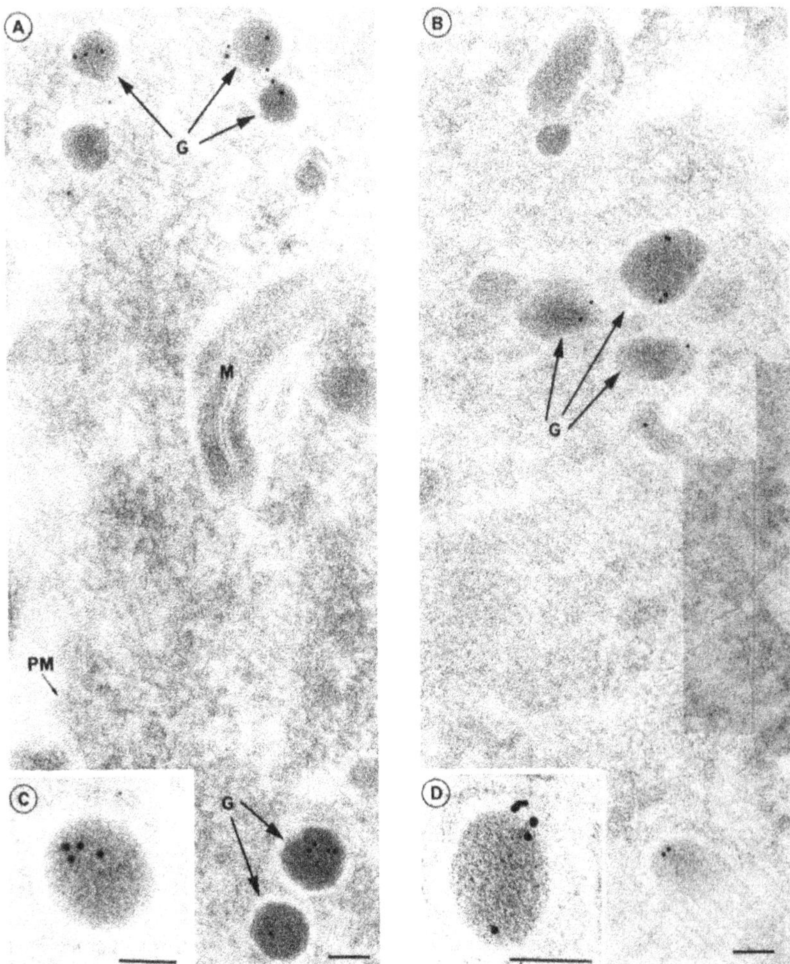

Figure 3. Electron micrograph of unstimulated AtT-20 cells that express P-selectin. A and C show immunogold labeling for ACTH, the endogenous hormone of AtT-20 cells; B and D for P-selectin of AtT-20 cells transfected with P-selectin cDNA. Labeling of both proteins was restricted to the dense core granules (G). Anti-ACTH antibody revealed a matricial labeling of the secretory granules. In contrast, P-selectin labeling was found near the granule membrane. M, mitochondria; PM, plasma membrane. Bars, 100nm. Reproduced with permission from Koedam J.A. et al., 1992.

selectin, when transfected into these cell types is stored in the absence of vWf (Koedam et al., 1992, Disdier et al., 1992).

WEIBEL-PALADE BODY FORMATION AND REPLENISHMENT

Weibel-Palade bodies are 0.1µm wide and upto 4um long and originate from the trans Golgi. Weibel-Palade bodies have been observed in endothelial cells of many blood vessel types originating from tissue of humans and other vertebrates. The tubular structure, longitudinally arranged in Weibel-Palade bodies, alpha granules and vWf containing storage granules formed in cells transfected with pro-vWf (Figure 1), probably represent vWf polymers. The compact tubular structure of vWf within the storage granules may consist of only mature polymers and similar to insulin granules, the propolypeptide may be distributed in the periphery of vWf containing storage granules (Wagner, 1990). The formation and unusual morphology of these vWf containing granules can be directly attributed to vWf since rod-shaped granules formed in heterologous cells transfected only with pro-vWf (Wagner et al., 1991).

The replenishment of Weibel-Palade bodies after their release could occur either through diversion of vWf from the constitutive to the regulated pathway, increased protein synthesis or at the same rate as that occuring in unstimulated endothelial cells. We found that Weibel-Palade body depletion as a result of thrombin stimulation does not serve as a signal for compensatory increase in vWf biosynthesis. Thrombin stimulation also did not affect the partitioning of vWf between the constitutive pathway and the regulated pathway. Instead, our data suggested that replenishment of Weibel-Palade bodies took place at a steady state rate similar to that of unstimulated cells (Mayadas et al., 1989). In addition, Reinders et al (1987) reported that phorbol myristate acetate or thrombin stimulation of endothelial cells did not result in an increase in vWf-specific mRNA. One might speculate that perhaps the immediate replenishment of Weibel-Palade bodies after their release is not desirable since the endothelial cells would then be in a position to be restimulated by physiological stimuli still present in the vicinity of the developing clot or at the site of inflammation. This would result in an uncontrolled release of biologically potent vWf multimers and P-selectin at the site of injury and could result in excessive platelet aggregation and phagocyte accumulation. One possible explanation for the progessively poorer responses observed in patients given successive infusions (three daily i.v. doses) of DDAVP (Mannucci et al., 1981) is that perhaps the vWf storage pools are being depleted since replenishment may not be occuring at an accelerated rate.

VON WILLEBRAND FACTOR AND P-SELECTIN SECRETION

Regulated secretion of these two proteins allows high concentration of protein to be available for interaction with platelets in the case of vWf and neutrophils and monocytes in the case of P-selectin. The multivalency of binding sites in vWf multimers explains the increased biological efficacy of large vWf multimers. It is possible that high membrane concentrations of P-selectin is required for avid interaction of P-selectin with white blood cells. The rapid endocytosis of P-selectin observed after its release (Hattori et al., 1989) may constitute a pathway to regulate P-selectin expression at sites of vascular injury. It is not known whether P-selectin is recycled from the plasma membrane by the sorting of endocytosed P-selectin into secretory granules.

Exocytosis of Weibel-Palade bodies occurs in a polarized manner when cells are stimulated with the calcium ionophore, A23187. Sporn et al (1989) demonstrated that regulated secretion occurs basolaterally whereas constitute secretion is not polarized. A proportion of basolaterally deposited vWf may interact with the vitronectin receptor and help anchor endothelial cells to the subendothelial matrix. Results from thrombin stimulation of endothelial cells were not as clear cut since thrombin causes endothelial cell retraction which would allow a possible basolateral pool of vWf to escape to the apical surface (Sporn et al., 1989). In cases where the secretagogue does not disturb the integrity of the endothelial monolayer, vWf may reach the apical surface by transendocytosis of the basolaterally deposited vWf across the cell layer. P-selectin may undergo a similar translocation. DDAVP mediated release of Weibel-Palade bodies may also be polarized to the basolateral direction. A polarized secretion of vWf could explain why circulating vWf levels increase in patients only 30-60 minutes after infusion with DDAVP (Manucci et al., 1976). DDAVP treated individuals had a higher level of vWf Antigen II (3-8 fold over resting values in healthy volunteers) relative to circulating vWf (2 fold over resting values in healthy volunteers) (Mannucci, 1986). The descrepancy in the levels of vWf and vWf Antigen II (the vWf propolypeptide) which are stored in 1:1 stoichiometric amounts in Weibel-Palade bodies (Wagner, 1987) may be explained if release of Weibel-Palade bodies in these patients occured in the basolateral direction. The basolateral deposition of vWf and vWf Antigen II could lead to a more efficient rerouting of vWf Antigen II to the luminal suface of endothelial cells in comparison to vWf, since vWf Antigen II does not bind to the subendothelium (Wagner et al, 1987).

Release of Weibel-Palade bodies has been demonstrated *in vitro* by exposing endothelial cells to various physiological secretagogues such as thrombin, histamine, fibrin and complement proteins C5b9 and non-physiological secretagogues such as A23187 and phorbol myristate acetate (Wagner, 1990). Release of Weibel-Palade bodies leads to the rapid release of vWf into the medium and the expression of P-selectin on the surfaces of activated endothelium. Although there is substantial evidence suggesting that DDAVP causes Weibel-Palade release *in vivo*, the mechanism of action of DDAVP has not been completely elucidated. Hashemi et al (1990) have reported that monocytes exposed to DDAVP secrete soluble factors which in turn were largely responsible for Weibel-Palade body release. The effectiveness of these soluble factors may be augmented by the presence of P-selectin. For instance, in the early response to DDAVP, stimulation of endothelial cells may be mediated by soluble factors secreted by circulating monocytes. However, P-selectin initally mobilized to the suface of the endothelium may then be availiable to recruit monocytes and bring them into close proximity to adjacent endothelial cell surfaces. This would allow more efficient exposure of the endothelial cells to soluble factors, secreted by monocytes, that would otherwise be rapidly diluted in the circulation. P-selectin interaction with monocytes and neutrophils does not require activation of the leukocytes and the interaction of neutrophils with P-selectin has been shown to be highly reversible: Under *in vitro* flow conditions unactivated neutrophils roll on a P-selectin coated suface (Lawrence and Springer, 1991) and are arrested only if a secondary activation-triggered attachment occurs between neutrophils and the endothelium. Since P-selectin function has only been assessed *in vitro* and since there are no cases where a clinical phenotype can be traced to a deficiency of this protein we are currently generating a mouse model for P-selectin deficiency by targeted disruption of the P-selectin gene by homologous recombination. In addition to elucidating the functions of P-selectin in inflammatory and wound healing processes in mice homozygous for the P-selectin mutation, it would be interesting to administer DDAVP to these mice to investigate the possibile involvement of P-selectin in potentiating the effects of DDAVP.

There may also be other factors or proteins secreted into the plasma of patients treated with DDAVP that could aid in the shortening of their bleeding times. Cattaneo et al (1989) reported that patients with severe von Willebrand disease, infused with cryoprecipitate, have a shortening but not always normalization of their bleeding times. Although these patients have no releasable vWf stores, DDAVP further shortened their bleeding times. Therefore, Weibel-Palade bodies may release other proteins or factors that have not yet been identified, that are important in hemostasis. To date, other components of Weibel-Palade bodies besides vWf and P-selectin have not been reported. In addition, the soluble factors originating from monocytes that are responsible for release of Weibel-Palade body release (Hashemi et al., 1990) may have other effects on the thrombogenic properties of the endothelium surface. Identification of other components of Weibel-Palade bodies and characterization of the monocyte derived soluble factor(s) could give further insight into the mechanism of DDAVP action both *in vivo* and *in vitro*.

ACKNOWLEDGEMENTS

I would like to thank Dr. Denisa Wagner for critical review of the manuscript. The work done in Dr. Wagner's laboratory was supported by grants from National Institute of Health (PO1 HL42443 and RO1 HL41002) and by an established investigatorship award from the American Heart Association.

REFERENCES

Berman, C.L., Yeo, E.L., Wencel-Drake, J.D., Furie, B.C., Ginsberg, M.H., and Furie, B., 1986, A platelet alpha granule membrane protein that is associated with the plasma membrane after activation. Characterization and subcellular localization of platelet activation-dependent granule-external membrane protein, Blood. 78:130.

Bevilacqua, M., Butcher, E., Furie, B.C., Furie, B., Gallatin, M., Gimbrone, M., et al., 1991, Cell 67:233.

Bonfanti, R., Furie, B.C., Furie, B., and Wagner, D.D., 1989, PADGEM (GMP140) is a component of Weibel-Palade bodies of human endothelial cells, Blood. 73:1109.

Cattaneo, M., Moia, M., Valle, P-D., Castellana, P., and Mannucci, P.M., 1989, DDAVP shortens the prolonged bleeding times of patients with severe von Willebrand disease treated with cryoprecipitate. Evidence for a mechanism independent of released von Willebrand factor, Blood 74:1972.

Corral, L., Singer, M.S., Macher, B.A., and Rosen, S.D., 1990, Requirement for sialic acid on neutrophils in a GMP-140 (PADGEM) mediated adhesive interaction with activated platelets, Biochem. Biophys. Res. Comm. 172:1349.

Disdier, M., Morrissey, J.H., Fugate, R.D., Bainton, D.F., and McEver, R.P., 1992, Cytoplasmic domain of P-selectin (CD62) contains the signal for sorting into the regulated secretory pathway, Mol. Biol. Cell. 3:309.

Ewenstein, B.M., Warhol, M.J., Handin, R.I., and Pober, J.S., 1987, Composition of the von Willebrand factor storage organelle (Weibel-Palade body) isolated from cultured human umbilical vein endothelial cells, J. Cell. Biol. 104:1423.

Fay, P.J., Kawai, Y., Wagner, D.D., Ginsberg, D., and Bonthron, D., et. al., 1986, Propolypeptide of von Willebrand factor circulates in blood and is identical to von Willebrand antigen II, Science 232:995.

Geng, J.-G., Bevilacqua, M.P., Moore, K.L., McIntyre, T.M., Prescott, S.M., Kim, J.M., Bliss, G.A., Zimmerman, G.A., and McEver, R.P., 1990, Rapid neutrophil adhesion to activated endothelium mediated by GMP-140. Nature 343:757.

Hamburger, S.A., and McEver, R.P., 1990, GMP-140 mediates adhesion of stimulated platelets to neutrophils, Blood. 75:550.

Hashemi, S., Tackaberry, E.S., Palmer, D.S., Rock, G., and Ganz, P.R., 1990, DDAVP-induced release of von Willebrand factor from endothelial cells *in vitro*: The effect of plasma and blood cells. Biochim. Biophys. Acta. 1052:63.

Hattori, R., Hamilton, K.K., Fugate, R.D., McEver, R.P., and Sims, P.J., 1989, Stimulated secretion of endothelial von Willebrand factor is accompanied by rapid redistribution to the cell surface of the intracellular granule membrane protein GMP-140, J. Biol. Chem. 264:7768.

Jackson, M.R., Nilsson, T., and Peterson, P.A., 1990, Identification of a consensus motif for retention of transmembrane proteins in the endoplasmic reticulum, EMBO J. 9:3153.

Jeanneau, C, Avner, P., and Sultan, Y., 1984, Use of monoclonal antibody and colloidal gold in E.M. localization of von Willebrand factor in megakaryocytes and platelets, Cell Biol. Int. Rep. 8:841.

Johnston, G.I., Cook, R.G., and McEver, R.P., 1989, Cloning of GMP-140, a granule membrane protein of platelets and endothelium: Sequence similarity to proteins involved in cell adhesion and inflammation, Cell. 56:1033.

Koedam, J.A., Cramer, E.M., Briend, E., Furie, B., Furie, B.C., and Wagner, D.D., 1992, P-Selectin, a granule membrane protein of platelets and endothelial cells, follows the regulated secretory pathway in AtT-20 cells, J. Cell Biol. 116:617.

Larsen, E., Celi, A., Gilbert, G.E., Furie, B.C., Erban, J.K., Bonfanti, R., Wagner, D.D., and Furie, B., 1989, PADGEM protein: a receptor that mediates the interaction of activated platelets with neutrophls and monocytes, Cell. 59:305.

Larsen, E., Palabrica, T., Sajer, S., Gilbert, G.E., Wagner, D.D., Furie, B.C., and Furie, B., 1990, PADGEM-dependent adhesion of platelets to monocytes and neutrophils is mediated by a lineage-specific carbohydrate, LNF III (CD15), Cell. 63:467.

Lawrence, M.B., and Springer, T.A., 1991, Leukocytes roll on a selectin at physiologic flow rates: Distinction from and prerequisite for adhesion through integrins, Cell 65:859.

Mannucci, P.M., 1986, Desmopressin (DDAVP) for treatment of disorders of hemostasis, Prog. Hem. Thromb. 8:19.

Mannucci, P.M., Canciani, M.T., Rota, L., and Donovan, B.S., 1981, Response of factor VIII/von Willebrand factor to DDAVP in healthy subjects and patients with Haemophilia A and von Willebrand's disease, Br. J. Haem. 47:283

Mannucci, P.M., Pareti, F.I., Holmberg, L., Nilsson, I.M., and Ruggeri, Z.M., 1976, Studies on the prolonged bleeding time in von Willebrand's disease, J. Lab. Clin. Med. 88:662.

Mayadas, T.N., and Wagner, D.D., 1989, *In vitro* multimerization of von Willebrand factor is triggered by low pH: Importance of the propolypeptide and free sulfhydryls, J. Biol. Chem. 264:13497.

Mayadas, T.N., and Wagner, D.D., 1992, Vicinal cysteines in the prosequence play a role in von Willebrand factor multimer assembly, Proc. Nalt. Acad. Sci. (in press).

Mayadas, T.N., Wagner, D.D., and Simpson, P.J., 1989, von Willebrand factor biosynthesis and partitioning between constitutive and regulated pathway of secretion after thrombin stimulation, Blood. 73:706.

McEver, R.P., Beckstead, J.H., Moore, K.L., Marshall-Carlson, L., and Bainton, D.F., 1989, GMP-140, a platelet alpha-granule membrane protein, is also synthesized by vascular endothelial cells and is localized in Weibel-Palade bodies, J. Clin. Invest. 84:92.

Peters, C., Braun, M., Weber, B., Wendland, M., Schmidt, B., Pohlmann, R., Waheed, A., and von Figura, K., 1990, Targeting of a lysosomal membrane protein: A tyrosine-containing endocytosis signal in the cytoplasmic tail of lysosomal acid phosphatase is necessary and sufficient for targeting to lysosomes, EMBO J. 9:3497.

Polley, M.J., Laurie Phillips, M., Wayner, E., Nudelman, E., Singhal, A.K., Hakomori, S-I., and Paulson, J.C., 1991, CD62 and endothelial cell-leukocyte adhesion molecule 1(ELAM1) recognize the same carbohydrate ligand, sialyl Lewis x, Proc. Natl. Acad Sci. 88:6224.

Prentice, C.R.M., Forbes, C.D., Smith, S.M., 1972, Rise of fVIII after exercise and adrenaline infusion measured by immunological and biological techniques, Thromb. Res. 1:493.

Reinders, J.H., Vervoorn, R.C., Verweij, C.L., van Mourik, J.A., and DeGroot, P.G., 1987, Perturbation of culture human vascular endothelial cells by phorbol ester or thrombin alters the cellular von Willebrand factor distribution, J. Cell. Physiol. 133:79.

Sevarino, K.A., Stork, P., Ventimiglia, R., Mandel, G., and Goodman, R.H., 1989, Amino-terminal sequences of prosomatostatin direct intracellular targeting but not processing specificity, Cell 57:11.

Sporn, L.A., Marder, V.J., and Wagner, D.D., 1989, Differing polarity of the constitutive and regulated secretory pathways of von Willebrand factor in endothelial cells, J. Cell Biol. 108: 1283.

Springer, T.A., 1990, Adhesion receptors of the immune system, Nature (Lond.) 346:425.

Stenberg, P.E., McEver, R.P., Schuman, M.A., Jacques, Y.V., and Bainton, D.F., 1985, A platelet alpha-granule membrane protein (GMP140) is expressed on the plasma membrane after activation, J. Cell Biol. 101:880.

Stoller, T.J., and Shields, D., 1989, The propeptide of prepromatostatin mediates intracellular transport and secretion of alpha-globin from mammalian cells, J. Cell. Biol. 108:1647.

Verweij, C.L., Hart, M., and Pannekoek, H., 1987, Expression of variant von Willebrand factor (vWf) cDNA in heterologous cells: Requirement of the propolypeptide in vWf multimer formation, EMBO J. 6:2885.

Wagner, D.D., 1990, Cell biology of von Willebrand factor, Ann. Rev. Cell Biol. 6:217.

Wagner, D.D., Fay, P.J., Sporn, L.A., Sinha, S., Lawrence, S.O., and Marder, V.J., 1987, Divergent fates of von Willebrand factor and its propolypeptide (von Willebrand antigen II) after secretion from endothelial cells, Proc. Natl. Acad. Sci. USA 84:1955.

Wagner, D.D., Olmsted, J.B. and Marder, V.J. 1982. Immunolocalization of von Willebrand protein in Weibel-Palade bodies of human endothelial cells, J.Cell Biol. 95:355.

Wagner, D.D., Saffaripour, S., Bonfanti, R., Sadler, J.E., Cramer, E.M., Chapman, B., and Mayadas, T.N., 1991, Induction of specific storage organelles by von Willebrand factor propolypeptide, Cell. 64:403.

Weibel, E.R., and Palade, G.E. 1964, New cytoplasmic components in arterial endothelia, J. Cell Biol. 23:101.

Williams, M.A., and Fukuda, M., 1990, Accumulation of membrane glycoproteins in lysosomes requires a tyrosine residue at a particular position in the cytoplasmic tail, J. Cell Biol. 111:955.

Wise , R.J., Pittman, D.D., Handin, R.I., Kaufman, R.J., and Orkin, S.H., 1988, The propeptide of von Willebrand factor independently mediates the assembly of von Willebrand multimers, Cell. 52:229.

Zucker, M.B., Broekman, M.J., and Kaplan, K.L., 1979, Factor VIII-related antigen in human blood platelets, J. Lab. Clin. Med. 94:675.

DISCUSSION

Bichet: Did you try to release granules formed in AtT-20 cells expressing pro-vWf by thrombin?
Mayadas-Norton: We tried thrombin and other secretogogues such as 8-bromocyclic AMP, but none caused release from the granules. But we thought perhaps the W-P bodies contain other components that may be important for their release such as proteins important for binding microtubules or other cellular machinery.

Kobrinsky: Is there storage of vWf and P-selectin in platelet alpha granules? Is the mechanism the same.
Mayadas-Norton: They both are stored. We presume the mechanism or the protein machinery is the same, since AtT-20 cells, a heterologous cell, store these proteins when each is independently transfected into AtT20 cells. But the signals for storage of these two proteins are different: the propolypeptide of vWF is important for vWF storage and the cytoplasmic tail of P-selectin is important for its storage.

Kobrinsky: Is there a similar role for P-selectin in releasing vWf from platelets?
Mayadas-Norton: P-selectin does not cause release of vWf. My hypothesis was that the initial expression of P-selectin may be potentiating release of Weibel-Palade bodies by DDAVP by

recruiting white blood cells to the endothelium, so that the monocyte-derived soluble factors hypothesized by Dr Hashemi may be in close contact, and therefore localized on the endothelium surface, causing enhanced release of weibel paladeo bodies which contain vWF and P-selectin.

Weinstein: Does P-selectin cause platelets to aggregate and adhere to vWf?
Mayadas-Norton: During longer aggregation of platelets, P-selectin may have homophilic binding which may aid in platelet-platelet interaction. This has not been rigorously proven. Of course it is known that GP IIb IIIa and its ligand are important in platelet-platelet interaction and aggregation.

FACTOR VIII IN MONKEYS, EFFECT OF DDAVP ANALOGUES

Hans Vilhardt [1] and Tomislav Barth[2]

[1]Medical Physiology C, Panum Institute,
Copenhagen University, Blegdamsvej 3c,
Copenhagen N, Denmark
[2]Institute of Organic Chemistry & Biochemistry,
Czechoslovak Academy of Sciences, 16610,
Prague 6, Czechoslovakia

INTRODUCTION

A synthetic analogue of vassopressin, [8 – D – arginine]deamino vasopressin (dDAVP), synthesized in the mid sixties[1], has become an important drug in the treatment of diabetes insipidus[2-4]. This peptide is so far the only vasopressin analogue which has been successfully used in patients with mild or moderate haemophilia A and von Willeb – rand's disease during bleeding episodes or prophylactically[5-7]. The pronounced and protracted antidiuretic effect is one of the side effects accompanying the use of dDAVP in treatment of haemophilia A, others such as tachycardia, feeling of pressure in the head, heat sensations and flacial flush have been reported in connection with dDAVP administration[8,9].

These findings initiated the structure – activity studies with vasopressin analogues on their Factor VIII activating properties. The results obtained in dogs[10] indicated different time courses of Factor VIII in dogs in comparison to man, the difference concerned also the level of maximal response obtained after the administration of dDAVP. Keeping in mind the species differences as far as the structure relationship is concerned we have established the basal structural features for preservation of Factor VIII activating properties of vasopressin analogues:

Desmopressin in Bleeding Disorders, Edited by G. Mariani *et al.*
Plenum Press, New York, 1993

a) the presence of β – mercaptopropionic acid instead of cysteine in position 1

b) the presence of a strongly positive charge on the amino acid in position 8 of the vasopressin molecule

c) the intact length of the amino acid chain potential metabolites [desGlyNH$_2$^{9}] – dDAVP and dDAVP with hydrolyzed bond between Tyr^2 and Phe^3 have eliminated Factor VIII activating properties[11].

At the same time we were looking for another animal model which would be more compatible with our demands (reproducibility of experiments, transfer of results from one species to another, economic cost of keeping the animals[12]). Such criteria were relatively well satisfied by squirrel monkeys. The increase of Factor VIII activating properties, after the administration of dDAVP were on the level found in man, further the basal conditions of structure – activity relationship corresponded with that found in dogs[11,12].

Here we present results obtained with several series of dDAVP analogues which were chosen to be synthesized because of the expected dissociation of their endocrine and Factor VIII activating properties.

EXPERIMENTAL

The peptides used in the study were prepared by Ferring Pharmaceuticals, Malmö, and by the Institute of Organic Chemistry and Biochemistry, Czech. Acad. Sci. in Prague.

Factor VIII estimation was performed using a method of Kabi Diagnostics employing a chromogenic substrate Bz – Ile – Glu(OR) – Gly – Arg – pNA.

Squirrel monkeys were used in our experiments. After being anesthetized with Ketalar (0.6 ml i.m.), the individual peptides were given i.m. in the front of the thigh. Blood (150 – 200 μl) was obtained before and 30 min after the injection of peptides through puncture of a popliteal vein and collected in Microvettes coated with EDTA. The samples were placed on ice and immediately centrifuged for 5 min at 4°C. Blood plasma was kept at - 80°C until assayed.

RESULTS AND DISCUSSION

We present the results with several series of dDAVP analogues:

a) analogues with replacement of amino acid in position 4 of the peptide

b) analogues with combined alterations in positions 4 and 7, 4 and 2

c) analogues with introduction of L – alanine in positions 2 – 5, 7 – 9 ($AlaNH_2^9$) of dDAVP

d) analogues with D – homoarginine in position 8 and modified position 2.

These peptides were chosen for their known or expected dissociation of antidiuretic and pressoric potencies with Factor VIII activating properties.

TABLE 1. Some biol. properties of dDAVP analogues modified in position 4.

Compound	Antidiuretic pot.*	Pressoric pot.	Factor VIII
dDAVP	1130 ± 107(7)^x	0.23 ± 0.035(6)^x	323 ± 53(4)^{xx}
[L – Val^4]dDAVP	575 ± 66(6)	< 0.187(6)	148 ± 36(3)
[L – Ala^4]dDAVP	645 ± 98(4)	< 0.041(4)	155 ± 36(4)
[L – Asn^4]dDAVP	608 ± 98(13)	< 0.070(6)	110 ± 7(5)
[L – Leu^4]dDAVP	50 ± 10(4)	< 0.100(5)	296 ± 65(3)
[Gly^4]dDAVP	19.2 ± 2(7)	< 0.004(5)	148 ± 34(4)
[D – Gln^4]dDAVP	< 0.008(9)	< 0.184(4)	90 ± 25(3)
[L – $Allo^4$]dDAVP	898 ± 99(6)	0.409 ± 0.05(7)	88(2)

^{x} – IU per μmol of peptide, ^{xx} – % increase, basal response equal to 100%, * – in brackets are numbers of experiments.

Table 1. represents the peptides incorporated in the group of dDAVP analogues with the replacement of amino acid in position 4. Here one of the candidates for further consideration is L – Leu^4dDAVP with 5% of dDAVP antidiuretic potency, but with preserved high Factor VIII activating properties.

The combination of substitutions in position 4 (Val) with those in positions 7 or 2 did not offer any promising results (Table 2.).

TABLE 2. Some biological properties of dDAVP analogues with combined modifica – tions.

Compound	Antidiuretic pot.*	Pressoric pot.	Factor VIII
dDAVP	1130 ± 107(7)^x	0.23 ± 0.035(6)^x	323 ± 53(4)^{xx}
[L – Val^4]dDAVP	575 ± 66(7)	< 0.187(6)	148 ± 36(3)
[Gly^7]dDAVP	41 ± 3(5)	< 0.13(4)	123 ± 36(3)
[L – Val^4, Gly^7] dDAVP	184 ± 18(6)	< 0.004(6)	88 ± 9(4)
[L – $OMeTyr^2$, L – Val^4]dDAVP	1011 ± 97(9)	< 0.07(10)	154(2)
[L – $OEtTyr^2$, L – Val^4]dDAVP	100 ± 14.1(8)	< 0.006(4)	95 ± 3(4)

x, xx, * – see footnotes under Table 1.

On the other hand the analogues of dDAVP with migrating alanine from positions 2 to 9 (alanineamide) gave some interesting results particularly related to substitution in position 5 (Table 3.).

We tried to develop another approach to the design of Factor VIII activating peptides. dDAVP being a peptide with a significantly lowered pressoric potency, the priority task would be to dissociate antidiuretic and Factor VIII activating properties. If one takes into consideration the basal structural requirements given above for Factor VIII activating properties, we come to a series of dDAVP analogues with homologues of D – amino acid in position 8. We extended the series of analogues for peptides with [D – $homoarginine^8$]deamino vasopressin, which already revealed only 5% of antidiuretic potency of dDAVP[13]. A series of [D – Har^8] analogues of dDAVP was synthesized[14] with the aim to dissociate the AD and Factor VIII activating properties more efficiently. The AD activity of the analogues presented in table 4 corresponded to the demand for elimination of antidiuretic potency, in comparison to [D-Har^8] de - amino vasopressin their AD potency is lowered by more than two orders of magnitude. Even their pressoric effect is eliminated and in some cases the peptides are inhibitory to AVP in the pressoric assay in rats.

TABLE 3. Some biological properties of L – alanine analogues of dDAVP.

Compound	Antidiuretic pot.*	Pressoric pot.	Factor VIII
dDAVP	1130 ± 107(7)[x]	0.23 ± 0.035(6)[x]	323 ± 53(4)[xx]
[L – Ala^2]dDAVP	0.35 ± 0.88(7)	< 0.036(6)	84.5(2)
[L – Ala^3]dDAVP	23.1 ± 7.5(7)	< 0.02(6)	112 ± 7(3)
[L – Ala^4]dDAVP	645 ± 98(4)	< 0.041(4)	155 ± 36(4)
[L – Ala^5]dDAVP	0.21 ± 0.02(7)	0.03 ± 0.01(4)	176 ± 37(3)
[L – Ala^7]dDAVP	111 ± 2.7(7)	< 0.004(4)	78.5(2)
[L – Ala^8]dDAVP	41.4 ± 5.9(4)	3.7 ± 0.53(4)	183 ± 76(3)
[L – AlaNH$_2$^{9}]dDAVP	115 ± 12(8)	0.24 ± 0.03(9)	102 ± 24(5)

x, xx, * – see footnotes under Table 1.

TABLE 4. Some biol. properties of dDAVP analogues modified in positions 2 and 8.

Compound	Antidiuretic pot.*	Pressoric pot.	Factor VIII
dDAVP	100%[xxx]	0.23 ± 0.035(6)[x]	323 ± 53(4)[xx]
[D-Har⁸]dVP	5%	0.28	127 ± 13(5)
[L-MePhe², D-Har⁸]dVP	0.02%	pA_2 6.2[a]	155 ± 35.6(4)
[D-MePhe², D-Har⁸]dVP	0.02%	0.0	112 ± 13(8)
[L-EtPhe², D-Har⁸]dVP	0.02%	pA_2 6.2	111.5 ± 18(3)
[D-EtPhe², D-Har⁸]dVP	0.02%	pA_2 6.35	96.5(2)
[L-OMeTyr², D-Har⁸]dVP	--	0.0	98.5(2)

[x], [xx], * - see footnotes under Table 1., [xxx] - potency of dDAVP laid equal to 100%, reference 13, [a] - see reference 15.

L-p-Methylphenylalanine derivatives of [D-Har[8]]deamino vasopressin preserved a substantial part of Factor VIII activating potency of dDAVP, the potency is higher than that of [D-Har[8]]deamino vasopressin. This derivative having L-p-methylphenylalanine in position 2 of [D-Har[8]]deamino vasopressin extended the number of compounds to be taken into consideration when new series of Factor VIII activating peptides are designed.

CONCLUSION

In the series of dDAVP analogues several peptides offer the possibility of further modification in the development of specific Factor VIII activating peptides. They are [L-Leu[4]]dDAVP, [L-Ala[5]]dDAVP and [L-p-MePhe[2], D-Har[8]]dVP.

REFERENCES

1. M. Zaoral, J. Kolc, and F. Sorm, Synthesis of 1 – deamino – 8 – D – aminobutyrine vasopressin, 1 – deamino – 8 – D – lysine vasopressin and 1 – deamino – 8 – D – arginine vasopressin, Collection Czechoslov. Chem. Commun. 32:1250 (1967).
2. I. Vavra, A. Machova, V. Holecek, J.H. Cort, M. Zaoral, and F. Sorm, Effects of a synthetic analogue of vasopressin in animals and in patients with diabetes insipidus, The Lancet I:948 (1968).
3. D.J. Becker and T.P. Foley, 1 – deamino – 8 – D – arginine in treatment of central diabetes insipidus in childhood, J. Pediatrics 92:1011 (1978).
4. J.P. Monson and P. Richard, Desmopressin urine concentration test, Brit. Med. J. 1:24 (1978).
5. P.M. Mannucci, M. Aberg, I.M. Nilsson, and B. Robertson, Mechanism of Plasminogen Activator and Factor VIII increase after vasoactive drugs, Brit. J. Haematol. 30:81 (1975).
6. J.D. Cash, A.M.A. Gader, and J. Da Costa, Release of Plasminogen activator and Factor VIII to lysine vasopressin, arginine vasopressin, 1 – desamino – 8 – D – arginine vasopressin, angiotensin and oxytocin in man., Brit. J. Haematol. 27:263 (1974).
7. A.I. Warrier and J.M. Lusher, DDAVP: A useful alternative to blood components in moderate haemophilia A and von Willebrands disease, J. Pediatrics 102:228 (1983).
8. H. Köstering, U. Ehrlich, J. Wiedig, and W. Wigger, Nebenwirkungen unter der Infusion von DDAVP (Mirinin R), in: "Mirinin," A.H. Sutor, ed., F.K. Schattauer Verlag, Stuttgart, New York (1980).
9. W. Blätter, Psychic effects of 1 – deamino – 8 – D – Arginine vasopressin (DDAVP), in: "Mirinin," A.H. Sutor, ed., F.K. Schattauer Verlag, Stuttgart, New York (1980).
10. H. Vilhardt, T. Barth, J. Falck, and I.M. Nilsson, Plasma concentrations of Factor VIII after administration of dDAVP to conscious dogs, Thrombosis Research 47:585 (1987).
11. H. Vilhardt and T. Barth, Structure – activity relationships of vasopressin analogues on release of Factor VIII in dogs, J. Receptor Research 11:233 (1991).
12. H. Vilhardt and T. Barth, Effect of desmopressin (DDAVP) on Factor VIII in various species, in: "Proceedings of Fourth International Conference on the Neurohypophysis," Copenhagen July 1989, Oxford University Press (1989).
13. J. Skopkova, P. Hrbas, J. Slaninova, and T. Barth, Prolonged antidiuretic action of vasopressin analogues in relation to their primary structure, Collection Czechoslov. Chem. Commun. 46:1850 (1981).
14. M. Zertova, Z. Prochazka, T. Barth, J. Slaninova, J. Skopkova, I. Blaha, and M. Lebl, Strong uterotonic inhibitors – analogs of 1 – deamino – 8 – D – homoarginine vasopressin with p – substituted phenylalanine in position 2, Collection zechoslov. Chem. Commun. 56:1761 (1991).
15. H.O. Schild, pA2 and competitive drug antagonism, Brit. J. Pharmacol. Chemotherap. 4:277 (1949).

POSSIBLE INVOLVEMENT OF SEROTONIN IN THE HAEMOSTATIC ACTION OF DDAVP IN PATIENTS WITH URAEMIA

Jacek Malyszko[1], Jolanta Malyszko[1], Michal Pietraszek[2],
Arsalan Azzadin[2], Michal Mysliwiec[1], Wlodzimierz Bucsko[2]

[1]Nephrology and [2]Pharmacodynamics Departments
Medical School
Bialystok, Poland

INTRODUCTION

The effect of DDAVP on some haemostatic and fibrinolytic parameters as well as on plasma and platelet serotonin was studied. DDAVP was administered intravenously in a dose of 0.4 µg/Kg b.w. to 16 uraemic patients maintained on chronic haemodialasys. The bleeding time was shortened significantly from 21.3 min + 8 to 11.5 min + 6($p < 0.001$), as was ECLT from 238 min +101 to 148 min + 84 ($p < 0.01$) after DDAVP administration. A significant rise in vWFR:Ag and vWF:RCof was found. We observed an increase in plasma tPA activity from 1.64 + 0.73 IU/ml to 3.09 + 0.76 IU/ml ($p < 0.01$) and a decrease in plasma PAI activity from 7.65 + 1.98 AU/ml to 4.28 + 0.72 AU/ml ($p < 0.01$). The plasma serotonin concentration rose significantly from 2.6 + 1.13 ng/ml to 4.25 + 1.04 ng/ml ($p < 0.05$) and platelet serotonin content was significantly reduced from 541.6 + 120 ng/10^9 platelets to 409 + 88 ng/10^9 platelets ($p < 0.05$). DDAVP inhibited ^{14}C serotonin uptake in a dose-dependent manner. After 2 hours of platelet incubation with DDAVP 15% of serotonin was released. We observed no changes in haematocrit, platelet count and factor VIII coagulant activity after DDAVP administration. We suggest that the serotoninergic mechanism may be involved in the haemostatic action of DDAVP on the shortening of the prolonged bleeding time.

Key-words: DDAVP, uraemia, bleeding time, vWf, serotonin, haemostasis, fibrinolysis.

Various haemostatic abnormalities are often associated with chronic renal failure. The most common feature is a prolongation of bleeding time, which is the laboratory parameter combining the best effects with the lowest risk of haemorrhage in uraemic patients. In spite of intensive research the pathogenesis of the bleeding tendency in uraemia is still not fully understood. It is suggested that lots of factors contribute to haemorrhagic diathesis in uraemia. They include metabolic changes in uraemic platelets and the von Willebrand factor (vWF)-platelet membrane interaction[1,2]. Anaemia itself may predispose to uraemic bleeding. The

Desmopressin in Bleeding Disorders, Edited by G. Mariani *et al.*
Plenum Press, New York, 1993

traditionally recommended therapy is dialysis intensification but it only partially corrects the prolonged bleeding time. Other possibilities include blood and cryoprecipitate transfusions, conjugated estrogens or desmopressin (1-deamino-8-D-arginine vasopressin, DDAVP).

DDAVP, the vasopressin analogue devoid of vasoconstrictory action, is known to shorten the prolonged bleeding time in uraemia[3], haemophilia[4], von Willebrand disease[4] and various platelet dysfunctions[5,6]. The haemostatic mechanism of action of this drug still remains unclear. It was found that DDAVP influenced von Willebrand factor but on the other hand it increased plasma fibrinolytic activity[7]. We have previously shown that desmopressin induces the release of serotonin from platelets in patients with chronic renal failure[8].

The aim of the study was further investigation of possible serotoninergic mechanisms in the action of DDAVP and their correlations with the bleeding time and the other haemostatic parameters.

MATERIALS AND METHODS

The studies were performed on 16 chronically haemodialyzed uraemic patients (11 females and 5 males, age range 33 - 66, mean 43.8 years). All the patients underwent regular dialyses three times a week for 4 - 5 hours (from 1 to 6 years, mean 3.5 years) using cuprophane dialysers. They were informed about the purpose of the study and gave their consent. None of the patients investigated had received blood transfusions for at least 1.5 months and apart from heparin during dialysis no drugs which could influence platelet function were administered for at least ten days before the study. They were given aluminium hydroxide, folic acid and vitamin supplements. The patients were in a stable clinical state, without infections. They were selected on the basis of having bleeding times over ten minutes. The normal values for uptake and release of ^{14}C serotonin from platelets were derived from the data in 16 healthy volunteers with similar ages to patients.

On the day of the study (between dialyses) patients received neither food nor morning drugs and after overnight fast and a rest period of 30 min in a supine position DDAVP (Adjuretin SD, Spofa, Czechoslovakia) was infused intravenously at a dose of 0.4 µg/kg body weight over 20 minutes. Blood was drawn from the venipuncture on the forearm both before and 90 min after DDAVP infusion. The first 0.5 ml was discarded. Blood was collected into 0.11 M sodium citrate in a 9:1 proportion. It was centrifuged at 200 g for 10 min to obtain platelet rich plasma addition, centrifuged further at 2500 g for 20 min at 20°C (in addition, centrifugation at 4°C was performed for vWFRCof and vWFR:Ag assays) to yield platelet poor plasma. Blood for the determination of tissue plasminogen activator (tPA) activity was immediately acidified by adding 1 volume of 0.2 M sodium acetate buffer pH 3.9 to 1 volume of citrated blood and centrifuged without delay. The samples were aliquotted and used immediately or stored at -25°C for a few days until assayed.

Bleeding time was measured by the Ivy method modified by Mielke[9]. Haematocrit was determined by a standard laboratory method. Platelets were counted using contrast-phase microscopy. vWF related antigen (vWFR:Ag) was determined by rocket immunoelectrophoresis using commercial antisera from Behringwerke, Germany[10]. Factor VIII coagulant activity (VIII:C) was measured by a one stage clotting assay. Deficient plasma was obtained from Bio-Merrieux. Ristocetin cofactor of vWF (vWF:RCoF) was assayed using commercial kits from "General Diagnostics", Morris Plains,USA. The fibrinolytic activity was measured as euglobin clot lysis time (ECLT)[11]. tPA and its inhibitor (PAI) activities were determined using the amidolytic method described by Chmielewska and Wiman[12]. Blood serotonin concentration was assayed according to Ashcroft and Crawford[13]. Platelet serotonin content was measured using the fluoroscopic method of Drummond and Gordon[14]. ^{14}C serotonin release from platelets was studied as described by Lingjaerde[15] and ^{14}C serotonin uptake was measured according to Gordon and Olverman[16]. The statistical analysis was performed by means of the student's t-test for paired data with p< 0.05 considered significant.

RESULTS

In the whole group of patients the bleeding time was significantly shortened from 21.3 + 8 min to 11.5 + 6 min (p < 0.001) 90 min after DDAVP infusion as well as ECLT from 238 +101 min to 148 +84 min (p <0.001). There was a parametric correlation between the bleeding time and ECRT (r = -0.43). There were no changes in haematocrit and platelet count following desmopressin administration. vWFR:Ag increased significantly as did vWF:RCof. We observed a small, not significant, rise in factor VIII coagulant activity after DDAVP infusion. Intravenously administered DDAVP caused a significant increase in plasma tPA activity and a significant decrease in plasma PAI activities. At the same time a significant fall in platelet serotonin content was observed. A fairly good correlation was found between tPA activity and platelet serotonin content (r = 0.8) as well as between PAI activity and platelet serotonin content (r = -0.6). A significant rise in plasma serotonin concentration was detected. All the above mentioned results are presented in Table 1. We observed a dose-dependent inhibition of ^{14}C serotonin uptake. The minimal concentration of the drug which significantly inhibited serotonin uptake was 1 ng/ml (the observed uptake was 146 + 12 pmol/108 platelets and 140 + 11 pmol/108 platelets in control and uraemic platelets, respectively). DDAVP concentrations of 2 and 4 ng/ml caused further uptake inhibition (128 + 7 pmol/108 platelets and 121 + 9 pmol/ 108 platelets respectively). There were no changes between ^{14}C serotonin uptake by control and uraemic platelets. We also investigated ^{14}C serotonin release after platelet incubation with DDAVP. We detected no alterations in ^{14}C serotonin release after 1 and 2 hours of platelet incubation with DDAVP at concentrations of 1 and 2 ng/ml while after 2 hours of platelet incubation with DDAVP at a concentration of 4 ng/ml 15% serotonin was released from platelets. Similar changes were observed between control and uraemic platelets. The results obtained are presented in Table 1.

DISCUSSION

We demonstrated that prolonged bleeding time in uraemic patients was markedly shortened by intravenous DDAVP administration. It reached the normal range in 7 and was shortened in 6 (without normalization) out of 16 patients. DDAVP had no effect on the prolonged bleeding time in 3 patients. The mechanism of the haemostatic action of DDAVP still remains unclear.

According to Yang et al [17] the shortening of the bleeding time by DDAVP in patients with primary platelet disorders is related to an indirect stimulatory effect of this drug on platelets. Escolar[18] and Grant[19] found an increase in noradrenaline levels following DDAVP administration. This may suggest a role of the activation of the noradrenergic system in the shortening of the bleeding time after DDAVP infusion. No changes in epinephrine and dopamine levels were observed after DDAVP administration[19]. Brommer and co-workers[20] found that desmopressin did not act by betaadrenoreceptor blockade.

There are some data that also serotonin in addition to causing vasoconstriction plays an important role in the interactions between platelets and the vessel wall[21]. In patients with chronic renal failure, decreased platelet serotonin level was observed simoultaneously with the prolongation of the bleeding time[22].

Table I. The effect of DDAVP on some haemostatic parameters in patients with chronic renal failure

	Before DDAVP	after DDAVP	
bleeding time (min)	21.3 ± 8	11.5 ± 6	***
haematocrit (1/1)	26.8 ± 3.1	26.4 ± 3.7	
platelets (x 109/1)	188.7 ± 101	173.9 ± 89	
ECLT (min)	238 ± 101	148 ± 84	**
vWFR:Ag (%)	239.1 ± 94	473.1 ± 293	**
vWF:RCoF (%)	231.1 ± 162	347.3 ± 176	**
VIII:C (%)	247.5 ± 84.5	297.7 ± 170	
tPA (IU/ml)	1.69 ± 0.73	3.09 ± 0.76	***
PAI (AU/ml)	7.65 ± 1.98	4.28 ± 0.72	**
plasma serotonin (ng/ml)	2.6 ± 1.13	4.25 ± 1.04	*
platelet serotonin (ng/109platelets)	541.6 ± 120	409 ± 88	*

Values given are means + SD

* $p < 0.05$ as compared with pre-treatment value
** $p < 0.01$ as compared with pre-treatment value
*** $p < 0.001$ as compared with pre-treatment value

We have previously shown that DDAVP caused a fall in platelet serotonin content in uraemic patients. In this study we confirmed our previous results and at the same time we observed a statistically significant rise in plasma serotonin concentration. Two mechanisms of such an action may be involved, either the release of serotonin from platelets or an impaired uptake of this amine from the blood.

We found a dose-dependent inhibition of ^{14}C serotonin uptake by DDAVP in contrast to Soslau et al[23] who showed a significant increase in platelet serotonin uptake caused by this drug in uraemic patients, using a different laboratory method. We were also able to demonstrate DDAVP-induced ^{14}C serotonin release from platelets. This phenomenon was also dose-dependent. There were no changes between uraemic and control platelets. It was hypothesized that platelets release serotonin and ATP at the site of injury modulated regional tone and haemostasis. Also ATP and serotonin helped to regulate cell/cell, cell/vessel wall interactions.

We observed a marked increase in vWFR:Ag, moderate in vWF:RCoF and not significant in factor VIII:C activity. Mannucci et al[3] reported a marked increase in all these parameters after intravenous administration of DDAVP in uraemics. Watson and Koegh[24] did not find any increase in either factor VIII:C activity or vWFR:Ag. In their studies, vWF:RCoF rose, but only two hours after DDAVP administration. It has been suggested that desmopressin acts by releasing vWF, particularly its high-molecular-weight multimers, from the endothelium25. Other studies have not confirmed these suggestions[1,23].

A counteracting mechanism in the shortening of the prolonged bleeding time is the activation of fibrinolysis. DDAVP is known to cause a marked increase in plasma fibrinolytic activity mainly due to the release of tPA from the endothelium. The possibility of desmopressin acting on fibrinolysis through the prostaglandin mechanism was excluded by Brommer et al[20]. We found a shortening of the ECLT and a rise in plasma tPA activity following DDAVP administration. We also observed a statistically significant fall in plasma PAI activity, probably secondary to the tPA rise. The fairly good, statistically significant, correlation between the fall in platelet serotonin content and the plasma tPA activity suggests a possible role of this amine in tPA release.

As a potent vasoconstrictor serotonin could mediate a shortening of prolonged bleeding time although we did not find a good correlation between platelet serotonin content and bleeding time ($r = -0.33$). A fairly good correlation between bleeding time and plasma serotonin concentration as well as between bleeding time and platelet serotonin content was found in those patients who responded to DDAVP by the shortening of bleeding time to the normal range. At the same time a good correlation observed between platelet serotonin content and tPA activity allowed us to take into account a possible serotoninergic mechanism of tPA release by DDAVP.

Our studies suggest that both a shortening of the bleeding time and an increase in fibrinolytic activity by DDAVP may be mediated by serotonin released from platelets.

REFERENCES

1. Gralnick H R, McKeown L P, Williams S B, Shafer B C, Pierce L. Plasma and platelet von Willebrand factor defects in uremia. Am J Med 1988; 85:806-810.
2. Escolar G, Cases A, Bastida E, Garrido M, Lopez J, Revert L, Castillo R, Ordinas A. Uremic platelets have a functional defect affecting the interaction of von Willebrand factor with glycoprotein IIb-IIIa. Blood 1990; 76:1336-1340.
3. Mannucci P M, Remuzzi G, Pusineri F, Lombardi R, Valsecchi C, Mecca G, Zimmerman T S. Deamino-8-D-arginine vasopressing shortens the bleeding time in uraemia. N Eng J Med 1983; 308:8-12.
4. Mannucci P M, Ruggeri Z M, Pareti F J, Capitanio A. 1 deamino-8-D-arginine vasopressin: a new pharmacological approach to the management of haemophilia and von Willebrand's disease. Lancet 1977; 1:869-872.
5. Kobrinski N L, Israels E D, Gerrard J M, Cheang M S, Watson C M, Bishop A J, Shroeder M L. Shortening of bleeding time by 1-deamino-8-D-arginine vasopressin in various bleeding disorders. Lancet 1984; 1:1145-1148.
6. Schulman S, Johnsson H, Edberg N, Blomback N. DDAVP induced correction of prolonged bleeding time in patients with congenital platelet defects. Thromb Res 1987; 45:165-174.
7. Mac Gregor I R, Roberts E M, Prowse C V, Bromhead A F, Ozolins M, Litka P. Fibrinolytic and haemostatic response to deamino-8-D-arginine vasopressin (DDAVP) administered by intravenous and subcutaneous routes in healthy subjects. Thromb Haemostas 1988; 59:34-39.

8. Malyszko J, Pietraszek M, Azzadin A, Buczko W, Mysliwiec M. Desmopressin induces decrease in platelet serotonin content in uremia. Thromb Haemostas 1989; 61:537.
9. Mielke C H, Kaneshiro MM, Maher J A, Wessler J M, Rapaport S I. The standardized normal Ivy bleeding time and its prolongation by aspirin. Blood 1969; 15:45-52.
10. Laurell C B. Quantitative estimation of proteins by electrophoresis in agarose gel containing antibodies. Anal Biochem 1966; 15:45-52.
11. Kowarzyk H, Buluk K. Postepy badan nad krzepnieciem krwi. Post Hig Med Dosw 1950; 2:1-76.
12. Chmielewska J, Wiman B. Determination of tissue plasminogen activator and its "fast" inhibitor in plasma. Clin Chem 1985; 32:482-485.
13. Ashcroft G, Crawford T B. Estimation of 5-hydroxytryptamine in human blood. Clin Chem Acta 1964; 9:364-369.
14. Drummond A H, Gordon J L. Rapid sensitive microassay for platelets 5 HT Thromb Diathes haemorrh. Stuttgart 1974;31:366.
15. Lingjaerde D. Inhibitory effect of ethanol of 5-hydroxytryptamide (serotonin) uptake in human blood platelets in vitro. Acta Pharmacol Toxicol 1979; 45:394-399.
16. Gordon J L,Olverman H J. 5-hydroxytryptamine and dopamine transport by rats and human blood platelets. Brit J Pharmacol 1978; 62:219.
17. Yang H, Jyoti D, Koneti R. Effect of 1-deamino-8-D-arginine vasopressin (DDAVP) on human platelets. Thromb Res 1990; 59:809-818.
18. Escolar G, Cases A, Monteguado J, Campistol M, Ordinas A, Lopez J, Revert J. Studies on the mechanisms of desmopressin (DDAVP)-induced hemostatic action in uremic patients. XXIVth Congress of the EDTBA-ERA, Berlin (west),1987,54.
19. Grant M B, Guay C, Lottenberg R. Desmopressin stimulates parallel norepinephrine and tissue plasminogen activator release in normal subjects and patients with diabetes mellitus. Thromb Haemostas 1988; 59:221-224.
20. Brommer E J P, Derkx F H M, Barret-Bergshoeff M M, Schalekamp M A D H . The inability of prophanol and aspirin to inhibit the response of fibrinolytic activity and factor VIII-antigen to infusion of DDAVP. Thromb Haemostas 1984; 51:42-44.
21. DeClerk T, Somers Y, Van Gorp L. Platelet-vessel wall interaction in haemostasis: implication of 5-hydroxytryptamine. Agents Actions 1984; 12:627-635.
22. Soslau G, Brodsky I, Putatunda B, Packer J, Schwartz A B. Selective reduction of serotonin storage and ATP release in chronic renal failure patient platelets. Am J Haematol 1990; 35:171-176.
23. Soslau G, Schwartz A B, Putatunda B, Conroy J D, Parker J, Abel R F, Brodsky I. Desmopressin-induced improvement in bleeding times in chronic renal failure patients correlates with platelet serotonin uptake and ATP release. Am J Med Sci 1990; 300:372-379.
24. Watson A J S, Koegh J A B. Effect of 1-deamino-8-d-arginine vasopressin on the prolonged bleeding time in chronic renal failure. Nephron 1982; 32:49-52.
25. Ruggeri Z M, Mannucci P M, Lombardi R, Federici A B, Zimmerman T S. Multimetric composition of factor VIII/von Willebrand factor following administration of DDAVP: implications for pathophysiology and therapy of von Willebrand's disease subtypes. Blood 1981; 59:1272-1278.

DISCUSSION

Kobrinsky: I am intrigued by the fall in PAI. Does this mean shortening of lysis time, and could it be part of the benefit?

Hashemi: PAF is a potent platelet activator, and fits very well with these results.
Kobrinsky: It could explain the flushing, headaches and other side effects. Desmopressin has an effect on amino acid transport, and this would support these findings.
Kinter: We could not block the flushing with ciproheptadine.
Malyszko: Ciproheptadine is not a selective serotonin blocker: there are others, such as ketanserin, and we intend to use it in future studies.

MOLECULAR MECHANISMS OF CELLULAR RESPONSES TO DDAVP

Sofia Hashemi[1], Douglas S. Palmer[1], Maung T. Aye[1,2] and Peter R. Ganz[1,3]

[1]Ottawa Centre, Canadian Red Cross, Blood Transfusion Service
Ottawa, Ontario, Canada

[2]Dept. of Medicine,[3]Dept. of Biochemistry, University of Ottawa, Ottawa
Ontario, Canada

INTRODUCTION

The synthetic vasopressin analogue 1-deamino-8-D-arginine vasopressin (DDAVP), which produces antidiuretic effects in diabetes insipidus patients without vasoactive side-effects,[1] also significantly increases plasma concentrations of von Willebrand factor (vWf), Factor VIII and tissue plasminogen activator (t-PA) in vivo in patients with mild or moderate Hemophilia A or Type I von Willebrand's disease. DDAVP treatment [2-4] is regarded as an important therapeutic alternative for Factor VIII- or vWf-deficient patients since the use of blood products is associated with a risk of transmitting infectious agents such as hepatitis B, hepatitis C and HIV. Given to healthy normal individuals prior to donation, it also increases plasma Factor VIII and vWf levels resulting in improved potency and purity of Factor VIII/vWf recovered after commercial fractionation.[5,6] However, its variable effects between individuals and within the same individual receiving repeated treatments [5,7] and unknown mechanism of action[3,4] have hindered the adoption of DDAVP on a more widespread basis even within the patient populations for which its use has been indicated.

An increasing body of evidence supports the hypothesis that DDAVP modulates certain endothelial cell (EC) hemostatic functions via some intermediary factor(s).[5,8-10] With respect to the enhancement of vWf levels following DDAVP treatment in vivo and the absence of direct effects of DDAVP on secretion of vWf by ECs in vitro, it would seem reasonable to hypothesize that these intermediaries might be secreted from other cells. Therefore, it is of paramount importance to identify the target cell(s) involved and once this has been achieved, to determine which of the various agents secreted by these cells might be responsible for enhancing vWf release from ECs. In this article, we will review current information concerning identification of one population of cells in the peripheral blood which, acting as target cells for DDAVP, secrete intermediaries that can augment vWf secretion from ECs.

DDAVP: AN OVERVIEW

DDAVP shares some characteristics of the natural hormone AVP (arginine vasopressin) including: a) low molecular weight (DDAVP = 1,069 daltons), b) ability to enhance secretion of Factor VIII, vWf and tissue plasminogen activator (t-PA),[11,12] c) potent activity at nanomolar concentrations [13,14] and d) interaction with high affinity V_2

Desmopressin in Bleeding Disorders, Edited by G. Mariani *et al.*
Plenum Press, New York, 1993

receptors.[15,16] Increases of Factor VIII, vWf and t-PA occur so rapidly and relatively transiently after DDAVP treatment that enhanced release rather than synthesis is now considered to be most likely to account for DDAVP's effects. Although vascular ECs are a major source of vWf and t-PA,[17] megakaryocytes and platelets might also release some vWf after DDAVP treatment.[18] The liver is the main organ responsible for the synthesis of Factor VIII [19,20] although other sites may be involved.[19] With regard to ECs isolated from human umbilical veins, there is no evidence of Factor VIII:Ag synthesis.[10] There is no significant release of vWf from DDAVP-treated cultured human ECs [9,10,21] or after direct perfusion of isolated human vessels.[22] The involvement of a secondary messenger in the hypothalamic areas of the CNS has been discounted and numerous other studies have failed to identify any putative second messengers, as reviewed by Mannucci.[23]

The natural hormone AVP may be involved in the regulation of circulating levels of Factor VIII and vWf [11,12] by exerting its effects through V_1 and V_2 receptors via different second messengers.[24] DDAVP might act through its strong V_2 agonist activity [25] as patients with nephrogenic diabetes insipidus (who lack V_2 receptors and are thus unresponsive to V_2 agonists) do not show the characteristic elevation of plasma Factor VIII and vWf after DDAVP treatment.[26] As AVP acts on both V_1 and V_2 receptors, it could cause release of Factor VIII directly from liver sinusoidal cells via V_1 receptors.[27] However, the greater potency of DDAVP over lysine vasopressin,[28] together with the results of structural specificity studies [29] strongly suggest that V_2 receptors are involved in both Factor VIII and vWf release. Given the primary sites of synthesis of vWf and Factor VIII,[24] we considered it likely that other target cells with V_2 receptors might secrete intermediaries that were responsible for some of DDAVP's indirect effects on ECs.

RELEASE OF vWf FROM ENDOTHELIAL CELLS

The vWf protein, which circulates as a non-covalent complex with Factor VIII and stabilizes its activity, promotes adhesion of platelets to exposed subendothelium with the subsequent formation of a platelet plug at the sites of vascular injuries. It behaves as an acute-phase reactant as its levels are raised in plasma in a wide variety of inflammatory disorders. The vWf required for primary hemostasis is found in the subendothelium, plasma, platelet α-granules [31] and ECs where, unlike platelets and megakaryocytes, it is both synthesized and stored.[18] ECs are involved in the production of and responses to various cytokines,[32,33] growth factors [34] and lipid mediators such as PAF [35,36] and there is evidence of an intimate relationship between PAF, cytokines and the mediators of coagulation on or in endothelial cells.[37-41] There are two pathways for vWf release from ECs: constitutive release, which is directly related to de novo synthesis, and the regulated pathway in which rapid release from Weibel-Palade bodies [42] can be stimulated by physiologic or exogenous agents. The vWf stored in Weibel-Palade bodies is composed of only the largest high molecular weight multimers without the pro-vWf subunit [43] whereas most constitutively released vWf multimers are dimeric and contain both the precursor (pro-vWf) and processed subunits.[44] The release of vWf from the regulated pathway occurs only following stimulation of ECs with an appropriate agonist. For example, thrombin which binds to high affinity receptors on ECs [45] induces the synthesis and release of prostacyclin (PGI_2),[46] adenine nucleotides [47] and vWf in a time- and dose-dependent manner.[21,45,48-50] In addition to the effects of exogenous agents such as calcium ionophore A23187 [48,50,51] or phorbol esters,[48,50-52] acute release of vWf from ECs has also been observed with such agents as plasmin, cytokines, adrenaline and bradykinin,[21,53,54] histamine,[55] endotoxin,[56] fibrin [49] and estrogen.[57] The secretion of vWf from ECs is bidirectional, being released both into the blood stream as well as incorporated into the subendothelial matrix [43] with the von Willebrand factor released from Weibel-Palade bodies binding more avidly to the extracellular matrix than that secreted constitutively.[58]

MECHANISM OF DDAVP INDUCED RELEASE OF vWf FROM ENDOTHELIAL CELLS

Although the regulated pathway of vWf release involves Weibel-Palade bodies in ECs,[5,42,56] many investigators have been unable to show that DDAVP stimulates the release

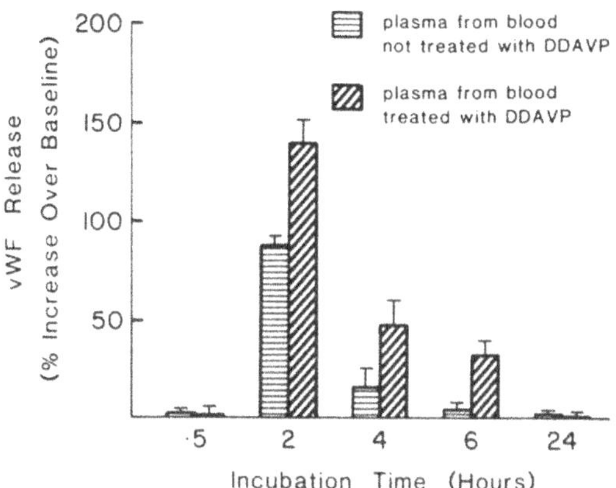

Figure 1. Release of vWf from cultured human umbilical vein endothelial cells (HUVECs) exposed to plasma from citrated whole blood which was either untreated or treated in vitro with 100 ng DDAVP/mL for 90 minutes at 37°C. The plasma was added in serum-free medium (1:1, v/v) to washed, confluent HUVECs which had been previously labelled for 24 hours with ^{35}S-methionine. After the designated incubation times at 37°C, the media were withdrawn and ^{35}S-vWf determined by immunoassay.[21] (Reprinted with permission from S. Hashemi, E.S. Tackaberry, D.S. Palmer, G. Rock, and P.R. Ganz, DDAVP-induced release of von Willebrand factor from endothelial cells in vitro: the effect of plasma and blood cells, Biochim. Biophys. Acta 1052:63, 1990, Elsevier Science Publishers BV).

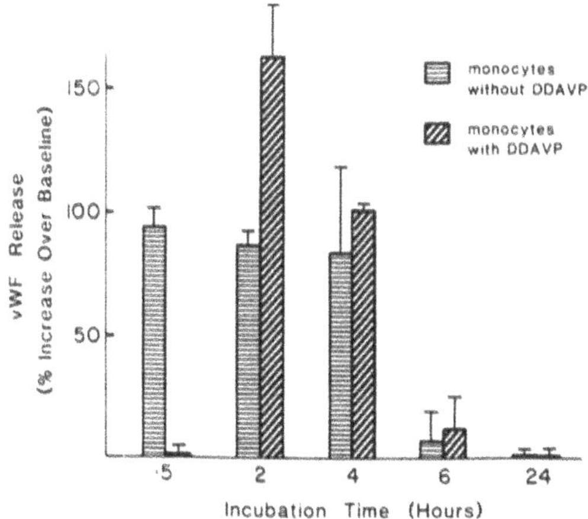

Figure 2. Release of vWf in response to fractionated monocytes prepared from normal individuals and added at 10^6 cells/mL to cultured HUVECs without or with 100 ng DDAVP/mL. After the indicated incubation times at 37°C, the medium was withdrawn and assayed for vWf by ELISA.[21] (Reproduced with permission as indicated in Fig. 1)

of vWf directly from ECs in vitro.[8,9,21,22,53] These observations have encouraged the hypothesis that DDAVP exerts its effects via the secretion of intermediaries, from cells other than ECs, which subsequently cause the release of vWf from ECs.[5,8,21,39] We have recently shown that plasma recovered from the whole blood of DDAVP-treated normal individuals could, following incubation with cultured human ECs, promote enhanced release of ^{35}S-labelled vWf compared to the effect of plasma from untreated individuals.[21] DDAVP added directly to cultured ECs had no demonstrable effect. Furthermore, when whole blood was treated with DDAVP in vitro and the plasma was subsequently added to cultured ECs, a significant increase in vWf release was also found (Fig. 1), suggesting that DDAVP's effects were mediated by a factor present in plasma which had been released from the cellular components of blood. Concerning the cell lineages involved in DDAVP's effects, we showed that coincubation of DDAVP and mononuclear cells with ECs increased the release of vWf.[21]

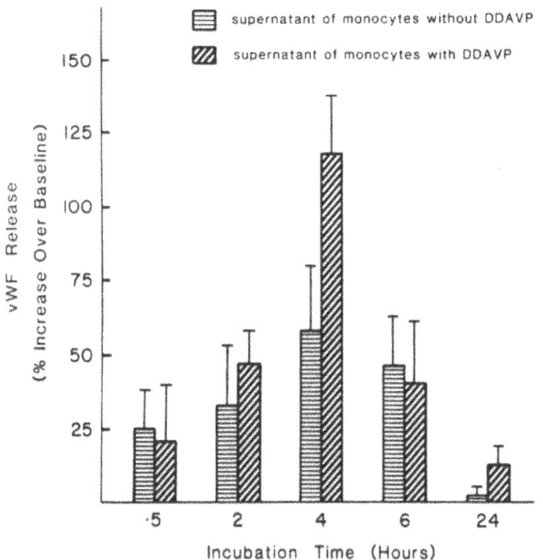

Figure 3. Release of vWf from cultured HUVECs in response to conditioned medium from untreated or DDAVP-treated monocytes (100 ng/mL). After incubation of 10^6 monocytes/mL with or without DDAVP for 30 minutes at 37°C, the monocytes were centrifuged and the supernatants were added to confluent HUVECs. Following incubation, the media were withdrawn and assayed for vWf by ELISA.[21] (Reproduced with permission as indicated in Fig. 1).

While T or B lymphocytes had marginal effects,[21] isolated monocytes were found to be the cells largely responsible (Fig. 2). In addition, when conditioned media isolated following incubation of monocytes with DDAVP were added to EC cultures, significant increases in vWf release from ECs were observed compared to conditioned medium from unstimulated monocytes (Fig. 3). These studies indicated that peripheral blood monocytes were intermediary target cells for DDAVP and that they produced some secreted factor(s) which could mediate the effects of DDAVP on EC release of vWf.

Block and coworkers [15] have studied the binding of AVP to circulating human blood cells and shown, following preparation of single cell types, that mononuclear phagocytes were almost entirely responsible for binding of the hormone and that DDAVP could effectively compete with AVP for its receptors on monocytes. Their findings are in agreement with our data showing that monocytes represent target cells for DDAVP. Results from our laboratory further showed that monocytes also secreted some factor(s) following DDAVP-treatment which stimulated vWf release from ECs.[21] Subsequent work in our laboratory directed to the identification of the monocyte-derived vWf-releasing activity has involved the ammonium sulphate fractionation or gel filtration of conditioned media recovered from DDAVP-stimulated monocytes. Results from these experiments as well as other data suggested to us that the secreted vWf-releasing activity was not proteinaceous. Moreover, exposure of monocytes to DDAVP did not increase the secretion of the following agonists, some of which have been previously shown to elicit vWf release from ECs: IL-1ß, IL-6, IL-8, tumor necrosis factor (TNF-α) or the growth factors G-CSF (granulocyte-) or GM-CSF (granulocyte, monocyte-colony stimulating factors). We further investigated the effects of DDAVP in enhancing the release of prostaglandins (PG) E_2, $PGF_{2\alpha}$ or PGI_2 and the purine nucleotides ATP and ADP from monocytes. These results were negative [60] (unpublished data). However, we were able to demonstrate a significant increase in the levels of PAF, a bioactive lipid, in conditioned media recovered from DDAVP-treated monocytes compared to untreated cells using a highly specific and sensitive radioimmunoassay (RIA) [61-64] (Table 1). Enhanced release of vWf from ECs could also be elicited with lipid extracts of conditioned media from DDAVP-treated monocytes (Unpublished).

Table 1. The Effect of DDAVP on the Secretion of PAF and vWf-Releasing Factor from Monocytes.

DDAVP (ng/mL)	Monocyte PAF Released (fmoles/mL)	% Increase in vWf Released from ECs
0	94 ± 14	104 ± 9
100	284 ± 50*	186 ± 18**

Conditioned media containing the indicated levels of PAF secreted from monocytes treated with DDAVP for 30 minutes or left untreated were incubated with confluent HUVECs for 4 hours. PAF secreted from the monocytes was determined by a highly specific and sensitive RIA following lipid extraction from the conditioned media. Release of vWf from endothelial cells was assayed by ELISA correcting for basal release in unconditioned medium. The data are presented as the means ± S.E.M. Statistical analysis (paired t-test): *$p<0.005$ and **$p<0.001$ ($n = 26$).

Table 2. The Effect of BTP-Dioxolane Treatment of Endothelial Cells in Blocking the Effect of Monocyte-Secreted vWf-Releasing Activity, Thrombin or PAF on vWf Release.

Agonist	Concentration	% Inhibition in vWf Release with BTP-Dioxolane	
Monocyte supernatant without DDAVP	0 ng/mL	67 ± 11	$p<0.005$
Monocyte supernatant with DDAVP	100 ng/mL	77 ± 8	$p<0.001$
Thrombin	5 units/mL	17 ± 12	N.S.
PAF	300 pM	88 ± 11	$p<0.005$

Confluent HUVECs were left untreated or incubated with each of the above agonists in the presence or absence of the specific PAF receptor antagonist BTP-dioxolane for 4 hours. The % inhibition in vWf released was computed from the % reduction in vWf released comparing antagonist treated to untreated cells. Statistical analyses were carried out by paired t-test ($n = 5$).

The effect of the vWf-releasing activity secreted from monocytes could be inhibited by the specific PAF-receptor antagonist (±)-trans-2,5-Bis(3,4,5-trimethoxyphenyl)-1,3-dioxolane [65-68] (Table 2). These data indicate that enhanced secretion of PAF from DDAVP-treated monocytes is one mechanism whereby DDAVP can indirectly provoke the increased release of vWf from ECs. Since PAF is a potent lipid mediator involved in many biological activities, we will briefly summarize below some of the multifunctional effects of PAF on various platelet, EC or monocyte responses.

MONOCYTES AS MEDIATORS OF ENDOTHELIAL CELL RESPONSES

Monocytes are derived from progenitor cells in bone marrow and play important functions through cell to cell contact in host defense, antigen presentation, tumor surveillance and destruction. The interaction between monocytes and ECs plays an important role in EC function in health and disease. For example, monocytes secrete various factors affecting hemostasis, thrombosis, fibrinolysis and inflammation such as lysozyme, elastase, complement components, leukotrienes, prostaglandins, fibronectin [69] various cytokines [37,70,71] and PAF.[72] They express TF [73] and secrete u-PA, PAI-1 and PAI-2.[69,74] Factors released from activated mononuclear cells, as in autoimmune diseases, might directly influence the synthesis and release of vWf.[33] Among the various substances secreted by monocytes, several have been shown to have short or long term effects on vWf release from ECs. For example, PAF studied in perfused rat hindleg was able to induce the release of vWf and of t-PA [41] within 2 minutes of stimulation. The time course of release of either protein was similar and the amounts of proteins secreted were closely correlated and dependent upon extracellular calcium. Previous studies by Tranquille and Emeis have shown that histamine, thrombin, adrenaline and bradykinin,[75] PAF [76] and leukotrienes C_4 and D_4 [77] all cause the acute release of t-PA in the perfused rat hindleg. PAF has also been shown to induce the release of t-PA in vivo [76,77] and within the first minute after injection in rats.[41]

PAF AS A MODULATOR OF ENDOTHELIAL CELL FUNCTION

Additional convincing evidence for the involvement of PAF in vWf release was obtained by incubating cultured ECs directly with purified PAF. The resulting data (Table 3) showed that PAF does indeed directly stimulate vWf release from ECs. It has been previously shown that ECs synthesize and secrete PGI_2, a potent inhibitor of platelet

Table 3. The Effect of Thrombin and PAF on vWf Release from Endothelial Cells.

Incubation Time (h)	% Increase in vWf Release	
	Thrombin (5 U/mL)	PAF (300 pM)
1	119 ± 33 [a]	94 ± 47
2	124 ± 26 [b]	42 ± 20
4	122 ± 32 [c]	131 ± 39 [f]
6	115 ± 28 [d]	69 ± 35
24	88 ± 22 [e]	79 ± 60

Confluent HUVECs were incubated with fresh medium with or without thrombin or PAF for the indicated times. The release of vWf was determined by a specific ELISA. The data are presented as the means ± S.E.M. Statistical analyses: p-values are from Student's t-test for paired data compared to the untreated cells (a,c,e: $p<0.025$; b: $p<0.005$; d: $p<0.01$; f: $p<0.05$) ($n = 6$).

aggregation following PAF treatment.[78,79] Since it is known that DDAVP given in vivo also increases PGI_2 production,[3] we determined its levels in conditioned media from monocytes before and after exposure to DDAVP as well as from ECs incubated with conditioned media from untreated or DDAVP-treated monocytes. When EC monolayers were incubated in conditioned media from DDAVP-treated monocytes, a 60% increase in PGI_2 release from ECs was observed compared to conditioned media from untreated monocytes (unpublished data, $p<0.05$ by Student's t-test). No change in the levels of PGI_2 in conditioned media from untreated monocytes was noted following DDAVP treatment so the changes were solely due to enhanced PGI_2 secretion from ECs. These observations collectively provide further evidence that PAF could serve as an intercellular second messenger in response to DDAVP treatment.

PAF: A MEDIATOR OF INFLAMMATORY AND HEMOSTATIC RESPONSES

PAF is produced by two independent pathways: i) the remodeling route which is triggered by cell activation and involves conversion of alkyl-acyl-glycerophosphocholine and lyso-PAF to PAF via phospholipase A_2 and acetyltransferase, and ii) de novo synthesis. Synthesized PAF is rapidly degraded by acetylhydrolase to lyso-PAF which is biologically inactive.[80,81] PAF is synthesized by neutrophils, platelets, monocytes and ECs.[82] Receptors for PAF have also been identified on these cells.[83] It is implicated in acute inflammation, endotoxic shock and anaphylaxis, initiation and progression of arthritis, cardiovascular disease, glomerulonephritis, arteriosclerosis, hyperacute graft rejection, asthma, shock, myocardial or cerebral ischemia as well as thrombosis.[37,84-86] PAF affects platelet or neutrophil aggregation and activation, vascular permeability and PMN adhesion to ECs.[37,84,87] It destabilizes the endothelium by the generation and release of leukotrienes, thromboxane, free radicals and other toxic products released from various blood cells.[37,86] Thrombin, histamine, bradykinin and peptidoleukotrienes all stimulate production of PAF as well as prostacyclin (PGI_2) [35] by ECs and monocytes.[36,82] PAF also causes superoxide formation, protein phosphorylation, activation of protein kinases and the generation of arachidonic acid and phosphoinositide metabolites.[40] TNF-α or Il-1ß cause synthesis and secretion of PAF by ECs.[88] TNF-α also primes the effects of PAF on EC walls [37] whereas PAF markedly alters the Il-1ß production by LPS-stimulated monocytes [89] and increases TNF-α production by peripheral blood monocytes.[90] Priming of monocytes by PAF may be an important step in the amplification of inflammatory and immune responses.[91,92]

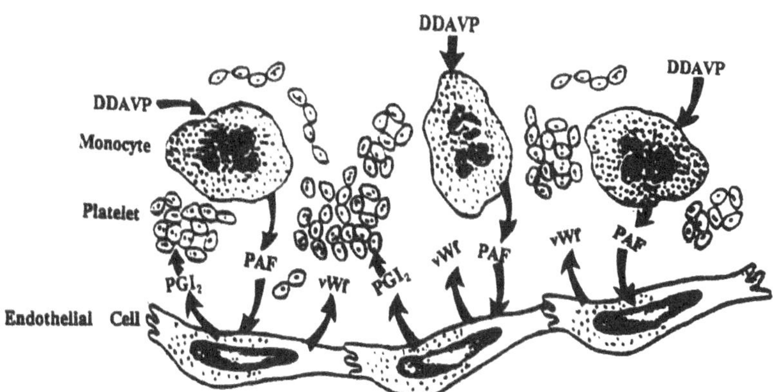

Figure 4. A proposed model indicating one mechanism by which DDAVP can indirectly affect endothelial cells and platelets. DDAVP treatment of monocytes causes increased secretion of PAF into the extracellular environment. Interaction of PAF with HUVECs induces increased release of vWf as well as PGI_2. PGI_2 is a potent inhibitor of platelet aggregation. The PGI_2 may also interfere with the procoagulant effects of PAF on platelets, monocytes and endothelial cells. The presence of such a feedback loop may be of physiological importance with respect to the specific and transitory effects of DDAVP.

A MODEL FOR CELLULAR RESPONSES TO DDAVP

The preceeding sections provide a review of the available evidence for the cellular mechanisms by which DDAVP might induce vWf release from ECs. A proposed model for PAF-dependent, cellular signalling by DDAVP is summarized schematically in Figure 4. The interaction of DDAVP with its receptor on monocytes may stimulate multiple pathways involved in intracellular signalling [15,16] such as increased adenylate cyclase activity and calcium mobilization. These events consequently lead to the rapid synthesis, probably by the remodelling pathway, and release of PAF [82] from monocytes. PAF in turn binds to its receptors on ECs and then initiates a myriad of intracellular events that contribute to the release of vWf and PGI_2.[21,93] The coinduction and release of PAF, PGI_2 and vWf in response to DDAVP can be added to a growing list of examples of crosstalk between different mediators through tightly controlled intracellular events. The production of PGI_2 may not only block platelet aggregation but also modulate further synthesis of PAF by ECs and monocytes, perhaps by interfering with the potential procoagulant effects of PAF on these cells. PGI_2 secretion may thus serve as a negative feedback stimulus to control the effects of DDAVP once enhanced PAF secretion and vWf release have occurred.

CONCLUDING REMARKS

In this review, we have summarized our current findings related to the effect of DDAVP in eliciting enhanced secretion of PAF from monocytes and of the role that PAF plays in intercellular signalling between monocytes and ECs causing the release of vWf from ECs. In studies reported here, DDAVP's in vitro effects on PAF release from monocytes and on vWf [21] and PGI_2 release from ECs respectively [21,94] were found to be similar to those of some cytokines which not only enhance PAF synthesis and release from monocytes [95] or ECs,[96] but also increase vWf [21,56] and PGI_2 release from ECs.[97] Since PAF has the ability to elicit its own release as well as affect the generation of cytokines and growth factors,[37] DDAVP can indirectly influence autokine feedback networks. It is generally known that PAF, which is produced by diverse types of cells, may function as an intermediary in the interaction of blood vessels and peripheral blood components. Our results provide further evidence for a previously undocumented functional role of PAF. Moreover, considering the fact that unlike PAF, there is no receptor for DDAVP on ECs, it seems reasonable that DDAVP's effects could be mediated by the secreted products from some other cells known to bind DDAVP, such as peripheral blood monocytes. The indirect mediation of vWf release from ECs by DDAVP via enhanced PAF secretion from monocytes is reflective of the effects of various cytokines and growth factors which can also act as mediators of various cellular activities.

While we provide a model for one mechanism by which DDAVP may induce vWf release, the means by which DDAVP elicits its other hemostatic or fibrinolytic effects remains unresolved. Preliminary results from additional studies indicate that there may be a different pathway for regulating t-PA release in response to DDAVP. We are currently investigating this possibility.

ACKNOWLEDGMENTS

These studies were funded by grants from the Canadian Red Cross Society Research and Development Program (#OT-01-88 and OT-01-90).

REFERENCES

1. D.W. Richardson and A.G. Robinson, Desmopressin, Ann. Intern. Med. 103:228 (1985).

2. F. Rodeghiero, G. Castaman, and P.M. Mannucci, Clinical indications for desmopressin (DDAVP) in congenital and acquired von Willebrand's disease, Blood Rev. 5:155 (1991).

3. S. Schulman, DDAVP-The multipotent drug in patients with coagulopathies, Transf. Med. Rev. V:132 (1991).

4. P.M. Mannucci, Desmopressin: A nontransfusional hemostatic agent, Annu. Rev. Med. 41:55 (1990).

5. P.M. Mannucci, Desmopressin (DDAVP) for treatment of disorders of hemostasis, in: Progress in Thrombosis and Hemostasis, B.S. Coller, ed., Grune and Stratton Inc., Volume 8, p. 19 (1986).

6. M. Mikaelsson, I.M. Nilsson, B. Cedergren, S. Jonsson, L. Rydberg, and B. Weichel, The use of desmopressin (DDAVP) in the preparation of improved factor VIII concentrate, Scand. J. Haematol. [Suppl.] 33:93 (1984).

7. P.M. Mannucci, M.T. Canciani, L. Rota, and B.S. Donovan, Response of factor VIII/von Willebrand factor to DDAVP in healthy subjects, and patients with hemophilia A and von Willebrand's disease, Br. J. Haematol. 47:283 (1981).

8. E.H. Moffat, J.C. Giddings, and A.L. Bloom, The effect of deamino-D-arginine vasopressin (DDAVP) and naloxone infusion on Factor VIII and possible endothelial cell related activities, Br. J. Haematol. 57:651 (1984).

9. F.M. Booyse, G. Osikowicz, and S. Feder, Effects of various agents on ristocetin-Willebrand factor activity in long-term cultures of von Willebrand and normal human umbilical vein endothelial cells, Thromb. Haemostas. 46:668 (1981).

10. E.G. Tuddenham, J. Lazarchick, and L. Hoyer, Synthesis and release of Factor VIII by cultured human endothelial cells, Br. J. Haematol. 47:617 (1981).

11. H. Vilhardt and T. Barth, The release of Factor VIII and tissue plasminogen activator can not be blocked by specific antagonists to vasopressin, J. Receptor Res. 11:239 (1991).

12. I.-M. Nilsson, H. Vilhardt, L. Holmberg, and B. Astedt, Association between factor VIII related antigen and plasminogen activator, Acta Med. Scand. 211:105 (1982).

13. C.D. Bolan and B.M. Alving, Pharmacologic agents in the management of bleeding disorders, Transfusion 30:541 (1990).

14. S. Lethagen, A.S. Harris, E. Sjorin, and I.M. Nilsson, Intranasal and intravenous administration of Desmopressin: Effect on F VIII/vWF, pharmacokinetics and reproducibility, Thromb. Haemostas. 58:1033 (1987).

15. L.H. Block, R. Locher, W. Tenschert, W. Siegenthaler, T. Hofmann, R. Mettler, and W. Vetter, ^{125}I-8-L-Arginine vasopressin binding to human mononuclear phagocytes, J. Clin. Invest. 68:374 (1981).

16. M.B. Vallottin, At the cutting edge. The multiple faces of the vasopressin receptors, Molec. and Cell. Endocrinol. 78:C73 (1991).

17. E.A. Jaffe, L.W. Hoyer, and R.L. Nachman, Synthesis of antihemophilic factor antigen by cultured human endothelial cells, J. Clin. Invest. 52:2757 (1973).

18. R.L. Nachman, R. Levine, and E.A. Jaffe, Synthesis of factor VIII antigen by cultured guinea-pig megakaryocytes, J. Clin. Invest. 52:2737 (1973).

19. N. Kadhom, C. Wolfrom, M. Gautier,, J.P. Allain, and D. Frommel, Factor VIII procoagulant antigen in human tissues, Thromb. Haemostas. 59:289 (1988).

20. H.V. Stel, Th. H. van der Kwast, and E.C. Veerman, Detection of factor VIII coagulant antigen in human liver tissue, Nature 303:530 (1983).

21. S. Hashemi, E.S. Tackaberry, D.S. Palmer, G. Rock, and P.R. Ganz, DDAVP-induced release of von Willebrand factor from endothelial cells in vitro: the effect of plasma and blood cells, Biochim. Biophys. Acta 1052:63 (1990).

22. M.I. Barnhardt, S.-T. Chen, and J.M. Lusher, DDAVP: Does the drug have a direct effect on the vessel wall ?, Thromb. Res. 31:239 (1983).

23. P.M. Mannucci, Desmopressin: A nontransfusional form of treatment for congenital and acquired bleeding disorders, Blood 72:1449 (1988).

24. V. Pliska, Pharmacology of deamino-D-arginine vasopressin, Frontiers in Hormone Res. 13:278 (1985).

25. F. Fahrenholz, R. Baer, P. Crause, G. Fritzsch, and Z. Grzonka, Interactions of vasopressin agonists and antagonists with membrane receptors, Eur. J. Pharmacol. 100:47 (1984).

26. D.G. Bichet, M. Razi, M. Lonergan, M.-F. Arthus, V. Papukna, C. Kortas, and J.-N. Barjon, Hemodynamic and coagulation responses to 1-desamino-8-D-arginine vasopressin in patients with congenital nephrogenic diabetes insipidus, N. Engl. J. Med. 318:881 (1988).

27. P.M. Mannucci, M. Aberg, I.M. Nilsson, and B. Robertson, Mechanism of plasminogen activator and Factor VIII increase after vasoactive drugs, Br. J. Haematol. 30:81 (1975).

28. C.V. Prowse, G. Sas, A.M.A. Gader, J.H. Cort, and J.D. Cash, Specificity in the Factor VIII response to vasopressin infusion in man, Br. J. Haematol. 41:437 (1979).

29. P. Meucci, I.R. Peake, and A.L. Bloom, Factor VIII-related activities in normal, haemophilic and von Willebrand's disease platelet fractions, Thromb. Haemostas. 40:288 (1978).

30. L.B. Rall, G.I. Bell, D. Caput, M.A. Truett, F.R. Masiarz, R.C. Najarian, P. Valenzuella, H.D. Anderson, N. Din, and B. Hansen, Factor VIII:C synthesis in the kidney, Lancet i:44 (1985).

31. D.D. Wagner, Cell biology of von Willebrand factor, Annu. Rev. Cell Biol. 6:217 (1990).

32. M.P. Bevilacqua, J.S. Pober, G.R. Majeau, R.S. Cotran, and M.A. Gimbrone, Interleukin-1 (IL-1) induces biosynthesis and cell surface expression of procoagulant activity in human vascular endothelial cells, J. Exp. Med. 160:618 (1984).

33. S.N. Breit and I. Green, Modulation of endothelial cell synthesis of von Willebrand factor by mononuclear cell products, Haemostas. 18:137 (1988).

34. D.K. Madtes, E.W. Raines, and R. Ross, Modulation of local concentrations of platelet-derived growth factor, Am. Rev. Respir. Dis. 140:1118 (1989).

35. R.E. Whatley, G.A. Zimmerman, T.M. McIntyre, R. Taylor, and S.M. Prescott, Production of platelet-activating factor by endothelial cells, Sem. Thromb. Haemostas. 13:445 (1987).

36. S.M. Prescott, T.M. McIntyre, and G.A. Zimmerman, The role of platelet-activating factor in endothelial cells, Thromb. Haemostas. 64:99 (1990).

37. P. Braquet, M. Paubert-Braquet, R.H. Bourgain, F. Bussolino, and D. Hosford, PAF/cytokine auto-generated feedback networks in microvascular immune injury: consequences in shock, ischemia and graft rejection, J. Lipid Mediators 1:75 (1989).

38. S.M. Prescott, G.A. Zimmerman, and T.M. McIntyre, Human endothelial cells in culture produce platelet-activating factor (1-alkyl-2-acetyl-sn-glycero-3-phosphocholine) when stimulated with thrombin, Proc. Natl. Acad. Sci. USA 81:3534 (1984).

39. J.J. Emeis and C.K. Luft, PAF-Acether-induced release of tissue-type plasminogen activator from vessel walls, Blood 66:86 (1985).

40. F. Snyder, Platelet-activating factor and related acetylated lipids as potent biologically active cellular mediators, Am. J. Physiol. 259 (Cell Physiol. 28):C697 (1990).

41. N. Tranquille and J.J. Emeis, The simultaneous release of tissue-type plasminogen activator and von Willebrand factor in the perfused rat hindleg region, Thromb. Haemostas. 63:454 (1990).

42. D.D. Wagner, J.B. Olmstead, and V.J. Marder, Immunolocalization of von Willebrand protein in Weibel-Palade bodies of human endothelial cells, J. Cell. Biol. 95:355 (1982).

43. L.A. Sporn, V. J. Marder, and D.D. Wagner, Inducible secretion of large biologically potent von Willebrand factor multimers, Cell 46:185 (1986).

44. D.D. Wagner, and V.J. Marder, Biosynthesis of von Willebrand protein by human endothelial cells: processing steps and their intracellular localization, J. Cell Biol. 99:2123 (1984).

45. B.J. Awbrey, J.C. Hoak, and W.G. Owen, Binding of human thrombin to cultured human endothelial cells, J. Biol. Chem. 254:4092 (1979).

46. B.B. Weksler, C.W. Ley, and E.A. Jaffe, Stimulation of endothelial cell prostacyclin (PGI_2) production by thrombin, trypsin, and the ionophore A23187, J. Clin. Invest. 62:923 (1978).

47. J.D. Pearson and J.L. Gordon, Vascular endothelial and smooth muscle cells in culture selectively release adenine nucleotides, Nature 281:384 (1979).

48. C. Loesberg, M.D. Gonsalves, J. Zandbergen, C. Willems, W.G. Van Aken, H.V. Stel, J.A. Van Mourik, and P.G. de Groot, The effect of calcium on the secretion of factor VIII-related antigen by cultured endothelial cells, Biochim. Biophys. Acta 763:160 (1983).

49. J.A. Ribes, C.W. Francis, and D.D. Wagner, Fibrin induces release of von Willebrand factor from endothelial cells, J. Clin. Invest. 79:117 (1987).

50. P.G. De Groot, M.D. Gonsalves, C. Loesberg, and M.F. Van Buul-Wortelboer, Thrombin-induced release of von Willebrand factor from endothelial cells is mediated by phospholipid methylation, J. Biol. Chem. 259:13329 (1984).

51. J.H. Reinders, P.G. De Groot, M.D. Gonsalves, J. Zandbergen, C. Loesberg, and J.A. Van Mourik, Isolation of a storage and secretory organelle containing von Willebrand protein from cultured human endothelial cells, Biochim. Biophys. Acta 804:361 (1984).

52. B.M. Ewenstein, M.J. Warhol, R.I. Handin, and J.S. Pober, Composition of the von Willebrand factor storage organelle (Weibel-Palade body) isolated from cultured human umbilical vein endothelial cells, J. Cell Biol. 104:1423 (1987).

53. F. Booth, M.J. Allington, and S.A. Cederholm-Williams, An in vitro model for the study of acute release of von Willebrand factor from human endothelial cells, Br. J. Haematol. 67:71 (1987).

54. F. Booth, J.M. Marshall, and S.A. Cederholm-Williams, Effect of bradykinin on the exposure of tissue plasminogen activator from human endothelial cells, Fibrinolysis 2:107 (1988).

55. K.K. Hamilton and P.J. Sims, Changes in cytosolic Ca^{++} associated with von Willebrand factor release in human endothelial cells exposed to histamine, J. Clin. Invest. 79:600 (1987).

56. A.E. Schorer, C.F. Moldow, and M.E. Rick, Interleukin 1 or endotoxin increases the release of von Willebrand factor from human endothelial cells, Br. J. Haematol. 67:193 (1987).

57. R.L. Harrison and P.A. McKee, Estrogen stimulated von Willebrand factor production by cultured endothelial cells, Blood 63:657 (1984).

58. L.A. Sporn, V.J. Marder, and D.D. Wagner, von Willebrand factor released from Weibel-Palade bodies binds more avidly to extracellular matrix than that secreted constitutively, Blood 69:1531 (1987).

59. V. Vicente, J. Corrales, J. Miralles, and I. Alberca, Normal response to DDAVP in patients with pathology of the hypothalamoneurohypophyseal axis, Thromb. Res. 45:695 (1987).

60. S. Hashemi, D. Palmer, P.R. Ganz, E. Trudel, and M.T. Aye, Effect of DDAVP and monocyte cytokines or growth factors on the release of von Willebrand factor from endothelial cells, Blood 76: [Suppl.1], p. 511a (Abstract).

61. M.A. Smal, B.A. Baldo, and D.G. Harle, The specificity of the binding of platelet-activating factor (PAF) to anti-PAF antibodies, J. Molec. Recognition 3:169 (1990).

62. M.A. Smal, B.A. Baldo, and A. McCaskill, A specific, sensitive radioimmunoassay for platelet-activating factor (PAF), J. Immunol. Methods 128:183 (1990).

63. M.A. Smal, B. A. Baldo, and J.W. Redmond, Production of antibodies to platelet activating factor, Molec. Immunol. 26:711 (1989).

64. M.A. Smal, M. Dziadek, S.J. Cooney, M. Attard, and B.A. Baldo, Examination for platelet-activating factor production by preimplantation mouse embryos using a specific radioimmunoassay, J. Reprod. Fert. 90:419 (1990).

65. E.J. Corey, R.K. Bakshi, S. Shibata, C.-P. Chen, and V.K. Singh, A stable and easily prepared catalyst for the enantioselective reduction of ketones. Applications to multistep synthesis, J. Am. Chem. Soc. 109:7925 (1987).

66. E.J. Corey, C.-P. Chen, and M.J. Parry, Dual binding modes to the receptor for platelet activating factor (PAF) of anti-PAF trans-2,5-diarylfurans, Tetrahedron Letters 29:2899 (1988).

67. S.-B. Hwang, M.-H. Lam, T. Biftu, T.R. Beattie, and T.-Y. Shen, Trans-2,5-Bis(3,4,5-trimethoxyphenyl)tetrahydrofuran: An orally active, specific and competitive receptor antagonist of platelet activating factor, J. Biol. Chem. 260:15639 (1985).

68. M.M. Ponpipom, S.-B. Hwang, T.W. Doebber, and J.J. Acton, (±)-Trans-2-(3-methoxy-5-methylsulfonyl-4-propoxyphenyl)-5-(3,4,5-trimethoxyphenyl)tetrahydrofuran (L-659,989), a novel, potent PAF receptor antagonist. Biochem. Biophys. Res. Commun. 150:1213 (1988).

69. S.D. Sharma, The Macrophages, in: Clinics in Immunology and Allergy: Immunological recognition of altered cell surfaces in infection and disease, Vol. 6, V. Britten and H.P.A. Hughes, eds., W.B. Saunders Co., London, p. 1 (1986).

70. S.D. Sisson and C.A. Dinarello, Production of interlukin-1α, interleukin-1ß and tumor necrosis factor by human mononuclear cells stimulated with granulocyte-macrophage colony-stimulating factor, Blood 72:1368 (1988).

71. J. Bauer, U. Ganter, T. Geiger, U. Jacobshagen, T. Hirano,, T. Matsuda,T. Kishimoto, T. Andus, G. Acs, W. Gerok, and G. Ciliberto, Regulation of interleukin-6 expression in cultured human blood monocytes and monocyte-derived macrophages, Blood 72:1134 (1988).

72. M.S. Crespo, J. Gomez-Cambronero, S. Fernandez-Gallardo, M.L. Nieto, and S. Velasco, Generation of platelet activating factor (PAF-Acether) from the mononuclear phagocytic system: Modulation and pathophysiological consequences, in: New Horizons in Platelet Activating Factor Research, C.M. Winslow, and M.L. Lee, eds., John Wiley and Sons, p. 73 (1987).

73. S.A. Gregory, R.S. Bornbluth, H. Helin, H.G. Remold, and T.S. edgington, Monocyte procoagulant inducing factor - a lymphokine involved in the T cell instructed monocyte procoagulant response to antigen, J. Immunol. 137:3231 (1986).

74. O. Saksela, T. Hovi, and A. Vaheri, Urokinase type plasminogen activator and its inhibitor secreted by cultured human monocytes-macrophages, J. Cell Physiol. 122:125 (1985).

75. J.J. Emeis, Perfused rat hindlegs. A model to study plasminogen activator release, Thromb. Res. 30: 195 (1983).

76. J.J. Emeis and C. Kluft, PAF-acether-induced release of tissue-type plasminogen activator from vessel walls, Blood 66:86 (1985).

77. N. Tranquille and J.J. Emeis, Release of tissue-type plasminogen activator is induced in rats by leukotrienes C_4 and D_4, but not by prostaglandins E_1, E_2 and I_2, Br. J. Pharmacol. 93:156 (1988).

78. G. Weigel, A. Griesmacher, and M.M. Muller, Regulation of eicosanoid release in human umbilical endothelial cells, Thromb. Res. 62:685 (1991).

79. S. D'Humieres, F. Russo-Marie, and B.B. Vargaftig. PAF-acether-induced synthesis of prostacyclin by human endothelial cells, Eur. J. Pharmacol. 131:13 (1986).

80. D.H. Albert and F. Snyder, Biosynthesis of 1-alkyl-2-acetyl-sn-glycero-3-phosphocholine (platelet-activating factor) from 1-alkyl-2-acyl-sn-glycero-3-phosphocholine by rat alveolar macrophages: Phospholipase A_2 and acetyltransferase during phagocytosis and ionophore stimulation, J.Biol. Chem. 258:97 (1983).

81. T.-C. Lee and F. Snyder, Overview of PAF synthesis and catabolism, in: Platelet Activating Factor and Human Disease, P.J. Barnes, C.P. Page, and P.M. Henson, eds., Blackwell Scientific Publ., Oxford, England, p. 1 (1989).

82. D. Bratton and P.M. Henson, Cellular origins of PAF, in: Platelet Activating Factor and Human Disease, P.J. Barnes, C.P. Page, and P.M. Henson, eds., Blackwell Scientific Publ., Oxford, England, p. 23 (1989).

83. G. Dent, D. Ukena, and P.J. Barnes, PAF receptors, in: Platelet Activating Factor and Human Disease, P.J. Barnes, C.P. Page, and P.M. Henson, eds., Blackwell Scientific Publ., Oxford, England, p. 58 (1989).

84. M.J. Mangino, C.B. Anderson, M.K. Murphy,, and J. Turk, Renal allograft platelet activating factor synthesis during acute cellular rejection, J. Lipid Med. 4:69 (1991).

85. J. Morley, S. Sanjar, and C.P. Page, Inflammatory features of asthma, in: New Horizons in Platelet Activating Factor Research, C.M. Winslow, M.L. Lee, eds., John Wiley and Sons, p. 317 (1987).

86. P. Braquet, L. Touqui, T.Y. Shen, and B.B. Vargaftig, Perspectives in platelet-activating factor research, Pharmacol. Rev. 39:97 (1987).

87. B.B. Vargaftig and P.G. Braquet, PAF-acether today-relevance for acute experimental anaphylaxis, Br. Med. Bull. 43:312 (1987).

88. F. Bussolino, G. Camussi, C. Baglioni, Synthesis and release of platelet-activating factor by human vascular endothelial cells treated with tumor necrosis factor or interleukin 1α, J. Biol. Chem. 263: 11856 (1988).

89. B. Pignol, S. Héhane, J.-M. Mencia-Huerta, M. Rola-Pleszczynski, and P. Braquet, Effect of platelet-activating factor (PAF-acether) and its specific receptor antagonist, BN-52021, on interleukin 1 (IL 1) release and synthesis by rat spleen adherent monocytes, Prostaglandins 33:931 (1987).

90. B. Bonavida, J.M. Mencia-Huerta, P. Braquet, Effect of platelet-activating factor (PAF) on monocyte activation and production of tumour necrosis factor (TNF), J. Allergy Appl. Immunol. 88:157 (1989).

91. M. Rola-Pleszczynski, Priming of human monocytes with PAF augments their production of tumor necrosis factor, J. Lipid Med. 2:S77 (1989).

92. M. Rola-Pleszcyznski, Immune modulation by PAF: effects on lymphocyte and monocyte functions, in: New Trends in Lipid Mediators Research, P. Braquet, ed., Karger, Basel, p. 30 (1987).

93. G.A. Zimmerman, R.E. Whatley, T.M. McIntyre, D.M. Benson, and S.M. Prescott, Endothelial cells for studies of platelet-activating factor and arachidonate metabolites, in: Arachidonate Related Lipid Mediators, R.C. Murphy, F.A. Fitzpatrick, eds., Methods in Enzymol. 187:520 (1990).

94. J.J.F. Belch, M. Small, F. McKenzie, P.A. Hill, G.D.O. Lowe, D.E. McIntyre, C.D. Forbes, and C.R.M. Prentice, DDAVP stimulates prostacyclin production, Thromb. Haemostas. 47:122 (1982).

95. G. Camussi, F. Bussolino, G. Salvidio, and C. Baglioni, Tumor necrosis factor/cachectin stimulates peritoneal macrophages, polymorphonuclear neutrophils and vascular endothelial cells to synthesize and release platelet-activating factor, J. Exp. Med. 166:1390 (1987).

96. F. Bussolino, C. Tetta, F. Breviario, M. Aglietta, A. Mantovani, and E. Dejana, Interleukin 1 stimulates platelet-activating factor production in cultured human endothelial cells., J. Clin. Invest. 77:2027 (1986).

97. V. Rossi, F. Breviario, P. Ghezzi, E. Dejana, and A. Mantovani, Prostacyclin synthesis induced in vascular endothelial cells by interleukin-1. Science 229:174 (1985).

DISCUSSION

Mayadas-Norton (United States): Why was there a lag time of 2-4 hours for maximum release in the presence of plasma? In vitro Weibel-Palade bodies release within 15 minutes, and in DDAVP patients vWf levels increase within 60 minutes.
Hashemi: There was an in vitro response after only 30 minutes incubation of endothelial cells with plasma from DDAVP-treated individuals with a maximum response observed after 2 hours incubation with normal donor plasma or after 2-4 hours in Type I or Type III vWD patients (Biochimica et Biophysica Acta, 1052:63-70, 1990). Our data do not rule out vWF release from endothelial cells after incubation periods shorter than 30 minutes. Concerning the difference in times at which maximum release of vWF from endothelial cells occurs in vivo and in vitro, this is presumably due to the absence of cells in the latter case. The data suggest that the response is in part dependent upon cell-to-cell interaction as well as upon the exposure of endothelial cells to the secreted products of monocytes or other peripheral blood cells. In the absence of these cells, the additional effects of a network of possible cell-to-cell interactions have not been accounted for. Also as we are dealing with a relatively small number of cells in tissue culture as compared with the number of cells involved in the vasculature and peripheral blood in vivo, the rates of reaction in vitro and in vivo are unlikely to be identical.

Weinstein: Did you see release of unusually large multimers?
Hashemi: We did not evaluate the size of the vWF multimers secreted by the endothelial cells. We assayed the quantity of vWF released with or without stimulation by an ELISA method and calculated the percentage increase in vWF secreted compared with release from endothelial cells exposed to unconditioned, fresh medium.

Bichet: It is not possible to demonstrate V2 receptors in monocytes: they possess V1 receptors only. The 1981 publication suggesting otherwise may have used a ''bad'' agonist, or there was platelet contamination.
Hashemi: We disagree with Dr. Bichet's criticism of the article published by Block et al. (J. Clin. Invest. 68:374-381,1981). The monocytes were purified as required to perform the reported studies. In any case, platelets do not have V2 receptors (Thomas et al., Thromb. Res. 32:557.566,1983; Yang et al., Thromb. Res. 32:809-818,1990). In our laboratory, further studies are being carried out to purify and characterize the monocyte receptors involved in binding DDAVP.

Bichet: The V2 receptor is already cloned. Did you test the viability of the endothelial cells after PAF activation at such doses? Could this be an anoxic/toxic phenomenon?
Hashemi: Yes, I am aware of that, however this comment is irrelevant to our study. We tested viability by the dye exclusion test and the cells remained 100% viable. There was no evidence of toxicity.

Mannucci: How did you distinguish vWF in plasma from vWF released form the cell surface?
Hashemi: By using 35S labelling of the endothelial cells to tag endogenous vWF prior to its release and detection using a dot-blot assay. Rabbit anti-human vWF immobilized on a nitrocellulose membrane was used to capture vWF present in endothelial cell conditioned media or plasma. The portion of vWF represented by secreted 35S-vWF was determined by autoradiography of the dot-blot and image analysis of the developed film. Please refer to our Biochimica et Biophysica Acta article (1052:63.70,1990) for details of our methodology.

SOME PHARMACOLOGICAL PROPERTIES OF DESMOPRESSIN

Hans Vilhardt

Department of Medical Physiology
University of Copenhagen
Blegdamsvej 3
DK-2200 Copenhagen
Denmark

BACKGROUND FOR THE DISCOVERY OF DESMOPRESSIN

Desmopressin (DDAVP) was originally designed and synthesized in an effort to create an analogue of the endogenous antidiuretic hormone, vasopressin, with selective antidiuretic properties (Zaoral et al., 1967). Vasopressin is a neuropeptide which functions as a hormone. Produced in the magnocellular cell bodies of the hypothalamic paraventricular and supraoptic nuclei, the precursor molecules containing vasopressin and the carrier protein neurophysin packed in secretory vesicles are transported intra-axonally to the nerve endings of the posterior pituitary gland. During the intravesicular transport in the neurons the precursor is processed both by cleavage of the peptide chain at appropriate positions and by carboxy terminal amidation to yield the nonapeptide vasopressin. On stimulation vasopressin is released through exocytosis, i.e. the secretory vesicles fuse with the axonal plasma membrane and thereby open up to the extracellular environment, so that vasopressin (and neurophysin) gain access to the blood circulation. There are several stimuli to the release of vasopressin, both physiological and pharmacological. In its function as an antidiuretic hormone vasopressin can be released by changes in the osmotic concentration of plasma, primarily by changes in the sodium concentration. Thus an increase in plasma sodium, such as that which takes place during dehydration will lead to an increased output of vasopressin while hydration will have the opposite effect. The changes in plasma osmolality are registered by osmoreceptors in the hypothalamus from where nervous messages are conveyed to the posterior pituitary gland. The precise location and physiology of the osmoreceptors still need clarification. It is unknown whether the massive discharge to the blood of pituitary vasopressin observed during hypovolemia due to hemorrhage stimulates the release of Factor VIII.

Impaired or absent production of vasopressin in the hypothalamus leads to a state of polyuria known as diabetes insipidus (diabetes refers to the rich flow of urine and insipidus means tasteless as opposed to the sweet taste of the urine in diabetes mellitus, Frank, 1794). In

Desmopressin in Bleeding Disorders, Edited by G. Mariani *et al.*
Plenum Press, New York, 1993

severe cases of the disease urine production may exceed 20 litres/24 hours. Since the beginning of this century diabetes insipidus has been treated with vasopressin in the form of posterior pituitary extracts (von den Velden, 1913; Kamm et al., 1928) and later with synthetically produced vasopressin (Chirman and Kinsel, 1964; Moses 1964). Three conditions, however, make vasopressin less suited for substitution therapy of diabetes insipidus. Firstly the peptide is a very potent stimulator of smooth muscle both in the vascular bed and in the intestines which may lead to increase in blood pressure and to intestinal colics. Secondly the half life of vasopressin in plasma is very short (approximately 5 minutes). To ensure a reasonable duration of effect the drug therefore has to be administered in fairly high doses, which, however, will augment the above mentioned side effects. Finally vasopressin has to be administered either as injections or as intranasal instillations, since like most peptides it is not absorbed folowing peroral administration. With the discovery of the chemical structure of vasopressin (du Vigneaud, 1954) it became possible to synthesize structural analogues of the peptide. This eventually led to the synthesis of DDAVP (1-deamino-8-D-arginine vasopressin, Zaoral et al., 1967). Because of its selective antidiuretic properties DDAVP quite soon became the drug of choice in the treatment of diabetes insipidus (Edwards et al., 1973). Some years later it was shown that DDAVP also possessed the ability of vasopressin to release Factor VIII to the blood (Mannucci et al., 1975). Eventually it was discovered that DDAVP can be administered perorally, e.g. as tablets (Vilhardt and Lundin, 1986).

CHEMISTRY OF DESMOPRESSIN

Vasopressin is a peptide chain made up of nine amino acids. Only two changes in the structure were made to yield DDAVP. Firstly the primary amino group at the amino terminal at position 1 of the peptide was removed and secondly the amino acid at position 8 of the chain, i.e. L-arginine, was substituted with the enanthiomer D-arginine (a synthetic variation of arginine not found in nature). Hence the name 1-deamino-8-D-arginine vasopressin, or DDAVP for short (Fig.1). According to proper chemical terminology the name should be [1-mercaptopropionic acid-8-D-arginine] vasopressin.

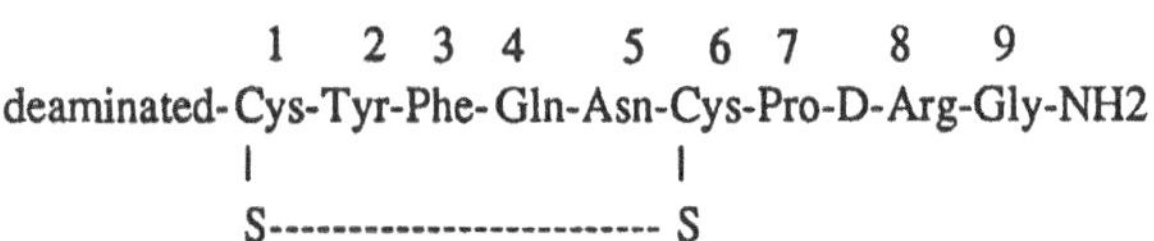

Fig.1: Chemical structure of Desmopressin

PHARMACOLOGICAL PROFILE OF DESMOPRESSIN

The structural modifications introduced in vasopressin to give DDAVP have changed the pharmacological profile of the peptide profoundly. Table I lists the biological effects of vasopressin. The main biological activities are the smooth muscle effects, which involve the so called V1-receptors and the antidiuretc effect expressed via V2-receptors. The activation of Factor VIII and tissue plasminogen activator seems to involve a class of receptors different from the V1- and V2-receptors (Vilhardt and Barth, 1991). Table II shows how the blood pressure action of vasopressin has been reduced to a minimum in DDAVP while the antidiuretic activity has been augmented. On a molar basis DDAVP is also a more powerful activator of Factor VIII and tissue plasminogen activator when compared to vasopressin (Cash et al., 1978).

PHARMACOKINETICS OF DESMOPRESSIN

Measurement of DDAVP in plasma, urine and other body fluids can only be performed using radioimmunoassays (RIA). In most studies antisera raised against arginine- or lysine vasopressin have been employed which may cause unwanted binding of endogenous plasma vasopressin to the antibodies. It is, however, not possible to raise antibodies against DDAVP using conventional immunisation techniques because of the lack of the amino terminal primary amino group in DDAVP. In the pharmacokinetic study performed by Vilhardt et al. (1986) antibodies were raised against 8-D-arginine vasopressin (synthesized by

Table I. Biological effects of vasopressin

1. Antidiuretic activity
2. Contraction of smooth muscle in intestinal wall and blood vessels
3. Contraction of the myometrium (uterotonic effect)
4. Release of pituitary ACTH
5. Release of Factor VIII
6. Activation of tissue plasminogen activator

Table II. Biological potencies of vasopressin (AVP) and Desmopressin (DDAVP)

	Activity (international units/mg peptide) Antidiuretic (AD)	Vasopressor (VP)	Ratio AD/VP
AVP	450	450	1.0
DDAVP	1200	0.5	2400

Ferring Pharmaceuticals, Malmö, Sweden). This antiserum cross reacted less than 0.008% with arginine vasopressin (Lundin et al., 1985).

After a single intravenous injection in man DDAVP is eliminated from the blood following a two phase pattern, the initial fast phase representing mainly the distribution of the peptide from the blood to the body volume of distribution, while the second, slower phase is regarded as reflecting the rate of elimination from the body by metabolic break down and excretion through the kidneys. When DDAVP was infused in humans over several hours to constant plasma concentrations the metabolic clearance was calculated as 2.6 ml x min-1 x kg-1 and the half life in plasma as 55 minutes. The apparent volume of distribution was 206 ml x kg-1 (Vilhardt et al., 1986). In uraemic patients Aunsholt et al. (1986) found that the metabolic clearance was reduced (1.4 ml x min-1 x kg-1) and the half life increased (200 minutes) possibly reflecting a reduced urinary excretion of DDAVP.

Burrow et al. (1981) assayed milk from a lactating woman treated with desmopressin for diabetes insipidus and found only minimal traces of the peptide. DDAVP appears not to pass the blood-brain barrier. When DDAVP was administered intravenously to plasma concentrations of approximately 1000 pg/ml in patients with non-high pressure hydrocephalus, analysis of cerebrospinal fluid sampled from the lateral ventricles showed no traces of DDAVP (S¨rensen et al., 1984). The uterotonic activity of DDAVP is ten times lower than that of vasopressin and the drug has been used in pregnant women without any side effects on either mother or fetus (Oravec and Lichardus, 1972; Burrow et al., 1981).

When administered perorally as tablets (Hammer and Vilhardt, 1985; Vilhardt and Lundin, 1986) or dissolved in water (Vilhardt and Bie, 1984) DDAVP can be absorbed from the gastrointestinal tract to the blood, although the bioavailability is approximately one order of magnitude smaller than after intranasal administration(Hammer and Vilhardt, 1985). Several studies report that patients with diabetes insipidus can successfully control their polyuria with desmopressin tablets(Hammer and Vilhardt, 1985; Fjellestad and Czernichow, 1986). The doses of DDAVP needed to increase Factor VIII and tissue plasminogen activator are higher than those required for inducing antidiuresis. Accordingly peroral ingestion of as much as 4 mg of DDAVP had no effect on the plasma level of these factors in man (H.Vilhardt and I.M.Nilsson, unpublished results).

Table III. Indications for Desmopressin.

1. Cranial diabetes insipidus.
   (Edwards et al., 1973; Aronson et al., 1973; Robinson, 1976; Becker and Foley, 1981)

2. Urine concentration test.
   (Aronson and Svenningsen, 1974; Delin et al., 1978; Curtis and Donovan, 1979; Tryding et al., 1987)

3. Nocturnal enuresis.
   (Pedersen et al., 1985; Belmaker and Bleich, 1986; Fjellestad-Paulsen et al., 1987; Rittig et al., 1989a,b)

4. Treatment of bleeding episodes in mild and moderate forms of haemophilia A and von Willebrand's disease.
   (Mannucci et al., 1977; Ockelford et al., 1980; Warrior and Lusher, 1983)

5. Prophylactic administration to patients with mild and moderate forms of haemophilia A and von Willebrand's disease prior to minor surgery.
   (Sweeney et al., 1980)

6. Administration to blood donors to increase the yield during Factor VIII production. (Vilhardt and Nilsson, 1981; Mikaelsson et al., 1982)

7. Reduction of bleeding during surgery such as coronary bypass operations and aorto-iliac grafting.
   (Saltzman et al., 1986; Lethagen et al., 1991)

INDICATIONS FOR DESMOPRESSIN

Although originally registered by Ferring Pharmaceuticals, Malmö, Sweden, as a drug to substitute for vasopressin in the treatment of patients with diabets insipidus, DDAVP has proven useful in the treatment of a number of other conditions, as listed in Table III.

ADMINISTRATION OF DESMOPRESSIN

The conventional form of administration of DDAVP is intranasally, either by spray or by drops (Harris et al., 1987). The bioavailability varies between 10 and 20% depending on the concentration of DDAVP and the volume of the dose (Harris et al., 1988). DDAVP may also be given as intravenous or subcutaneous injections or as tablets for peroral use. Antidiuretic doses are 10 to 40 µg intranasally once or twice daily or 100 to 400 µg perorally once or twice daily. Optimal haemostatic doses are 0.3-0.4 µg/kg bodyweight infused intravenously over 10-20 minutes (Åberg et al., 1979; Lethagen et al., 1991).

SIDE EFFECTS OF DESMOPRESSIN

Since desmopressin is a strong antidiuretic agent, there is a hypothetical risk of water retention during desmopressin treatment. Fluid retention has, however, never been reported in patients with diabetes insipidus on chronic treatment, but there are a few reports of water retention in infants after administration of DDAVP in the urine concentration test. Consequently fluid intake in infants should be reduced to 50% for 12 hours after administration of desmopressin. Following infusion of DDAVP in haemostatic doses facial flush and slight tachycardia are often observed. These effects are rarely seen after intranasal administration and never after antidiuretic doses.

ACKNOWLEDGMENTS

This work was supported by the Danish Medical Research Council, the Danish Biotechnology Programme and Ferring Pharmaceuticals.

REFERENCES

Åberg,M., Nilsson,I.M., and Vilhardt,H., 1979, the release of fibrinolytic activator and factor VIII after injection of DDAVP, in: Progress in chemical fibrinolysis and thrombolysis, J.F.Davidson,ed., Churchill Livingstone, London and New York.

Aronson,A.S., Andersson,K.E., Bergstrand,C.G., and Mulder,J.L., 1973, Treatment of diabetes insipidus in children with DDAVP, a synthetic analogue of vasopressin, Acta Pædiat. Scand. 62:133.

Aronson, A.S., and Svenningsen,N.W., 1974, DDAVP test for estimation of renal concentrating capacity in infants and children, Arch. Disease in Childhood 49:654.

Aunsholt,N.A., Vilhardt,H., and Schmidt,E.B., 1986, Plasma half-life of DDAVP in uraemic patients, Acta Pharmacol. Toxicol. 59:332.

Becker,D.J., and Foley,T.P., 1981, The effect of water deprivation and water loading during treatment with 1-deamino-8-D-arginine vasopressin in central diabetes insipidus in children, Acta Endocrinol. 97:538.

Belmaker, R.H., and Bleich,A., 1986, The use of desmopressin in adult enuresis, Military Med. 151:660.

Burrow,G.N., Wassenaar,W., Robertson,G.L., and Sehl,H., 1981, Treatment of diabetes insipidus during pregnancy, Acta Endocrinol. 97:23.

Cash,J.D., Gader,A.M., Mulder, J.L., and Cort,J.H., 1978, Structure-activity relations of the fibrinolytic response to vasopressins in man, Clin. Sci. Mol. Med. 54:403.

Chirman,S.B., and Kinsell,L.W., 1964, Diabetes insipidus. Treatment with 8-lysine vasopressin in a nasal spray, California Medicine 101:1.

Curtis, J.R., and Donovan,B.A., 1979, Assessment of renal concentrating ability, Br. Med. Journal 1: 304.

Delin,K., Aurell,M., and Ewald,J., 1978, Urinary concentration test with desmopressin, Br. Med. Journal I:757.

du Vigneaud,V., Gish,D.T., and Katsoyannis,P.G., 1954, A synthetic preparation possessing biological properties associated with arginine vasopressin, Am. Chem. Soc. 76:4751.

Edwards,C.R.W., Kitau,M.J., Chard,T., and Besser,G.M., 1973, Vasopressin analogue DDAVP in diabetes insipidus; clinical and laboratory studies, Br. Med. Journal 3:375.

Fjellestad, A., and Czernichow, P., 1986, Central diabetes insipidus in children. V. Oral treatment with a vasopressin analogue (DDAVP), Acta Pædiat. Scand. 75:605.

Fjellestad-Paulsen,A., Wille,S., and Harris,A., 1987, Comparison of intranasal and oral desmopressin for nocturnal enuresis, Arch. Disease in Childhood 62:674.

Frank,J.P., 1794, De curandis hominum morbis, III, classis V (profluvia), ordo I (profluvia serosa), genus II (diabetes), Caen et socios, Firenze.

Hammer, M., and Vilhardt,H., 1985, Peroral treatment of diabetes insipidus with a polypeptide analogue, desmopressin, Journal Pharmacol. Expmt. Ther. 234:754.

Harris,A., Hedner,P., and Vilhardt,H., 1987, Nasal administration of desmopressin by spray and drops, Journal Pharmaceut. Pharmacol. 39:932.

Harris,A.S., Ohlin,M., Lethagen,S, and Nilsson,I.M., 1988, Effects of concentration and volume on nasal bioavailability and biological response of desmopressin, Journal Pharmaceut. Sci. 77:337.

Kamm,O., Aldrich,T.B., Grote,I.W., Rowe,L.W., and Bugbee,E.P., 1928, The active principle of the posterior lobe of the pituitary gland, I the demonstration of the presence of two active principles, II the separation of the two principles and their concentration in the form of potent solid preparations, Journal Am. Chem. Soc. 50:573.

Lethagen,S., Rugarn,P., and Bergqvist,D., 1991, Blood loss and safety of desmopressin or placebo during aorto-iliac graft surgery, Eur. Journal Vascular Surgery 5:173.

Lundin,S., Melin,P., and Vilhardt,H., 1985, Use of three specific radioimmunoassays in measuring neurohypophysial hormone content and plasma concentrations of vasopressin, oxytocin and DDAVP in rats after prolonged infusion of DDAVP, Experientia 41:933.

Mannucci,P.M., Ruggeri,Z.M., Pareti,F.I., and Capitano,A., 1977, DDAVP in haemophilia, Lancet 2:1171.

Mannucci,P.M., Åberg,M., Nilsson,I.M., and Robertson,B., 1975, Mechanism of plasminogen activator and factor VIII increase after vasoactive drugs, Br. Journal Haematol. 30:81.

Mikaelsson,M., Nilsson,I.M., Vilhardt,H., and Weichel,B., 1982, Factor VIII concentrate prepared from blood donors stimulated with intranasal administration of a vasopressin analogue, Transfusion 22:229.

Moses,A.M., 1964, Synthetic vasopressin nasal spray in the treatment of diabetes insipidus, Clin. Pharmacol. Ther. 5:422.

Ockelford,P.A., Chandrasekhara,M.N., and Berry,E.W., 1980, Clinical experience with arginine vasopressin (DDAVP) in von Willebrand's disease and mild haemophilia, New Zealand Med. Journal 92:3375.

Pedersen,P.S., Hejl,M., and Kjoller, S.S., 1985, Desamino D arginine vasopressin in childhood nocturnal enuresis, Journal Urol. 133:65.

Rittig,S., Knudsen, U.B., Jonler,M., Norgaard,J.P., and Pedersen,E.B., 1989a, Adult enuresis. The role of vasopressin and atrial natriuretic peptide, Scand. Journal Urol. Nephrol., suppl. 125:79.

Rittig,S., Knurgaard,J.P., Pedersen,E.B., and Djurhus,J.C.,1989b, Abnormal diurnal rythm of plasma vasopressin and urinary output in patients with enuresis, Am. Journal Physiol. 256:664.

Robinson,A.G., 1976, DDAVP in the treatment of central diabetes insipidus, New Engl. Journal Med. 294:507.

Salzman,E.W., Weinstein,M.J., Weintraub,R.M., Ware,J.A., and Thurer,R.L., 1986, Treatment with desmopressin acetate to reduce blood loss after cardiac surgery, New Engl. Journal Med. 324:1402.

Sorensen,P.S., Vilhardt,H., Gjerris,F., and Warberg,J.,1984, Impermeability of the blood-cerebrospinal fluid barrier to 1-deamino-8-D-arginine vasopressin (DDAVP) in patients with acquired, communicating hydrocephalus, Eur. Journal Clin. Invest. 14:435.

Tryding,N., Sterner, G., Berg,B., Harris,A., and Lundin,S., 1987, Subcutaneous and intranasal administration of 1-deamino-8-D-arginine vasopressin in assessment of renal concentration capacity, Nephron 45:27.

Vilhardt,H., and Barth,T., 1991, The release of factor VIII and tissue plasminogen activator can not be blocked by specific antagonists to vasopressin, Journal Receptor Research 11:1.

Vilhardt,H., and Bie,P., 1984, Antidiuretic effect of perorally administered DDAVP in hydrated humans, Acta Endocrinol. 105:474.

Vilhardt,H., and Lundin,S., 1986, Biological effect and plasma concentrations of DDAVP after intranasal and peroral administration to humans, Gen. Pharmacol. 17:481.

Vilhardt,H., Lundin,S., and Falch,J., 1986, Plasma kinetics of DDAVP in man, Acta Pharmacol.Toxicol. 58:379.

Vilhardt,H., and Nilsson,I.M., 1981, Further studies on the use of DDAVP in blood donors, in: DDAVP in bleeding disorders, A.H.Sutor,ed., F.K.Schattaur Verlag, Stuttgart and New York.

von den Velden,R., 1913, Die Nierenwirkung von Hypophysenextrakten beim Menschen, Berliner Klinische Wochenschrift, 2:3083.

Warrior, A.I., and Lusher,J.M., 1983, DDAVP: A useful alternative to blood components in moderate haemophilia A and von Willebrand's disease, Journal Pediat. 102:228.

Sweeney,J.D., Crosby,P., McCann,S.R., and Temperley,I.J., 1980, Clinical experience with deamino-8-D-arg-vasopressin (DDAVP) in patients with factor VIII deficiency, Irish Journal Med. Sci. 150:236.

Zaoral,M., Kolc,J., and Sorm,F., 1967, Amino acids and peptides LXXI. Synthesis of 1-deamino-8-D-aminino-butyrine vasopressin, 1-deamino-8-D-lysine vasopressin and 1-deamino-8-D-arginine vasopressin, Collection Czech. Chem. Commun. 32:1250.

DISCUSSION

Bichet: Your last slide can be explained by there being the same receptor, but with different affinities.
Vilhardt: I agree. There is a similar example in the human uterus. In women the uterine receptors are far more sensitive to vasopressin than oxytocin, but at term pregnancy, oxytocin is far more dominant. The receptor seems to change its affinity.

Mannucci: Why were you disappointed with the analogues? Several showed they have Factor VIII activity and no ADH activity. Also, the double peak may not be real, as in a range of 100 to 150% there is little weight in changes from 110 to 120%.
Vilhardt: I agree about the double peaks. Only similar results have been obtained in sheep. We were not satisfied with the analogues because they had their effects in supramaximal doses. It may not be possible to increase the response by increasing the dose.
Mannucci: As a clinician I would be satisfied with an analogue raising FVIII by 200%.

Brommer: May I comment on the biphasic response? In our institute we looked at the rat hind leg, and failed to see a response until we examined the first minutes, when we saw an acute response. Perhaps DDAVP has both acute and "normal" effects.

Kinter (United States): I encourage you to continue with your analogues. We looked at the rhesus monkey dose response to DDAVP and found that we did not get a maximum response until we reached a dose 10 times the considered maximum.

Lusher: Even though the response in dogs is suboptimal, does it still correct bleeding?
Vilhardt: We do not know. It takes skill to venepuncture in the monkeys, which only weigh 300 grams, and we can only withdraw 200 microlitres of blood at a time, so the study was restricted. We are waiting for a more satisfactory analogue before we do such work.
Kinter: DDAVP has been used to manage prolonged bleeding times in strains of bleeding dogs.

PHARMACOKINETICS OF DESMOPRESSIN

Michael Köhler[1] and Alan Harris[2]

[1]Department of Transfusion Medicine
University of Göttingen
3400 Göttingen
Germany

[2]Ferring Pharmaceuticals
200 62 Malmö
Sweden

INTRODUCTION

In 1967 Zaoral and coworkers synthesized several analogues of vasopressin. One of these derivatives, 1-deamino-8-D-arginine vasopressin (DDAVP, desmopressin), soon became the treatment of choice for diabetes insipidus centralis. DDAVP has a prolonged half-life and a decreased pressor activity when compared with the parent hormone vasopressin (VP). This allows the use of significantly higher dosages without the cardiovascular side effects of VP. Gader et al. (1973), Cash (1974) and Mannucci (1977) observed that DDAVP increases Factor VIII (FVIII) and von Willebrand Factor (vVF) in healthy subjects and patients with bleeding disorders such as milder forms of haemophilia A and von Willebrand's disease.In these disorders, desmopressin proved not only to be a substitute for blood products, but also the most effective treatment.

For treatment of diabetes insipidus centralis, DDAVP was administered intranasally in a highly concentrated solution, while in bleeding disorders desmopressin had to be infused intravenously, since approximately 10-fold higher dosages are required to exert significant haemostatic effects in comparison with the antidiuretic activity. Optimistic reports of Kobayashi (1979) with i.n. administration of DDAVP in patients with haemophilia could not be confirmed by other groups. Thus, in the mid 1980's, when desmopressin was already established as a haemostatic agent, interest focused on improvement of treatment. Mannucci's group (1981) evaluated optimal dosing schemes for intravenous (i.v.) infusion. Our group investigated subcutaneous (s.c.) injection of desmopressin (Köhler et al., 1984). The aim of our studies was to compare the different routes of administration available at that time.

METHODS

We report on 2 studies, which have been already described in detail (Köhler et al., 1986, 1989, Köhler and Harris 1988). The first study compared 0.4 µg DDAVP per kg body weight

Desmopressin in Bleeding Disorders, Edited by G. Mariani *et al.*
Plenum Press, New York, 1993

(b.w.), either infused i.v. or injected s.c., and 300 µg DDAVP, administered intranasally using a single dose pipette (Octostim[R], Ferring Pharmaceuticals) in 10 healthy subjects in a randomized, cross-over design. In the second study, a more concentrated compound (40 µg/ml) was compared with placebo in a double blind study.

DDAVP-levels were determined using a highly sensitive radio immuno assay (RIA) as described by Harris et al. (1986). The cross-reactivities with arginine-vasopressin and oxytocin were 0.8 and 0.1%, respectively.

The results of DDAVP plasma levels were normally distributed and are expressed as mean values and standard deviation.

The pharmacodynamic effects of desmopressin, especially on the coagulation parameters, did not always lead to normally distributed values, and thus the results are expressed as median and ranges (minima-maxima).

Mean arterial pressure (MAP) was calculated by the formula:

MAP= 1/3 systolic pressure + 2/3 diastolic blood pressure.

FVIII:Cag and vWF:Ag were determined as described elsewhere in detail (Köhler et al., 1986).

The area under the curve (AUC) was calculated by the trapezoidal rule and data obtained between t=0 (before DDAVP) and 24 h after administration of desmopressin.

RESULTS

Pharmacokinetics

The plasma DDAVP levels are shown in fig.1. The peak concentrations after s.c. and i.n. desmopressin were observed 60 min after administration (range 15 to 240 min). 24 hours after desmopressin administration, median DDAVP levels were 9.5 and 6.1 pg/ml after s.c. injection and i.v. infusion, respectively. The mean elimination half-life was 3.5 hours and did not vary between routes of administration.

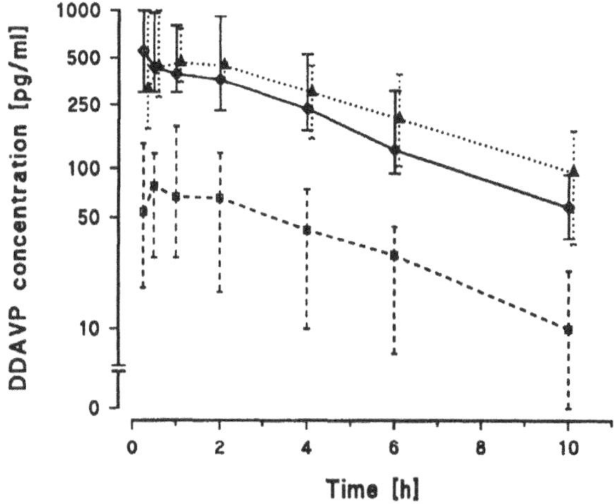

Figure 1. Mean DDAVP levels after different routes of administration.
Median values and ranges (minima and maxima). Solid lines and diamonds represent i.v. infusion, dotted lines and triangles s.c. injection and dashed lines and squares i.n. administration.

The more concentrated preparation (40 µg/ml) had a peak level of 544 pg/ml, while 12 h after the injection 50 pg/ml DDAVP were present. Based on the AUC data, s.c. injection appeared to be equivalent to i.v. infusion. No significant differences between the two preparations (4 µg/ml and 40 µg/ml DDAVP) became apparent. The peak levels of i.v. infused DDAVP were not detected, since the first blood sample was obtained 15 min after the end of the infusion. Thus, the distribution phase of desmopressin could not be recorded.
The pharmacokinetic data are summarized in table 1.

Pharmacodynamics

Immediately after DDAVP, a decrease of blood pressure, dependent on the route of administration was observed (see fig.2).

Table 1. Pharmacokinetics of DDAVP after different routes of administration.

Dose and route of administration	AUC (pg/ml*h)	maximum concentration (pg/ml)	half-life (min)
0.4 g/ml i.v.	3109±1056 (34%)		217±25 (12%)
0.4 µg/ml s.c. (4 µg/ml ampoule)	3492±659 (19%)	568±203 (36%)	210±23 (11%)
0.4 µg/ml s.c. (40 µg/ml ampoule)	3164±393 (12%)	544±46 (8%)	190±19.8 (10%)
300 µg/ml i.n. (pipette)	483±225 (47%)	98±48 (49%)	

Mean values and standard deviation from ten healthy volunteers. Coefficients of variation are in parentheses.

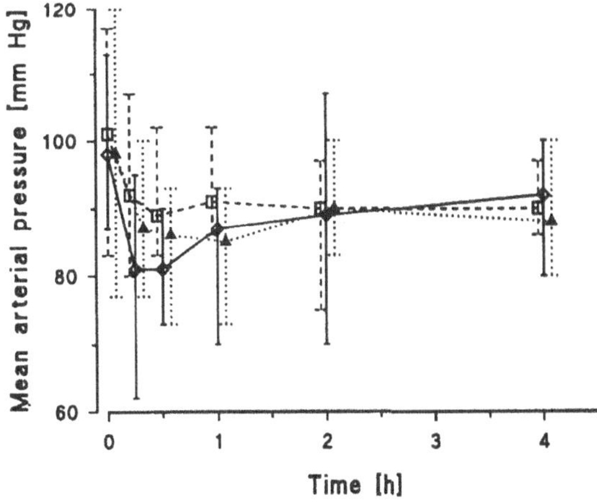

Figure 2. Mean arterial pressure after DDAVP.
Median values and ranges (minima and maxima). Solid lines and diamonds represent i.v. infusion, dotted lines and triangles s.c. injection and dashed lines and squares i.n. administration.

The factor VIII release after desmopressin is shown in fig.3. The maxima after i.v. DDAVP were higher after i.v. infusion when compared with s.c. injection (4.0 vs. 2.9), however, when the AUC of FVIII increase was compared, the difference was minimal (26.5 vs. 22.8 U*h/ml).

The maximum concentrations and activities of FVIII were reached in most volunteers 60 min after DDAVP administration.

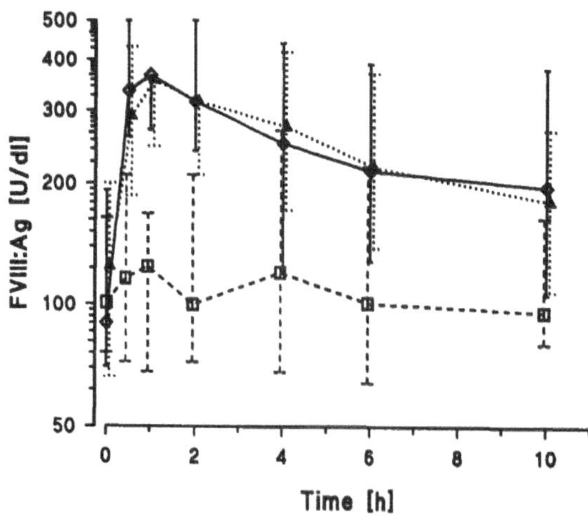

Figure 3. Factor VIII:Ag after DDAVP.
Median values and ranges(minima and maxima). Solid lines and diamonds represent i.v.infusion dotted lines and triangles s.c. injection and dashed lines and squares i.n. administration.

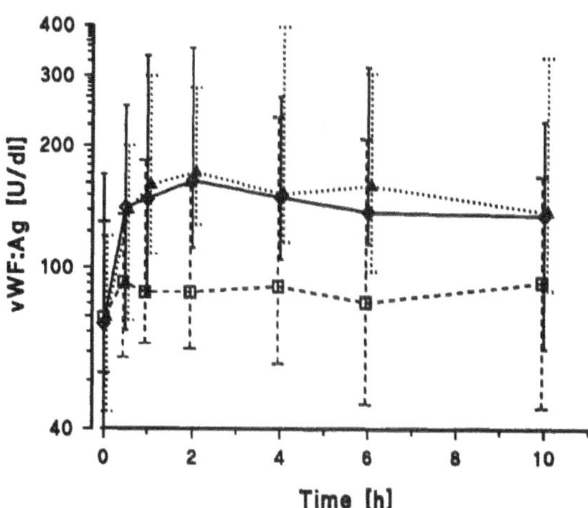

Figure 4. von Willebrand Factor antigen after DDAVP.
Median values and ranges(minima and maxima). Solid lines and diamonds represent i.v.infusion dotted lines and triangles s.c. injection and dashed lines and squares i.n. administration.

The rate of increase of vWF:Ag was somewhat slower (see fig. 4). The AUC data were 12,5 U*h/ml for i.v. and 13,9 U*h/ml for s.c. DDAVP, respectively.

Additionally, serum protein levels decreased by 9% one hour after DDAVP. The leucocyte count was increased by 40 to 80% of initial values 4 hours after i.v. and s.c., but not after i.n. desmopressin.

The haematological effects of DDAVP are summarized in table 2.

The scatterplot of peak DDAVP concentrations and FVIII:C increase is shown in fig.5. It appears that no correlation exists between the amount of FVIII increase and plasma levels of DDAVP at concentrations above 300 pg/ml, i.e. when the i.n. data are excluded.

Table 2. Haematological effects of DDAVP after different routes of administration.

Parameter*	i.v.	s.c. (4 μg/ml ampoule)	s.c. (40 μg/ml ampoule)	i.n.
FVIII:Ag	4.0 (60)	2.9 (60)	3.1 (60)	1.2 (60)
FVIII:C	3.1 (30)	2.3 (60)	2.4 (60)	1.3 (60)
vWF:Ag	2.5 (120)	2.3 (120)	2.0 (120)	1.2 (120)
RCof	3.1 (120)	2.0 (120)	2.3 (120)	1.2 (120)
t-PA	1.9 (15)	1.4 (60)	2.1 (60)	0
Leucocyte count	1.8 (240)	1.4 (240)	1.5 (240)	0

* Mean increase (expressed as a ratio) and median time to peak (min) in parentheses from ten healthy volunteers.

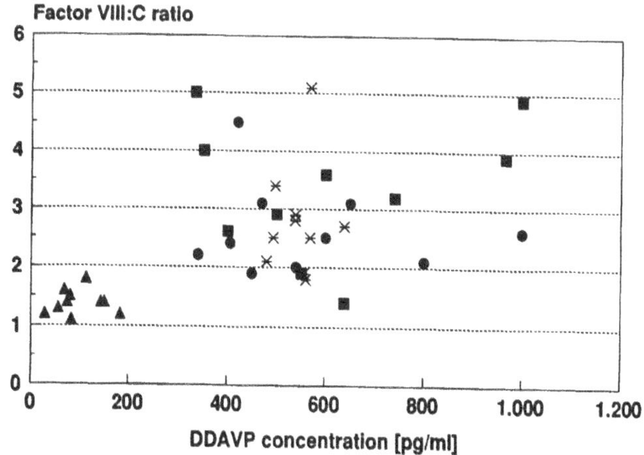

Figure 5. Scatterplot of Factor VIII:Ag increase and maximum DDAVP concentration in plasma. Intranasal administration: triangles, s.c. injection circles (4 μg/ml ampoule) and asterisks (40 μg/ml ampoule) and squares i.v. infusion.

CONCLUSION

From earlier reports, using a less specific RIA, a distribution half-life of 7.8 min and an elimination half-life ranging from 30 min to 158 min was calculated (Edwards et al., 1973). Using a sensitive RIA, a sufficient number of subjects, a longer period of observation and dosages utilized for treatment of bleeding disorders, we found an elimination half-life of approximately 3.5 h. These results are in agreement with the results obtained in patients (Mannucci et al., 1987). In 14 patients, the bioavailability of s.c. injected DDAVP was 82% of i.v. infused DDAVP, and the elimination half-life was 4.4 h. Additionally, no significant correlation between peak (or AUC) levels of DDAVP and peak FVIII levels (Mannucci et al., 1987) could be observed. Lethagen et al. (1987) studied the pharmacokinetics and pharmacodynamics of different dosages of desmopressin infused intravenously. In agreement with earlier studies of Mannucci and coworkers (1981), a maximum effect on FVIII release (3.6 x the initial activity) was observed at a dosage of 0.3 µg/kg body weight. The half-life ranged between 2.3 and 2.7 h. In this investigation a new nasal spray was evaluated. The results obtained with this new preparation appear promising, with plasma concentrations and effects in the magnitude of i.v. or s.c. administration (Harris et al., 1986; Lethagen et al., 1987, Rose and Aledort, 1991).

From these studies it can be concluded, that a dosage of 0.3 µg/kg b.w. DDAVP should be sufficient to obtain a maximum effect on haemostasis. Although s.c. and i.v. administration appear to be bioequivalent in terms of AUC data, i.v. infusion exerts higher peak levels and these peaks are reached earlier. A 12 hour dosage interval should be the regular lower limit, in order to avoid accumulation of antidiuretic activity. The effects of i.v. and s.c. DDAVP should be monitored between 1 and 2 hours after injection or infusion.

REFERENCES

Cash, J. D., A. M. A. Gader, and J. DaCosta. 1974. The release of plasminogen activator and factor VIII to lysine vasopressin, arginine vasopressin, 1-desamino-8-D vasopressin, angotensin and oxytocin in man (Abstr.). Br. J. Haematol. 15:363-364.

Edwards, C.R.W., M.J. Kitau, and G.M. Besser. 1973. Vasopressin analogue DDAVP in diabetes insipidus: Clinical and laboratory studies. Br. Med. J. 3: 375-378.

Gader, A. M. A., J. DaCosta, and J. D. Cash. 1973. A new vasopressin analogue and fibrinolysis. Lancet 2:978-979.

Harris, A. S., I. M. Nilsson, Z. G. Wagner, and U. Alkner. 1986. Intranasal administration of peptides: nasal deposition, biological response, and absorption of desmopressin. J. Pharm. Sci. 75:1085-1088.

Kobayashi, I. 1979. Treatment of haemophilia and von Willebrand's disease patients with an intranasal dripping of DDAVP. Thromb. Res. 16:775-779.

Köhler, M. and A. Harris. 1988. Pharmacokinetics and haematological effects of desmopressin. Eur. J. Clin. Pharmacol. 35:281-285.

Köhler, M., P. Hellstern, C. Miyashita, G. von-Blohn, and E. Wenzel. 1986. Comparative study of intranasal, subcutaneous and intravenous administration of desamino-D-arginine vasopressin (DDAVP). Thromb. Haemost. 55:108-111.

Köhler, M., P. Hellstern, B. Reiter, G. von Blohn, and E. Wenzel. 1984. The subcutaneous administration of the vasopressin analogue 1-desamino-8-D-arginine vasopressin in patients with von Willebrand's disease and hemophilia. Klin Wschr 63:543-548.

Köhler, M., P. Hellstern, H. Tarrach, R. Bambauer, E. Wenzel, and G. A. Jutzler. 1989. Subcutaneous injection of desmopressin (DDAVP): Evaluation of a new, more concentrated preparation. Haemostas 19:38-44.

Lethagen, S., A. S. Harris, E. Sjörin, and I. M. Nilsson. 1987. Intranasal and intravenous administration of desmopressin: Effect on FVIII/vWF, pharmacokinetics and reproducibility. Thromb Haemostas 58:1033-1036.

Mannucci, P. M., M. T. Canciani, L. Rota, and B. S. Donovan. 1981. Response of factor VIII/von Willebrand factor to DDAVP in healthy subjects and patients with haemophilia A and von Willebrand's disease. Br. J. Haematol. 47:283-293.

Mannucci, P. M., Z. M. Ruggeri, F. I. Pareti, and A. Capitanio. 1977. DDAVP: A new pharmazeutical approach to the management of haemophilia and von Willebrand's disease. Lancet 1:869-872.

Mannucci, P. M., V. Vicente, I. Alberca, E. Sacchi, G. Longo, A. S. Harris, and A. Lindquist. 1987. Intravenous and subcutaneous administration of desmopressin (DDAVP) to haemophiliacs: Pharmacokinetics and factor VIII responses. Thromb Haemostas 58:1037-1039.

Rose, E.H. and L.M. Aledort. 1991. Nasal spray desmopressin for mild hemophilia A and von Willebrand disease. Ann. Int. Med. 114: 563-568.

Zaoral, M., J. Kolc, and F. Sorm. 1967. Synthesis of 1-deamino-8-D-aminobutyrine vasopressin, 1-deamino-8-D-lysine vasopressin and 1-deamino-8-D arginine vasopressin. Collect. Czech. Chem. Commun. 32:1250-1257.

DISCUSSION

Mannucci: You showed that the response in terms of peak level after s.c. DDAVP was somewhat better than that after i.v. administration. We found the two responses the same. Do you think that in terms of peak levels they are bioequivalent?

Kohler: I have the impression that they are. We may be giving too high a dose at 0.4 µg/kg body weight. An increase above 0.3 µg/kg causes Factor VIII levels to decline. Some papers have shown better results with 0.3 µg/kg when standardization was better than in the initial studies. We now recommend a decrease of dose to 0.3 µg/kg .

Mannucci: You also showed that there was less variance in response with s.c. dosing than with i.v. Why?

Kohler: I cannot answer. DDAVP plasma levels after i.v. administration do not have the same quality as the i.c. levels. There may be small errors in the blood sampling, so that the s.c. samples may be more true.

Mannucci: The increase of Factor VIIIc was earlier than that of vWf. This is interesting as we have been discussing vWf release and fibrinogen activation, and we believe that Factor VIIIc is released as a consequence of vWf. Surely this must be reviewed?

Kohler: This is not a new finding. I wished to mention it because of the morning's discussion. I have no explanation.

Kobrinsky: Could the variations of s.c. and i.v. routes be due to dilution, or because of short and long tubing (and therefore binding to plastics)?

Kohler: Diluting the material further may lower the effect, and with smaller volumes the coefficient of variation after s.c. injection of DDAVP is smaller. I favour use of a more concentrated compound. The intranasal variation is explained by the vagaries of absorption of the compound used at the time, which may not be the problem, and may be overcome by the modern compound.

FALL OFF OF FACTOR VIII ELICITED BY DESMOPRESSIN ADMINISTRATION IN HEMOPHILIACS AND von WILLEBRAND'S DISEASE PATIENTS

Massimo Morfini,[1] Francesco Rodeghiero, [2] Giovanni Longo,[1] Giancarlo Castaman,[2] and Sandro Cinotti[1]

[1] Hematology Department and Hemophilia Center, Ospedale di Careggi, USL 10/D, Florence, Italy
[2] Hematology Department & Hemophilia and Thrombosis Center, Ospedale San Bortolo, USL 8, Vicenza, Italy

INTRODUCTION

The decay of factor VIII:C elicited by Desmopressin (DDAVP) administration has been one of the first topics addressed by investigators[1,2] since the discovery of the effects of this new compound in normal subjects, hemophiliacs and patients with von Willebrand's disease (vWD).

In 1979, Ludlam and coworkers assayed the Factor VIII:C and vWF:Ag during the first 5 hours after the beginning of DDAVP infusion in 5 normal subjects, in 6 hemophiliacs (only 4 responders to DDAVP) and in 12 vWD patients of different subtypes[1]. They found a Factor VIII:C half life of 4.5 hrs in normal subjects and 3 hrs in hemophiliacs. No data were reported on vWD patients, but a very short half life, about 1 or 2 hours, can be argued from graphical evaluation of the plots displaying the increase and decay of Factor VIII:C in these patients.

In 1980, Mannucci and coworkers[2] designed a study aimed not only at assessing the dose-response relationship between Factor VIII:C and DDAVP administration but also at evaluating the disappearance time of Factor VIII:C and vWF:Ag. Also in this study the timing of Factor VIII:C assay was very short (not more than 6 hours). The half life was evaluated by least square regression analysis. This method can be considered suitable only for cases with a clearly monophasic decay. Nevertheless, these Authors found a significant difference between normal subjects, who showed a very short half life (about 4.5 hrs), and hemophiliacs, who displayed a half life of about 11 hrs. This last figure is very similar to the generally well accepted values found after the infusion of FVIII concentrates in hemophiliacs. On the contrary, the half life of Factor VIII:C in vWD patients was found to be similar to that observed in normal subjects (5 hrs)[2]. In subsequent studies, a shorter half-life (about 70 minutes) was calculated in patients with type I vWD[3,4].

Desmopressin in Bleeding Disorders, Edited by G. Mariani *et al.*
Plenum Press, New York, 1993

During the last 10 years we have applied general pharmacokinetic methodology to the study of in vivo behavior of FVIII or FIX concentrates. The aim was to establish an objective procedure for the evaluation of FVIII/vWF complex pharmacokinetics.

The aim of the present study was to evaluate the decay of Factor VIII in hemophiliacs A (HA) and VWD patients after intravenous DDAVP according to the most suitable pharmacokinetic analysis.

MATERIAL AND METHODS

Study design

12 vWD patients and 8 HA were enrolled at the Vicenza and Florence Haemophilia Center. DDAVP was infused at a dosageof 0.3 mcg/kg body weight, diluted in 100ml of isotonic saline, over 30 min. Blood samples have been drawn before and 0.25, 0.5, 1, 3, 6, 9, 12 and 24 hours after the end of infusion in HA. In VWD patients the time of study was slightly different because of poor compliance of these patients to the protocol: the samples have been drawn before and 0.5, 1, 2, 4, 8, 24 hours after the end of infusion.

Factor VIII:C assay:

The Factor VIII:C was measured by one-stage clotting assay, APTT, using as substrate plasma a FVIII/vWF:Ag immunodepleted human plasma (Dade-Mertz) and partial thromboplastin Actin FS (Dade-Mertz) [4]. Three dilutions of the sample and three of the Reference 100% (Immuno), calibrated against the 2nd International Factor VIII standard 87/718, were tested in duplicate, in a balanced order. Factor VIII:C potency has been evaluated according to the mathematical procedure (Parallel lines assay) of Ingram et al.[5].

Pharmacokinetic analysis:

The decay of VIII:C, elicited after DDAVP infusion, was analyzed according to the model independent method [6,7,8]. The model-independent method does not require a best-fitting procedure and the Area Under the Curve (AUC) can be easily evaluated by the trapezoidal rule. According to this method, the most reliable parameters are the Clearance (Cl) and the Mean Residence Time (MRT). We added to these parameters also the Terminal Half Life (THL), which is the half life of the right portion of the curve, i.e. the half life after the distribution phase.

RESULTS AND DISCUSSION

Table 1 reports the findings observed in hemophiliacs and Table 2 those observed in VWD patients, both after treatment with DDAVP. The findings substantially confirm those reported by Ludlam[1] and by Mannucci[2]. In VWD patients Mean Residence Time or Terminal Half Life resulted clearly shorter in comparison to HA [Student 2-tailed t-test for unpaired data 2.413 ($p=0.027$) and 2.204 ($p=0.042$) respectively]. The differences between the mean values of Cl did not, however, give significant results (2-tailed t.1.189, p=0.25). The kinetic parameters observed in HA are also shorter than those reported in hemophiliacs infused with traditional FVIII concentrates, where the MRT is 15.9 hrs and half life 11.0 hrs at least[9]. Even much longer values have been estimated with some pasteurized concentrates[10,11]. This difference is one of the parameters that must be taken into account in deciding which type of therapy (FVIII concentrates or DDAVP) is more suitable for the HA affected by bleedings or undergoing surgery.

In vWD patients instead, the MRT and Terminal Half Life were clearly shorter (4.5 and 3.9 hrs respectively). A poor increase or a shorter half-life of vWF:Ag after DDAVP in these patients can explain this finding[1,2]. The reason for

Table 1. Factor VIII kinetic parameters in hemophiliacs A after DDAVP i.v. administration.

	Patient	Cl (ml/h/kg)	MRT (h)	THL (h)
	C.G.	0.076	27.37	20.34
	P.L.	0.308	23.55	20.00
	C.C.	0.168	10.43	8.92
	C.N.	0.155	9.13	6.76
	P.M.	0.754	6.87	5.81
	F.G.	0.621	6.58	5.01
	F.L.	1.084	4.08	1.44
	M.A.	0.326	5.51	6.71
Mean		0.436	11.69	9.37
95% Conf.	Upper Limit	0.740	19.30	15.43
	Lower Limit	0.133	4.09	3.32

Table 2. Factor VIII kinetic parameters in VWD patients after DDAVP i.v. administration.

	Patient	Cl (ml/h/kg)	MRT (h)	THL (h)	TYPE
	B.L.	0.161	7.84	7.71	II I
	B.P.	0.165	9.81	6.46	I A
	DL.MG.	0.434	1.91	1.92	I A
	F.A.	0.369	6.08	8.66	I A
	M.R.	0.560	1.99	1.51	I A
	P.M.J.	0.062	11.57	8.75	I A
	F.P.	0.448	1.87	1.04	I Vicenza
	G.D.I.	0.243	2.36	1.39	I Vicenza
	G.P.	0.202	3.38	4.95	I Vicenza
	G.P.	0.203	2.25	1.62	I Vicenza
	T.S.	0.407	2.25	1.47	I Vicenza
Mean		0.296	4.62	3.91	
95% Conf.	Upper Limit	0.492	7.10	5.94	
	Lower Limit	0.191	2.23	1.87	

this result is unknown and more investigations are needed to fully addresses this issue. We did not investigate Factor VIII:C behavior in normal subjects but the observation of Mannucci et al.[2] of shorter half life in this group as well as in vWD patients in comparison to that of hemophilia A, makes the topic intriguing. Probably another variable, the increase of fibrinolytic activity, should be taken into account. As a matter of fact, the release of tissue plasminogen activator from endothelial cells after DDAVP infusion may be the reason for vWF proteolysis in normal subjects as well as in vWD patients[13,14].

CONCLUSION

In conclusion, a carefully standardized pharmacokinetic approach confirms the difference between the Factor VIII:C decay in classical hemophiliacs and in vWD patients, and between the Factor VIII:C elicited after DDAVP and after FVIII concentrate in both diseases.

REFERENCES

1. C.A.Ludlam, I.R.Peake, N.Allen, B.L.Davies, R.A.Furlong and A.L.Bloom, Factor VIII and fibrinolytic response to Deamino-8-D-Argenine Vasopressin in normal subjects and dissociate response in some patients with Haemophilia and von Willebrand's disease, Br J Haematol. 45:499 (1980).
2. P.M.Mannucci, M.T.Canciani, L.Rota, and B.S.Donovan, Response of Factor VIII/vov Willebrand Factor to DDAVP in healthy subjects and patients with Haemophilia A and von Willebrand's disease. Br J Haematol.47:283(1981).
3. P.M.Mannucci, R.Lombardi, R.Bader, M.H.Horellou, G.Finazzi, C.Besana, J.Conard, and M.Samama, Studies of the pathophysiology of acquired von Willebrand's disease in seven patients with linphoproliferative disorders or benign monoclonal gammopathies, Blood 64:614(1984).
4. F.Rodeghiero, G.Castaman, E.Di Bona, M.Ruggieri, R.Lombardi, and P.M.Mannucci, Hype-responsiveness to DDAVP for patients with type I von Willebrand's disease and normal intraplatelet von Willebrand Factor, Eur J Haematol.40:163(1988).
5. R.D.Langdell, R.H.Wagner, and K.M.Brinkhous, Effect of antihaemophilic factor on one-stage clotting test, J Lab Clin Med.41:637 (1953).
6. K.N.Williams, J.M.F.Davidson, and G.I.C.Ingram, A computer program for the analysis of parallel-line bioassay of clotting factors, Br J Haematol.31:13(1975).
7. M.Matucci, A.Messori, G.Donati-Cori, G.Longo, S.Vannini, M. Morfini, E.Tendi, and P.Rossi Ferrini, Kinetic evaluation of four Factor VIII concentrates by model-independent methods, Scand J Haematol.34:22 (1985).
8. G.Longo, M.Matucci, A.Messori, M.Morfini, and P.Rossi Ferrini, Pharmacokinetics of a new heat-treated concentrate of Factor VIII estimated by model-independent methods, Thromb Res.42:471(1986).

9. A.Messori, G.Longo, M.Matucci, M.Morfini, and P.Rossi Ferrini, Clinical pharmacokinetics of Factor VIII in patients with classic hemophilia, Clin Pharmacokinet. 13:365(1987).
10. M.Morfini, A.Messori, S.Cinotti, D.Rafanelli, E.Filimberti, E. Boni, and G.Longo, Comparative studies on available clotting factor concentrates, in:"Hemophilia and von Willebrand 's Disease in the 1990s" J.M. Luscher and C.M. Kessler, ed., Elsevier Science Publisher B.V., Amsterdam(1991).
11. K.Schimpf, and T.Reis, Comparison of recovery and half-life of a new factor VIII high-purity concentrate (FVIII C HS) with a factor VIII HS (Haemate P), Ricerca Clin Lab.16: 231(1986).
12. A.Messori, M.Morfini, M.Blomback, S.Cinotti, G.Longo, K.Schimpf, K.Schumaker, A.Novakova-Banet, U.Delvos, and H.Kjellman, Pharmacokinetics of two pasteurized factor VIII concentrates by different and multicenter assays of Factor VIII activity, Thromb Res.65:699(1992).
13. J.Battle, M.F.Lopez-Fernandez, C.Lopez Berges, J.Dent, S.D. Berkowitz, and T.S.Zimmerman, Proteolytic degradation of von Willebrand Factor after DDAVP administration in normal individuals, Blood 70:173(1987).
14. M.F.Lopez-Fernandez, R.Gonzalez-Boulosa, M.J.Blanco-Lopez, M.Perez, and J.Battle, Abnormal proteolytic degradation of von Willebrand Factor after Desmopressin infusion in a new subtype of von Willebrand disease, Amer J Hematol.36:163 (1991).

DISCUSSION

Kobrinski: Five years ago we studied 10 severely Factor VIII deficient patients. We had the idea that vWf as a carrier might prolong Factor VIII activity, and we also gave desmopressin on the grounds that it might prolong the activity of vWf. However, we found no difference in response among the 8 patients who were HIV negative. In the 2 HIV positive patients, who had high endogenous vWf levels, the half life of Factor VIII rose from 8 to 15 hours. Because they were only two patients, we dismissed the finding, but patients with high baseline vWf levels may have a prolonged Factor VIII half life.
Morfini: I agree that vWf is very much a carrier of Factor VIIIc.

TOXICITY OF DESMOPRESSIN AND RELATED PEPTIDES

Lewis B. Kinter, Dennis J. Murphy, Richard A. Macia, William A. Mann and Henk A. Solleveld

Department of Toxicology - U.S.
SmithKline Beecham Pharmaceuticals
P.O. Box 1539
King of Prussia, PA 19405-0939
(215) 270-7613

Introduction

The first recorded use of the antidiuretic (V_2) activity of pituitary extracts to treat polyuria was in 1913 (Heller 1974). Forty years later, the structure of the antidiuretic hormone, arginine vasopressin (AVP), was established (Acher and Chauvet, 1953). As peptide synthesis techniques improved synthetic AVP replaced the use of pituitary extracts in antidiuretic therapy. In 1972, the use of a synthetic antidiuretic analog of AVP, deamino-8D arginine vasopressin (dDAVP), to treat polyuria was described (Anderson and Arner, 1972) and dDAVP rapidly eclipsed AVP to become the drug of choice for treatment of vasopressin-sensitive polyuria (Ziai et al., 1978; Harris, 1989). In 1975 Mannucci and colleagues published the unexpected activity of dDAVP to stimulate plasma concentrations of clotting factors. The subsequent use of dDAVP, at doses 10-fold or more those associated with maximal antidiuresis, in the management of clotting disorders and in the production of clotting factor concentrates has resulted in much larger drug exposures than those associated with the treatment of diabetes insipidus.

In the last 20 years additional agonists and antagonists of V_1 and V_2 receptors have been developed as potential therapeutic agents (see Kinter et al., 1988ab; Huffman et al., 1988). In this chapter the toxicity of dDAVP and 2 additional vasopressin analogues, SK&F 101926 and SK&F 105494 (Table 1), having antidiuretic activity in humans are briefly reviewed.

TOXICITY OF dDAVP, SK&F 101926 AND SK&F 105494

Water Intoxication and Hyponatremia: DDAVP stimulates renal water reabsorption (antidiuresis) by activating adenylate cyclase-coupled V_2 receptors in the distal nephron (Hays, 1976) and water intoxication and hyponatremia may result from exposure to large doses of dDAVP and other antidiuretic drugs. In practice, water intoxication rarely occurs in otherwise healthy laboratory animals or humans given large doses of dDAVP (Kinter and Beeuwkes, 1982; Mannucci, 1986; Shulman et al., 1990). Oral administration of up to 0.2 mg/kg dDAVP per day to rats for 30 days was associated with a near-maximal antidiuretic state without evidence of fluid-electrolyte imbalance; however, oral administration of 2 to 2.5 mg/kg per day was associated with a delayed maximal antidiuretic state, similar to that previously reported in rats given very large daily subcutaneous

Table 1. Structures and Activities of Vasopressin Analogs [1]

Compound	Structure	K_{bind}[2] [pig] (nM)	K_i[3] [pig] (nM)	K_i[4] [human] (nM)	Activity[5] [human] (In Vivo)
AVP	arginine vasopressin	1.7	1.0(K_{act})	1.7(K_{act})	antidiuresis
dDAVP	1-deamino-8-D-arginine vasopressin	385.	100.(K_{act})	24.(K_{act})	antidiuresis
SK&F 105494	O-ethyl-D-tyrosyl-L-phenylalanyl-L-valyl-L-asparaginyl-5-[1-(carboxymethyl) cyclohexyl]-L-norvalyl-L-arginyl-D-argininamide, cyclic (5→1) peptide	5.1	--	3.9	antidiuresis
SK&F 101926	desGly(CH_2)$_5$D-Tyr(O-ethyl)-4-valine-8-arginine-vasopressin	11.8	3.6	3.6	antidiuresis

[1] Kinter et al. 1992; [2] binding constants (K_{bind}) for pig V_2 receptors (Kinter et al, 1991a); [3], [4] inhibition (K_i) and activation (K_{act}) constants for pig and human vasopressin-stimulated renal adenylate cyclase activity, respectively (Kinter et al., 1991a, Brooks et al., 1988a); [5] human data from Allison et al., 1988 and Kinter et al., 1991b.

doses of vasopressin, and is suggestive of water intoxication (Kinter and Beeuwkes, 1982; Kinter, 1982). On the other hand, administration of even pharmacologic doses of dDAVP to laboratory animals or humans whose fluid-electrolyte regulatory mechanisms have been compromised can result in water intoxication and hyponatremia. Combination of dDAVP infusion (5 ng/hr, s.c.) and food administration as a liquid diet produces a stable state of profound hyponatremia (plasma [Na^+] = 110 mmol/l) in rats (Verbalis and Martinez, 1991). Combination of dDAVP administration, uninephrectomy, desoxycorticosterone acetate (DOCA) and 0.6% saline administration produces volume expansion and hypertension in rats (Zicha et al., 1989). It has been suggested that chronic dDAVP treatment results in renal hypertrophy in rats and may contribute to the progression of renal failure (Bankir et al., 1991). Hyponatremia is thought to be a relatively common hospital-acquired electrolyte disturbance resulting from non-osmotic secretion and/or iatrogenic stimulation of vasopressin in patients in advanced stages of cardiac or liver failure, primary volume contraction, and other conditions (Anderson et al., 1985; Gross, et al., 1987). Collectively, these results indicate that water intoxication and hyponatremia are much more likely to be associated with dDAVP administration in subjects with compromised thirst, cardiovascular, hepatic and renal functions.

Chronic administration of SK&F 101926 and related peptides produces an antidiuretic effect in rats that is distinct from that produced by dDAVP (Figure 1). SK&F 101926 is an analog of $d(CH_2)_5$-D-Tyr(Et)^2-Val^4-Arg^8 vasopressin and has high affinity for both V_1 and V_2 receptors (Huffman et al., 1988, Kinter et al., 1991a). This compound is a potent antagonist of V_1 receptors in vitro and in vivo, and is also a potent antagonist of V_2 receptors in vitro (Table 1). In vivo however, the activity SK&F 101926 is species-dependent (Kinter et al., 1988a, 1988b, 1990).

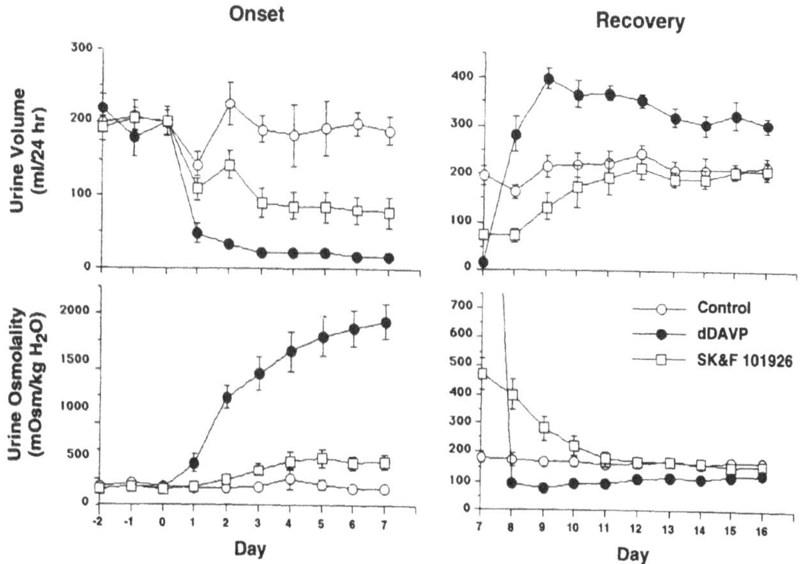

Figure 1 Comparison of the antidiuretic effects of dDAVP and SK&F 101926 in Brattleboro strain diabetes insipidus rats (n=5/group). Rats were housed individually in metabolism cages with free access to food and water. Following establishment of baseline (days -2 thru 0) daily urine flow rates (ml/24 hr) and urine osmolality (mOsm/kg H_2O), miniature osmotic pumps (Alzet 2001) loaded to deliver 0.9% NaCl (1 µl/hr, Control, open circle), dDAVP (2 ng/day, closed circle), or SK&F 101926 (12 µg/day, open square) were inserted subcutaneously and urine volume and osmolality monitored daily for days 1 thru 7 (left-hand panels). On day 7 all the pumps were removed and the rats monitored daily for an additional 9 days (right-hand panels). See Caltabiano and Kinter (1991) for additional details.

In the rat, SK&F 101926 is a potent antidiuretic antagonist (aquaretic), while in the dog, rhesus monkey and human it is an antidiuretic agonist (Allison et al., 1988; Brooks et al., 1988a; Kinter et al., 1990). SK&F 105494 is another vasopressin antagonist that is aquaretic in rats, dogs, and monkeys, but, like SK&F 101926, is antidiuretic in humans (Kinter et al., 1991b). When given to rats, SK&F 101926 and SK&F 105494 produce a massive water diuresis over the first 24 hours, as anticipated from their activities in vitro. However, after additional daily dosing the aquaresis is replaced with a gradually-developing antidiuresis (Caltabiano and Kinter, 1991). Similar observations have been made after repeated administration in dogs (unpublished observations). The antidiuresis is not associated with disturbances in body weight gain, food consumption, or evidence of water intoxication or hyponatremia. The most striking feature of this 'antagonist-associated antidiuretic response' is that it may persist for days to weeks following cessation of dosing, long after the drug has cleared from the circulation (Figure 1; Caltabiano and Kinter, 1991). The antidiuretic effect associated with chronic administration of vasopressin antagonists appears to be the result of up-regulation of renal V_2 receptors in the treated animals. There is no evidence that similar administration of dDAVP or AVP results in up-regulation of V_2 receptors, indeed, several lines of evidence suggests that down-regulation of V_2 receptors occurs (Caltabiano and Kinter, 1991).

Flushing: Flushing of the face and thorax has been associated with administration of dDAVP and SK&F 101926 in laboratory animals and humans (Williams et al., 1986; Pigache, 1984; Allison et al., 1988; Brooks et al., 1988b). Desensitization to the flushing response may occur with repeated administration of dDAVP (Yokota et al., 1982; Brooks et al., 1988b). Mast cell stabilization and repeated administration of dDAVP will reduce flushing associated with dDAVP and other V_2 agonists in rhesus monkeys. Flushing associated with non-vasopressin peptides has been associated with histamine release (Roy et al., 1980; Lorenz et al., 1981; Wilkin, 1981; Foreman and Jordan, 1983; Morgan, et al., 1986). However, administration of cyproheptadine (a mixed serotonin/histamine receptor antagonist, 8 mg) did not effect SK&F 101926-associated flushing in humans (unreported data). Whether direct dDAVP-stimulated vasodilation (see below) also contributes to flushing is unknown. Collectively, due to the auto- and cross-desensitization phenomena, and the fact that dDAVP-stimulated flushing is most evident in humans and other primates, reliable characterizations of the mechanisms involved have proved time-consuming and difficult.

Hypotension: DDAVP, SK&F 101926 and SK&F 105494 cause vasodilation and hypotension (with reflex tachycardia) and stimulate plasma renin activity in laboratory animals and humans (Harris, 1989; Schwartz, 1989; Kinter et al., 1992; Table 2). Hypotension occurs following intravenous doses of ≥1.0 mg/kg in rats and dogs, ≥.003 mg/kg in rhesus monkeys, and ≥0.0003 mg/kg in humans. Rats and dogs surviving a hypotensive episode following the first dose of peptide exhibit tolerance to subsequent doses (unreported findings). The hypotensive action of these peptides in rats is prevented by prior administration of cyproheptadine (Macia et al., 1990b). The hypotensive action of a structurally unrelated growth-hormone-releasing peptide is also prevented by cyproheptadine or ketanserin, or by prior degranulation of mast cells with compound 48/80 (Macia et al., 1990a). The hypotensive activity of other peptides in dogs is prevented by the H_1 antagonist, clemastine (Lorenz et al., 1981). The hypotensive effect of dDAVP in humans is associated with an increase in arterial plasma histamine concentrations (Jahr et al., 1991). On the other hand, the hypotensive effect of dDAVP and SK&F 101926 in rhesus monkeys is not diminished by prior administration of the mast cell stabilizer, SK&F 78729-A (Brooks et al., 1988b).

Selective V_2 agonists produce peripheral vasodilation in dogs by a mechanism independent of the kidney and the central nervous system (Liard 1988; 1989). Direct vasodilator effects of both AVP and dDAVP have been reported in human forearm vasculature in vivo (Suzuki et al., 1989; Hirsch et al., 1989). DDAVP ($>7.5\times10^{-9}$ M) relaxes phenylephrine-contracted rat and rabbit aorta in vitro and the effect appears to depend upon an intact endothelium and cyclooxygenase pathway (Johns, 1990). The vasodilator effect of dDAVP is distinct from the well known vasoconstrictor (V_1) effect of AVP. It is not apparent in patients with congenital X-linked nephrogenic diabetes insipidus (Bichet et al., 1988), suggesting that vasodilation is mediated by an extra-renal V_2-like receptor mechanism. SK&F 105494 prevents the hypotension associated with dDAVP administration in the rhesus monkey, an observation consistent with the V_2 receptor hypothesis (Kinter et al., 1992).

Collectively, these results suggest that the hypotensive action of dDAVP and other peptides occurs as a result of mast cell degranulation in some, but perhaps not all species. In those species in which mast cell degranulation is indicated, histamine and/or serotonin, and perhaps other autocoids, may mediate the vasodilatory response. In those species in which mast cells are not indicated, the hypotensive activity of dDAVP may be the result of a direct drug-induced vasodilation via an extra-renal V_2-like receptor mechanism. By either mechanism, dDAVP-induced hypotension may be potentially dangerous in some patients (Salmenpera et al., 1991). The effects of dDAVP on renin release are most likely secondary to vasodilation and hypotension (Kinter et al., 1992).

Death: SK&F 101926 and SK&F 105494 caused death in rats when given intravenously at doses of approximately 5 mg/kg (Table 2). Death occurred within 5 to 60 minutes of dosing. Dogs appeared to be less susceptible to lethality associated with these peptides than rats. Dogs and rats that collapsed following the first dose of peptide and survived, exhibited tolerance to subsequent daily doses (unreported findings). At necropsy, rats dying after a single dose exhibited right-sided heart dilation. Rats which died 24 hours or longer after the initial dose had clinical and histologic evidence of renal tubular degeneration, consistent with a prolonged hypotensive episode.

Peptide-related death in rats can be prevented by either prior mast cell degranulation or mast cell stabilization (Murphy and Joran, 1992); death may also be prevented by prior administration of a serotonin receptor blocker, but not by either H_1 or H_2 receptor blockers (Macia et al., 1990b). The mechanism of vasopressin-peptide-induced death in rats has been further characterized as more closely associated with respiratory failure than cardiovascular collapse (Murphy and Joran, 1992). Collectively, the data suggest that peptide-induced degranulation of mast cells and serotonin release results in acute hypertension and respiratory failure in rats.

DISCUSSION

DDAVP is a potent pharmacologically-active drug that has been in clinical use for nearly 20 years for the treatment of polyuria and has proved to have a substantial safety margin. Indeed, had it not been for the unexpected discovery of the clinical utility of dDAVP in the management of clotting disorders a discussion of the toxicity of dDAVP would be nearly moot. DDAVP is a V_2 agonist which has little or no activity at vascular (V_1) vasopressin receptors (Harris, 1989). Once thought to be a 'super agonist', dDAVP actually has reduced affinity for renal V_2 receptors, and lower activity to stimulate cAMP or water flux in vitro than the endogenous agonists (Table 1; Mann et al., 1985). The superior efficacy of dDAVP over AVP is

Table 2. Summary of Toxicology of Sk&f 101926 & Sk&f 105494

	RAT Single and Multiple Doses		DOG Single and Multiple Doses		RHESUS MONKEY Single Doses	
Clinical Observations	SK&F 105494	SK&F 101926	SK&F 105494	SK&F 101926	SK&F 105494	SK&F 101026
Flushing	≥1.0	≥0.5	≥3.0	≥0.025	0.03	0.01
Hypotension	≥1.0	≥3.0	≥3.0	≥7.5	0.03	0.01
Cyanosis/Prostation	≥1.0	≥2.0	≥3.0	≥7.5	NO	≥0.01
Death	≥1.0	≥3.0	NO	10.0	NO	NO
Azotemia (moderate)	≥1.0	2.0	NO	NO	--	--
Elevated ALT (Moderate)	≥1.0	NO	≥8.0	8.0	--	--
Pathology						
Increased Kidney Weights	≥0.3	NO	NO	NO	--	--
Renal Tubular Degeneration	≥0.3	3.0	NO	NO	--	--
Right-Sided Heart Dilation	≥1.5	3.0	NO	NO	--	--
Testicular Degeneration	NO	NO	10	NO	--	--

Values are mg/kg administered intravenously; NO, not observed; monkeys were not necropsied.

due to (1) dDAVP's enhanced metabolic stability, resulting in improved absorption (when administered subcutaneously, intranasally, or orally) and prolonged duration of action, and (2) dDAVP's V_2 receptor specificity, resulting in elimination of side-effects related to V_1 activity (including splanchnic and coronary ischemia and peripheral vasoconstriction/gangrene, and nausea; see Kinter et al., 1988b). In the treatment of diabetes insipidus and nocturia, therapeutic plasma drug concentrations are approximately 10 pg/ml. These doses are associated with minor side-effects (notably flushing) which decrease with repeated dosing. Some tolerance to the antidiuretic effect of dDAVP may occur with repeated dosing; this may be the result of homologous down-regulation of renal V_2 receptors. Evidence of development of neutralizing antibodies or anaphylactic reactions following prolonged administration of even very large doses of dDAVP, SK&F 101926, SK&F 105494 or other vasopressin peptides has not been reported or observed. Nausea appears to be much less frequently reported with dDAVP than AVP. Recently, it has been reported that V_1 activity (present with AVP but not dDAVP) may directly stimulate emesis in primates (Kinter and Kohl, 1991). Finally, the lack of water intoxication associated with dDAVP, SK&F 101926, and SK&F 105494 is consistent with recent studies showing that much of physiological regulation of renal water reabsorption occurs along the V_2-effector pathway, following the agonist-V_2 receptor interaction (see Kinter et al., 1990).

Clinical and veterinary use of dDAVP in the management of clotting disorders has been reported (Mannucci, 1986; Mansell and Parry, 1991). In the treatment of clotting disorders, therapeutic plasma concentrations of dDAVP are approximately 1 ng/ml (Bichet et al., 1988), and are 10 to 100-fold those required for antidiuresis. In studies of SK&F 101926 and SK&F 105494, peak plasma concentrations were 100 ng/ml or more in laboratory animals and humans. These exposures may produce an acute allergic-like, or anaphylactoid (Lorenz et al., 1981), reaction associated with flushing and/or hypotension and tachycardia and, in the rat, collapse and death from respiratory failure. This reaction is distinguished from an anaphylactic reaction in that (1) it occurs immediately with the first dose of peptide in otherwise naive animals or subjects, and (2) that tolerance rapidly develops with repeated dosing. This phenomenon is described for a large number of small peptides, and appears to result from massive degranulation of one or more populations of mast cells, which likely explains the subsequent tolerance.

On the other hand, dDAVP and other agonists may also dilate vascular smooth muscle directly via a V_2-like receptor pathway. While the location of this receptor pathway is not precisely known, several lines of evidence implicate the vascular endothelial cells (Schwartz, 1989; Johns, 1990). The vascular endothelial cells are also implicated as a source of dDAVP-released clotting factors (Hashemi et al., 1990). It is tempting to speculate that both vasodilatory autocoids and clotting factors are co-released from endothelial cells by the same V_2 receptor mechanism.

ACKNOWLEDGEMENTS

The authors acknowledge the contributions of the Toxicology Department staff who conducted the studies of SK&F 101926 and SK&F 105494 and DJ Passerin for assistance in preparing this manuscript.

REFERENCES

Acher, R. and Chauvet, J., 1953, La structure de la vasopressine de boeuf. Biochim. Biophys. Acta 12:487-488.

Andersson, K.E. and Arner, B., 1972, Effects of DDAVP, a synthetic analogue of vasopressin, in patients with cranial diabetes insipidus. Acta Med. Scand. 192:21-27.

Anderson, R.J., Chung, H-M., Kluge, R., and Schrier, R.W., 1985, Hyponatremia: a prospective analysis of its epidemiology and the pathogenic role of vasopressin. Ann. Inter. Med. 102:164-168.

Allison, N.L., Albrightson-Winslow, C.R., Brooks, D.P., Stassen, F.L., Huffman, W.F., Stote, R.M., and Kinter, L.B., 1988, Species heterogeneity and antidiuretic hormone antagonists: what are the predictors? In: Vasopressin: Cellular and Integrative Aspects, edited by A.W. Cowley, J-F. Liard, and D.A. Ausiello, Raven Press, Ltd., New York, pp.207-214.

Bankir, L. Bouby, N., and Trinh-Trang-Tan, M-M., 1991, Vasopressin-dependent kidney hypertrophy: role of urinary concentration in protein-induced hypertrophy and in the progression of chronic renal failure. Am. J. Kidney Dis. 17:661-665.

Bichet, D.G., Razi, M., Lonergan, M., Arthus, M-F., Papukna, V., Kortas, C., and Barjon, J-N., 1988, Hemodynamic and coagulation responses to 1-desamino[8-D-arginine] vasopressin in patients with congenital nephrogenic diabetes insipidus. N. Engl. J. Med. 318:881-887.

Brooks, D.P., Koster, P.F., Albrightson-Winslow, C.R., Stassen, F.L., Huffman, W.F., and Kinter, L.B., 1922a, SK&F 105494 is a potent antidiuretic hormone antagonist in the rhesus monkey (Macaca mulatta). J. Pharmacol. Expl. Ther. 245:211-215.

Brooks, D.P., Koster, P.F., Stassen, F.L., Albrightson, C.R., Huffman, W.F., Wasserman, M.A., and Kinter, L.B., 1988b, Flushing and haemodynamic responses to vasopressin peptides in the rhesus monkey. Br. J. Pharmacol. 94:759-764.

Caltabiano, S. and Kinter, L.B., 1991, Up-regulation of renal adenylate cyclase-coupled vasopressin receptors after chronic administration of vasopressin antagonists to rats. J. Pharmacol. Expl. Ther. 258:1046-1054.

Foreman, J. and Jordan, C., 1983, Histamine release and vascular changes induced by neuropeptides. Agents Actions 13:105-116.

Gross, P.A., Pehrisch, H., Rascher, W., Schomig, A., Hackenthal, E., and Ritz, E., 1987, Pathogenesis of clinical hyponatremia: observations of vasopressin and fluid intake in 100 hyponatremic medical patients. European J. Clin. Invest. 17, 123-129.

Harris, A.S., 1989, Clinical experience with desmopressin: efficacy and safety in central diabetes insipidus and other conditions. J. Pediatrics 114:711-718.

Hays, R.M., 1976, Antidiuretic Hormone. N. Eng. J. Med. 295:659-665.

Heller, H., 1974, History of neurohypophysial research. In Handbook of Physiology, Section 7, Endocrinology, Volume IV, Part 1, ed. by E. Knobil and W.H. Sawyer, Am. Physiol. Soc. Wash. DC, pp. 103-117.

Hirsch, A.T., Dzau, V.J., Majzoub, J.A., and Creager, M.A., 1989, Vasopressin-mediated forearm vasodilation in normal humans: evidence for a vascular vasopressin V2 receptor. J. Clin. Invest. 84:418-426.

Huffman, W.F., Kinter, L.B., Moore, M.L., Stassen, F.L., 1988, Vasopressin antagonists. Annual Reports in Med. Chem. 23:91-99.

Jahr, J.S., Marques, J., Cottington, E., and Cook, D.R., 1991, Hemodynamic performance and histamine levels after desmopressin acetate administration following coronary bypass in adult patients. J. Cardiothorac. Vasc. Anesth. 5:139-141.

Johns, R.A., 1990, Desmopressin is a potent vasorelaxant of aorta and pulmonary artery isolated from rabbit and rat. Anesthesiology 72:858-864.

Kinter, L.B., 1982, Water balance in the brattleboro rat: considerations for hormone replacement therapy. Ann. N.Y. Acad. Sci. 394:448-463.

Kinter, L.B. and Beeuwkes, R. III., 1982, Oral antidiuretic therapy: studies in the diabetes insipidus rat. Am. J. Physiol. 243:R-491-R499.

Kinter, L.B., Caldwell, N., Caltabiano, S., Winslow, C., Brooks, D.P., and Huffman, W.F., 1990, Physiological regulation of the renal vasopressin receptor-effector pathway in dogs. Am. J. Physiol. 258:R763-R769.

Kinter, L.B., Caltabiano, S., and Huffman, W.F., 1991a, Vasopressin Receptors. In Receptor Data for Biological Experiments: A Guide to Drug Selectivity, edited by H.N. Doods and J.C.A. van Meel, Ellis Horwood, Ltd, New York, pp.62-68.

Kinter, L.B., Huffman, L.B., and Stassen, F.L., 1988a, Antagonists of the antidiuretic activity of vasopressin. Am. J. Physiol. 254:F165-F177.

Kinter, L.B., Ilson, B.E., Brooks, D.P., Albrightson-Winslow, C., Stassen, F., and Huffman, W., 1988b, Clinical pharmacology of agonists and antagonists of vasopressin. Exerpta Medica 797:167-175.

Kinter, L.B., Ilson, B.E., Caltabiano, S., Jorkasky, D.K., Murphy, Solleveld, H.A., D.J., Rhodes, G.R., Brooks, D.P., Albrightson-Winslow, C.R., Stote, R.M., and Huffman, W.F., 1991b, Antidiuretic hormone antagonism in humans: are there predictors? In Vasopressin, ed. by S. Jard and R.L. Jameson, Colloque INSERM/John Libby Eurotext Ltd. Vol. 208:321-329.

Kinter, L.B. and Kohl, R.L., 1991, Method of treating nausea and emesis related to motion sickness with vasopressin antagonists. United States Patent No. 5,051,400, September 24.

Kinter, L.B., McConnell, I., Goodwin, B.T., Campbell, S., Huffman, W.F., Arthus, M-F., Lonergan, M., and Bichet, D.G., 1992, Vasopressin antagonist inhibition of clotting factor release in the rhesus monkey (Macaca mulatta). J. Pharmacol. Expl. Ther. 261:(in press).

Liard, J-F., 1989, Peripheral vasodilation induced by a vasopressin analogue with selective V_2-agonism in dogs. Am. J. Physiol. 256:H1621-H1626.

Liard, J-F., 1988, Effects of a specific antidiuretic agonist on cardiac output and its distribution in intact and anephric dogs. Clin. Sci. 74:293-299.

Lorenz, W., Doenicke, A., Schoning, B., Karges, H., and Schmal, A., 1981, Incidence and mechanisms of adverse reactions to polypeptides in man and dog. Develop. Biol. Standard. 48:207-234.

Macia, R.A., Gabel, R.A., Reginato, M.J., and Matthews, W.D., 1990a, Hypotension induced by growth-hormone-releasing peptide is mediated by mast cell serotonin release in the rat. Toxicol. Appl. Pharacol. 104:403-410.

Macia, R.A., Silver, A.C., Gabel, R.A., Campbell, G.K., Hanna, N., and DiMartino, M.J., 1990b, Hypotension induced by vasopressin antagonists in rats: role of mast cell degranulation. Toxicol. Appl. Pharmacol. 102:117-127.

Mann, W.A., Kinter, L.B., Stassen, F., and Huffman, W., 1986, Mechanism of action and structural requirements of vasopressin analog inhibition of transepithelial water flow in toad urinary bladder. J. Pharmacol. Expl. Ther. 238:401-406.
Mannucci, P.M., 1986, Desmopressin (DDAVP) for the treatment of disorders of hemostasis. Prog. Hemost. Thromb. 8:19-45.
Mannucci, P.M., Aberg, M., Nilsson, I.M., and Robertson, B., 1975, Mechanism of plasminogen activator and factor VIII increase after vasoactive drugs. Brit. J. Haematol 30:81-93.
Mansell, P.D. and Parry, B.W., 1991, Changes in Factor VIII:coagulant activity and von Willebrand factor antigen concentration after subcutaneous injection of desmopressin in dogs with mild hemophilia A. J. Vet. Intern. Med. 5:191-194.
Morgan, J.E., O'Neil, C.E., Coy, D.H., Hocart, S.J., and Nekola, M.V., 1986, Antagonistic analogs of leuteinizing hormone-releasing hormone are mast cell secretagogues. Int. Archs. Allergy appl. Immun. 80:70-75.
Murphy, D.J. and Joran, M.E., 1992, Respiratory and cardiovascular changes associated with toxic doses of a peptide antagonist of vasopressin in the rat. Fundamental Appl. Toxicol. 18:307-313.
Pigache, R.M., 1984, Facial flushing induced by vasopressin-like peptides lacking pressor activity. Br. J. Clin. Pharmacol. 17:309-310.
Roy, P.D., Moran, D.M., Bryant, V., Stevenson, R., and Stanworth, D.R., 1980, Further studies on histamine release from rat mast cells in vitro induced by peptides. Biochem. J. 191:233-237.
Salmenpera, M., Kuitunen, A., Hynynen, M., and Heinonen, J., 1991, Hemodynamic responses to desmopressin acetate after CABG: a double-blind trial. J. Cardiothorac. Vasc. Anesth. 5:146-149.
Schwartz, J., 1989, Vasodilation associated with V_2-type vasopressin activity: findings and implications. Mol. Cell. Endocrinol. 64:133-136.
Shulman, L.H., Miller, J.L., and Rose, L.I., 1990, Desmopressin for diabetes insipidus, hemostatic disorders and enuresis. Am. Fam. Phys. 42:1051-1057.
Suzuki, S., Tsutomu, T., Hirooka, Y., Yoshida, M., Ando, S., and Nakamura, M. 1989, Biphasic forearm vascular responses to intraarterial arginine vasopressin. J. Clin. Invest. 84:427-434.
Verbalis, J.G. and Martinez, A.J., 1991, Neurological and neuropathological sequelae of correction of chronic hyponatremia. Kidney Int. 39:1274-1282.
Walker, B.R., 1986, Evidence for a vasodilatory effect of vasopressin in the conscious rat. Am. J. Physiol. 251:H34-H39.
Wilkin, J.K., 1981, Flushing reactions: consequences and mechanisms. Ann Int. Med. 95:468-476.
Williams, T.D.M., Lightman, S.L., and Leadbeater, M.J., 1986, Hormonal and cardiovascular responses to DDAVP in man. Clin. Endocrinol. 24:89-96.
Yokota, M., Matsukura, S., Kaji, H., Taminato, T. and Fujita, T., 1982, Allergic reaction to DDAVP in diabetes insipidus: successful treatment with its graded doses. Endocrinol. Japan 29:467-477.
Ziai, F., Walter, R., and Rosenthal, I.M., 1978, Treatment of central diabetes insipidus in adults and children with desmopressin. Arch. Intern. Med. 138:1382-1385.
Zicha, J., Klunes, J., Pohlova, I., Slaninova, J., and Jelinek, J., 1989, Antidiuretic and pressor actions of vasopressin in age-dependent DOCA-salt hypertension. Am. J. Physiol. 256:R138-R145.

DISCUSSION

Brommer: We saw in 2 healthy volunteers and 2 patients very fast developing hypotension, within 2-3 minutes, which reversed as quickly when the infusion was stopped. Would you explain this by an anaphylactoid reaction?

Kinter: In humans there is not enough data to separate two possible mechanisms:
- an anaphylactoid reaction, which was either over when the pump is turned off, or disappeared purely coincidentally
- or a drug related vasodilation, which needs an intact endothelium and is related to the same mechanism that releases clotting factors, perhaps via an unidentified autocoid.

THE HEMODYNAMIC AND COAGULANT EFFECTS OF dDAVP ARE SPECIFIC EXTRARENAL V_2- RECEPTOR RESPONSES

Daniel G. Bichet, Marie-Françoise Arthus, and
Michèle Lonergan

Service de néphrologie, Unité de recherche clinique
et Département de médecine, Université de Montréal
Hôpital du Sacré-Coeur de Montréal
5400, boulevard Gouin Ouest
Montreal (Quebec) Canada H4J 1C5

The mechanisms of the stimulation of coagulation factor release and of the vasodilating properties of 1-desamino[8-D-arginine]vasopressin (dDAVP) have similarities and our laboratory (Bichet et al., 1988, 1989, 1991) and others (Mannucci et al., 1975; Liard, 1988a, 1988b; Hirsch et al., 1989) have pioneered the concept of extrarenal V_2 receptors.

THE VASOPRESSIN ISORECEPTORS

The vasopressor and antidiuretic properties of AVP

Although vasopressin was extracted as a pressor substance from the neurohypophysis by Oliver and Schäffer in 1895, its renal antidiuretic property, masked by its vascular action, was only revealed some 30 years later by Starling and Verney (1924). Hence, it was renamed antidiuretic hormone. This name has been used interchangeably with AVP ever since its structure was characterized. Soon after its characterization, it became the first peptide hormone to be synthesized, for which du Vigneaud won the Nobel Prize in 1954 (du Vigneaud, 1954, 1955).

The multiple "other" actions of AVP

There is evidence that vasopressin: 1) partricipates in the short-term regulation of arterial blood pressure by its direct vascular action, and that it interacts with the central nervous system baroreceptor pathways; 2) is one component of the multifactorial regulation of adrenocorticotropin release by the adenohypophysis; 3) acts specifically on anterior pituitary cells to enhance the release of the thyroid-stimulating

Desmopressin in Bleeding Disorders, Edited by G. Mariani *et al.*
Plenum Press, New York, 1993

hormone; 4) induces contraction of glomerular mesangial cells; 5) increases prostaglandin synthesis by medullarky interstitial cells; 6) causes platelet aggregation and the release of at least three coagulation factors: Factor VIIIc, vWF and t-PA: 7) has a mitogenic effect on several cell types; and 8) increases the firing rate of the hippocampal neurons and affects several brain functions such as memory consolidation (for a review, see Jard, 1985; Lumpkin et al., 1987; Kovacs and Lichardus 1989a and b).

V_1 and V_2 receptors

The multiple actions of AVP could be explained by the interaction of AVP with at least two types of membrane receptors. It was first established that cyclic AMP mediated the effects of AVP on the renal tubules. However, in 1974, Kirk and Hems reported that the glycogenolytic effect of vasopressin in rat liver was not accompanied by an increase in the intracellular concentration of cyclic AMP. Rather, a role for calcium was demonstrated in the mechanism of vasopressin stimulation of the liver and smooth muscle. On this functional basis, Michell et al. (1979) proposed that two types of vasopressin receptor lead to an increase in intracellular calcium concentration: V_2 receptors coupled to adenylate cyclase and V_1 receptors coupled to various mechanisms (hydrolysis of phosphatidyl-inositol-4,5-biphosphate and the formation of diacyl-glycerol). As yet, the cloning of the vasopressin receptors has not been published, but they are most probably guanine-nucleotide (G) protein-coupled receptors with seven transmembrane domains (Lefkowitz 1991; Simon et al., 1991)

A VASOPRESSIN V_2-SPECIFIC RECEPTOR MECHANISM IS INVOLVED IN HUMANS IN THE VASODILATING PROPERTIES OF dDAVP

Since the antidiuretic-pressure ratio of dDAVP is 4000:1, it is classified as a strong V_2 (antidiuretic) agonist with a minimal V_1 (pressor) activity (Pliska, 1985). It was first introduced in 1977 in the treatment of patients with central (or vasopressin-sensitive) diabetes insipidus and is now preferred to AVP for two reasons: 1) it does not increase blood pressure nor contract the uterus or the gastrointestinal tract (these effects are related to the stimulation of V_1-pressor-receptors); and 2) its biological half-life in plasma is much longer (55 minutes vs 5 minutes).

After the administration of dDAVP, mean arterial blood pressure decreased by 10 to 15 percent (Fig. 1), pulse rate increased by 20 to 25 percent and plasma renin activity increased by 65 percent in normal subjects (Bichet et al., 1988). These "hemodynamic" effects are not secondary to the presumed "antagonistic" effect of dDAVP on endogenous AVP bound to vascular V_1-receptors, since the vasodilating effects of dDAVP administration have been described in patients with untreated central diabetes insipidus who characteristically lack endogenous AVP (Williams et al., 1986; Bichet et al., 1988). Nor are the vasodilating effects of dDAVP administration secondary to the release of a mediator from the central nervous system, since they have been observed in dogs in which the central nervous system had been destroyed (Liard, 1989). The rapid changes in mean arterial blood pressure, pulse rate and plasma renin activity observed after dDAVP infusion would exclude the possible involvement of inhibition of water excretion; similar hemodynamic effects have been observed in anephric animals (Liard, 1988a). Furthermore, these vasodilating effects are not mediated by beta-adrenergic receptors (Schwartz et al., 1985), by sympathetic withdrawal (Hirsch et al, 1989, (Fig. 2)) nor by the release of prostaglandins (Liard 1988b). Measurements of PGE_2 and 6-keto-$PGH_{1\alpha}$ concentrations also failed to demonstrate a relationship between the peripheral vasodilatory action of AVP and the plasma concentrations of these compounds (Hirsch et al., 1989). The endothelium-derived relaxing factor, a compound released by a V_1 mechanism, is not involved (Katusic, 1984; VanHoutte, 1987). Finally, the above vasodilating effects were not observed in male patients with congenital nephrogenic diabetes insipidus (Bichet et al., 1988) (Fig. 1).

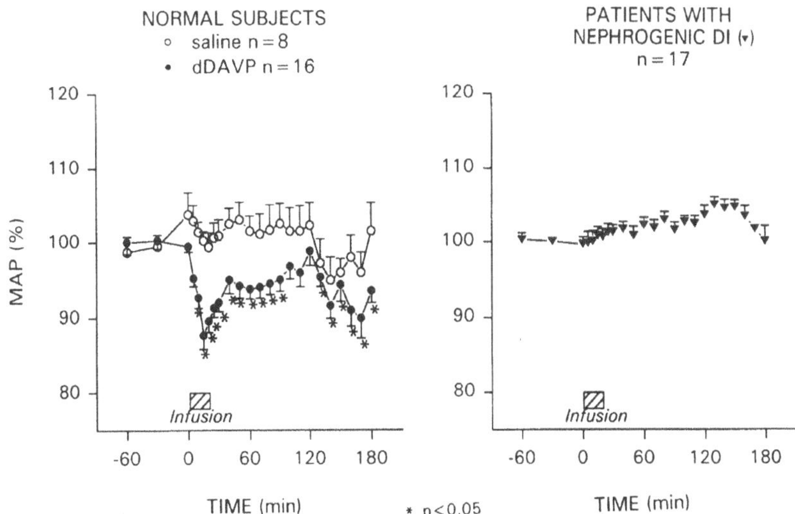

Figure 1: Mean arterial blood pressure (MAP) response to dDAVP infusion (0.3 μg/kg of body weight up to a maximum of 24 μg infused from 0 to 20 minutes) in 16 normal subjects and in 17 male patients with congenital nephrogenic diabetes insipidus. Eight saline infusion studies were also done in normal subjects (control). Results are reported as the mean ± SEM of per cent of the baseline values observed at -60, -30 and 0 minutes. The responses observed in male patients with congenital nephrogenic diabetes insipidus were significantly different from those of the normal subjects infused with dDAVP (variance and Newman-Keul's analysis). Error bars are contained within the symbol when not visible.

Congenital nephrogenic diabetes insipidus (CNDI) is usually a rare X-linked disorder associated with tubular resistance to arginine-vasopressin (AVP) (Reeves and Andreoli, 1989) but normal V_1-receptor responses (Bichet et al., 1991). In affected families, 50 per cent of the males are symptomatic and completely unresponsive to vasopressin. Polyuria and polydipsic measurements are usually larger than 8 liters/day in adult patients. During their early years, the affected male patients have repeated episodes of dehydration and hypernatremia as a consequence of the severe polyuria. These episodes could lead to severe and definitive physical and mental retardation. Early recognition and the subsequent treatment of CNDI with an abundant intake of water leads to a normal life span with normal physical and mental development (Niaudet et al., 1985). In a large study (Crawford and Bode, 1975), 39 out of 44 affected male patients had some degree of mental retardation. In Montreal, Halifax and Toronto, we have examined 19 affected males, 13 of whom had some degree of mental retardation. In these latter patients, the diagnosis was not made during their first year of life.

Female patients can also be afflicted with variable degrees of polyuria and polydipsia. This variable expression is secondary to the phenomenon of X chromosome inactivation. Early in the development of the female embryo, one of the two X chromosomes in every cell becomes permanently inactivated in a random process known as lyonization (Ohno, 1967). All mature cell lineages in the females are thus expected to be composed of a mixture of cells in which only one of the X chromosomes is active. In female carriers of the nephrogenic diabetes insipidus gene, the X chromosome carrying the defective gene could be randomly activated in the majority of the renal collecting duct cells. These females will then be polyuro-polydipsic, however, they maintain a limited capacity to concentrate their urine. Thus, they are usually protected against dehydration episodes, and their physical and mental development is entirely normal.

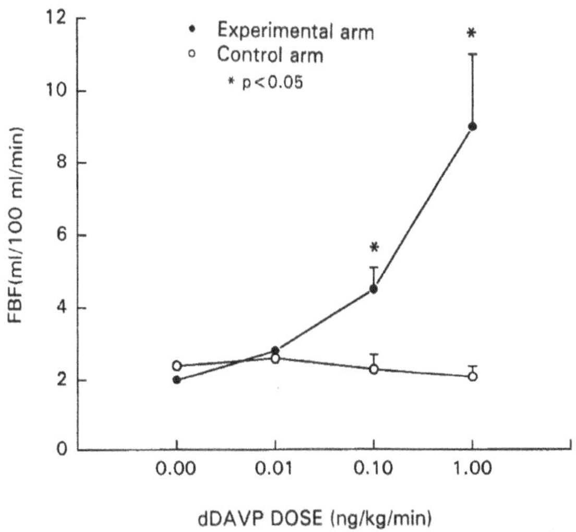

Figure 2. The dose-response relationship of forearm blood flow (FBF) to intraarterial dDAVP administration in normal subjects. Data are presented as mean ± SEM, FBF was equal in both arms at baseline but increased significantly in experimental arm when dDAVP was infused. FBF in the control arm was unchanged at all infusion rates. Figure adapted from Hirsch et al., 1989, Reprinted from J. Clin. Invest., with permission.

Jans et al. (1990) demonstrated that derivatives of somatic cell hybrids that carry the human gene locus for nephrogenic diabetes insipidus express functional vasopressin V_2 receptors. The gene coding for the V_2 receptor is thus most probably localized in the distal part of the X chromosome (Xq28) (Bichet et al., 1990b), and alterations of this gene are likely to be the molecular basis of congenital nephrogenic diabetes insipidus. Male patients with this disease offer the unique opportunity to test directly for the physiological importance of extrarenal V_2 receptor. Recent experiments performed in the Rhesus Monkey (*Macaca mulatta*) also demonstrated that the tachycardia and renin release associated with dDAVP administration were most likely secondary to vasodilation, also mediated by a V_2-like mechanism (Kinter et al., 1992). In these experiments, the V_2 receptor antagonist, SK&F 105494 (30 μg/kg, i.v.) had no effect on heart rate or blood pressure, but prevented the tachycardia induced by dDAVP. A similar demonstration is not possible in humans since SK&F 105494 is a full V_2 agonist in humans (Kinter et al., 1991).

A VASOPRESSIN V_2-SPECIFIC RECEPTOR MECHANISM INVOLVED IN HUMANS IN THE STIMULATION OF COAGULATION FACTORS IDUCED BY dDAVP.

Holemans (1967) initially thought that there was a close correlation between the activity of some drugs on vascular motility and their activity on fibrinolysis and coagulation. In their experiments, blood fibrinolytic activity was enhanced and clotting time was shortened by vasodilator drugs, whereas vasoconstrictor drugs caused little change. In contrast, in 1975, Mannucci et al. showed that a strong vasoconstrictor drug such as lysine-vasopressin very effectively stimulated the release of t-PA and FVIIIc from the vascular cells. Strong vasodilator drugs like histamine, theophylline and cyclic AMP did not have this effect. Furthermore, dDAVP, a synthetic analogue of AVP was more effective than lysine-vasopressin in stimulating the release of t-PA and FVIIIc from the endothelial vascular cells (Mannucci, 1975).

Since the responses of FVIIIc and VWF to dDAVP administration appear too rapidly to be accounted for by an accelerated synthesis, it is postulated that a release mechanism is involved (Mannucci, 1988). The mechanisms by which DDAVP releases FVIIIc and vWF from the vascular endothelium are not well understood. In 1975, Mannucci et al. suggested that specific receptors are involved in the response of FVIIIc to dDAVP administration. It is not likely that beta-adrenergic mechanisms, prostaglandins or beta-endorphin mediators are involved, since the coagulation-factor responses observed after dDAVP administration are not modified by propranolol, aspirin or naloxone administration. Furthermore, the putative receptors are V_2-like rather than V_1-like, since they require the levo-stereoisomer at position 8 for their activation. They are also extrarenal, since in two anephric patients (regularly undergoing hemodialysis) given dDAVP, the increases in both plasma t-PA and FVIIIc concentrations were similar in magnitude to those observed in normal subjects treated with the same dose of dDAVP (Mannucci, 1975). In addition similar changes in the plasma ratios of FVIIIc:vWF were induced by the administration of dDAVP to patients with uremia and to normal subjects (Mannucci et al., 1983).

Earlier claims that dDAVP may act indirectly through the release of a putative hypothalamic mediator (Cort et al., 1981) have not been confirmed (Budiansky, 1983). Nor does dDAVP stimulate the release of the coagulation factors by displacing endogenous AVP from its receptor (an antagonistic effect), since the stimulating properties of dDAVP on the release of the coagulation factors have been described in patients with untreated central diabetes insipidus who characteristically lack endogenous AVP (Bichet et al., 1988). The hypothesis that dDAVP stimulates the release of the coagulation factors directly through a V_2-receptor specific mechanism has received strong support from our studies in male patients with congenital nephrogenic diabetes insipidus (Bichet et al., 1988). In these male patients the antidiuretic response to AVP

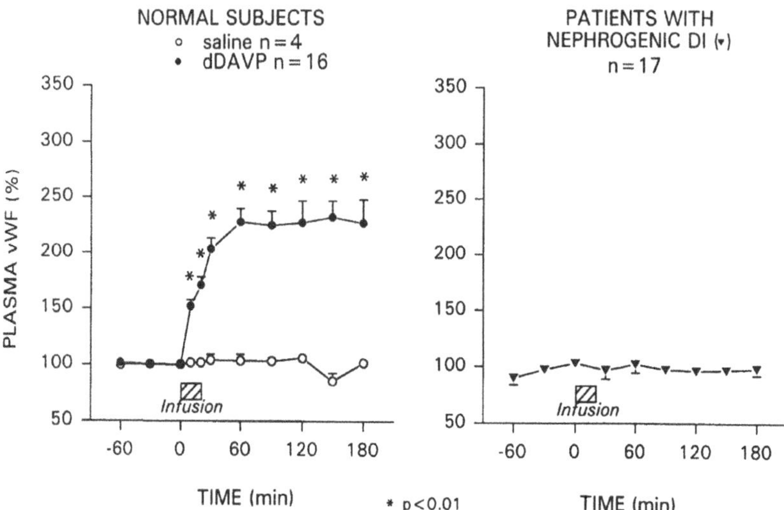

Figure 3. von Willebrand factor (vWF) responses to dDAVP infusion (0.3 μg/kg of body weight up to a maximum of 24 μg infused from 0 to 20 minutes) in 17 male patients with congenital nephrogenic diabetes insipidus. Four saline infusion studies were also done in normal subjects (control). Results ar reported as the mean $\pm$ SEM of per cent of the baseline values observed at -60, -30 and 0 minutes. The responses observed in male patients with congenital nephrogenic diabetes insipidus were significantly diferent from those of the normal subjects infused with dDAVP (variance and Newman-Keul's analysis). Error bars are contained within the symbol when not visible.

or dDAVP administration is absent due to abnormal renal V_2 receptor responses. Their extrarenal V_2 receptor responses are also defective, since the release of the coagulation factors (FVIIIc and vWF) did not increase in response to the administration of dDAVP (Fig. 3). The abnormal coagulant responses in patients with congenital nephrogenic diabetes insipidus are specific, since the releases of factor VIIIc, vWF and t-PA were normally stimulated by epinephrine administration (Bichet 1989). Additional arguments in favor of the specificity of these responses have been presented by Brommer et al. (1990). They observed no increases in the releases of factor VIIIc, the vWF or the t-PA in response to dDAVP infusion in three patients with congenital nephrogenic diabetes insipidus. However, they did observe an increase in the plasma concentration of tissue plasminogen antigen and in tissue plasminogen activity during venous occlusion. Finally, we recently demonstrated that, in anesthetized female rhesus monkeys, dDAVP (3.0 μg per kilogram) given intravenously stimulated the release of vWF, Factor VIIIc and renin and was associated with tachycardia and hypotension. The V_2 receptor antagonist, SK&F 105494 (30 μg per kilogram) given intravenously, had no effect on clotting factor or renin release, heart rate, or arterial blood pressure, but it did prevent dDAVP-induced stimulation of clotting factor release and tachycardia (Fig. 4). The stimulation of the release of the clotting factor by dDAVP administration seems, then, to be mediated by a low-affinity, extrarenal, V_2-like receptor mechanism in this species (Kinter et al., 1992). Endothelial vascular cells could bear these putative V_2 receptors. Alternatively, dDAVP may act through a V_2 receptor specific mechanism, to stimulate the release of an unknown mediator which itself acts on the release of FVIIIc and vWF (Hashemi et al., 1990).

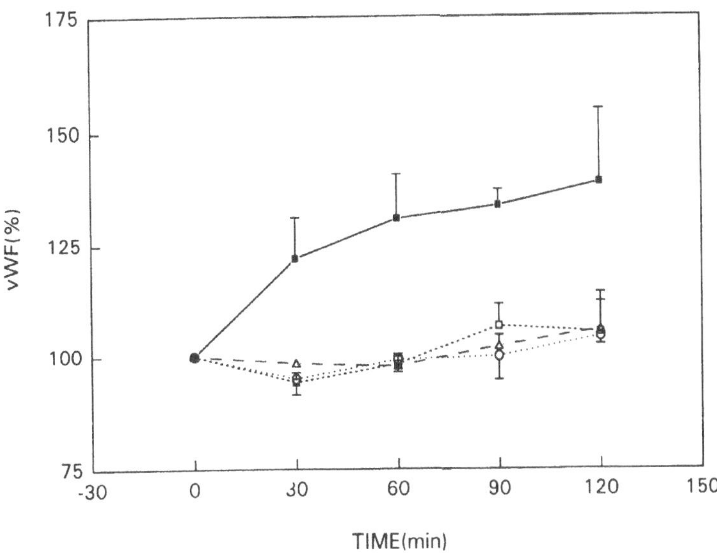

Figure 4. Effect of the V_2 receptor antagonist SK&F 105494 (30 μg/kg) alone (▵) or in the presence of dDAVP (3 μg/kg) (□) on plasma concentrations of vWF measured in Rhesus Monkeys. The dDAVP (3 μg/kg) induced stimulation of vWF (■) was prevented by the V_2 receptor antagonist (▵ 105494 alone, □ dDAVP + 105494), Saline infusion (○).

In summary the stimulation of coagulation-factor release and the vasodilating properties of dDAVP are likely mediated by specific V_2-like receptors. The localization of these receptors is unknown. Neither animal nor in vitro studies are likely to supply the answers, since FVIIIc release after the administration of DDAVP is less marked in dogs than in humans, and rats and rabbits do not respond to dDAVP administration (Mannucci, 1988). The V_2 receptors in the central nervous system cannot be involved, since a pronounced fall in blood pressure was observed in decapitated dogs infused with dDAVP (Liard, 1989). However, myocardial receptors could be involved, since there was a greater increase in cardiac output and a greater decrease in total peripheral resistance after intracoronary than after intravenous infusion (Liard, 1989). Vascular endothelial cells could also bear these hypothetical receptors and release FVIIIc, VWF and t-PA in response to appropriate stimuli. However, DDAVP perfused through umbilical veins (an in vitro preparation of human endothelial cells) was not effective in releasing FVIIIc (Booyse et al., 1981). The vascular beds responsible for the "coagulant" properties of DDAVP could thus be selective and the releasing properties of DDAVP may not be expressed in in vitro perfused human umbilical veins.

THE V_2 RECEPTOR ABNORMAL RESPONSES OBSERVED IN PATIENTS WITH CONGENITAL NEPHROGENIC DIABETES INSIPIDUS ARE PRECYCLIC-AMP DEFECTS

We observed that dDAVP administration increased plasma cyclic AMP concentrations in normal subjects, but had no effect in 14 male patients with CNDI (Fig. 5) (Bichet et al., 1989). In the obligatory carriers the responses were intermediate which possibly represented a normal response by half of the receptors (carriers have one normal and one defective gene). Thus, the altered interaction between vasopressin and its V_2 receptor occurs at a step which precedes the stimulation of cyclic AMP. The receptor-adenylate cyclase complex appears to have three components: 1) the receptor that recognizes the hormone, 2) a regulatory subunit which is a guanine nucleotide-binding protein(G), and 3) the catalytic subunit (Hanley and Steiner, 1989). The administration of parathyroid hormone stimulated the urinary excretion of cyclic AMP in two male patients with CNDI (Moses and Coulson, 1982), therefore, an alteration of a transduction G-type protein is unlikely. The mechanism underlying the hormonal resistance in patients with CNDI seems then to be different from that in patients with pseudohypoparathyroidism type Ia (PHP-Ia) which is characterized by a reduced expression of messenger ribonucleic acid for the G alpha subunit (Gs) (Van Dop, 1989). This molecular difference is not surprising, since the phenotypic characteristics of PHP-Ia do not include a concentrating defect, and since the hereditary transmission is autosomal dominant (Moses et al., 1986; Spiegel, 1989).

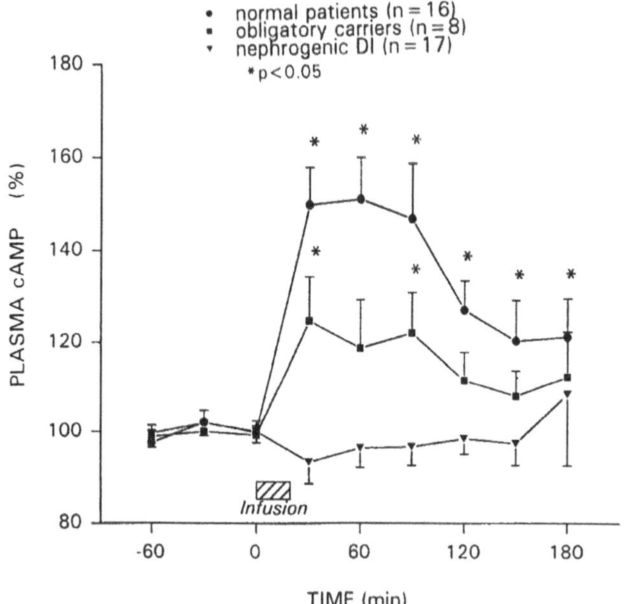

Figure 5. Plasma cyclic AMP responses to DDAVP infusion in the three groups of subjects. Symbols: (■) normal, (▲) obl. carriers, (●) nephrog. DI. Asterisks indicate significant differences from baseline values (at -60, -30 and 0 minute). Figure adapted from Bichet et al., 1989. Reprinted from Kidney International, with permission).

In mice with congenital nephrogenic diabetes insipidus, there is an inadequate increase in the water permeability of the collecting duct system in response to AVP administration (Kusano et al., 1986). There is also an increased catabolism of renal medullary cyclic AMP by phosphodiesterases. In this animal model, the concomitant administration of two inhibitors of cyclic AMP-phosphodiesterase isoenzyme type IV (Rolipram and Cilostamide), completely restored cyclic AMP accumulation in response to AVP administration (Coffey et al., 1988), and increased urinary osmolality and corrected the high fluid turnover (Coffey et al., 1989). The physiopathological defect present in mice with HNDI is probably not present in humans with HNDI, since in humans the disease is an X-linked inheritance rather than a non-X-linked trait as in mice. Furthermore, we have unsuccessfully used Rolipram for 7 days in two patients with HNDI. In these patients, urinary osmolality was unchanged (less than 200 mmol/kg) as were free water and osmolar clearances, urinary cyclic AMP excretion rates and plasma cyclic AMP concentrations (Bichet et al., 1990a). In recent experiments, we demonstrated that dDAVP administration induced an increase in the plasma concentrations of guanosine 3',5'-cyclic monophosphate (cyclic GMP) (Kluge et al., 1991). This increase was not observed in male patients with congenital nephrogenic diabetes insipidus nor in anephric patients. The hemodynamic and coagulant extrarenal responses to dDAVP administration are possibly related to the stimulation of the release of cyclic GMP.

ACKNOWLEDGEMENTS

These studies were supported by the Canadian Kidney Foundation, the Medical Research Council of Canada (MT-8126) and the Canadian Heart Foundation. Dr. Daniel G. Bichet is a senior scholar of Le Fonds de la recherche en santé du Québec. The manuscript was prepared by Ms. Diane Dugas.

REFERENCES

D.G. Bichet, M. Razi, M. Lonergan, M.F. Arthus, V. Papukna, C. Kortas, and J.N. Barjon, Hemodynamic and coagulation responses to 1-desamino[8-D-arginine]vasopressin in patients with congenital nephrogenic diabetes insipidus. *N. Engl. J. Med.* 318:881(1988).

D.G. Bichet, M. Razi, M.F. Arthus, M. Lonergan, P. Tittley, R.K. Smiley, G. Rock, and D.J. Hirsch, Epinephrine and dDAVP administration in patients with congenital nephrogenic diabetes insipidus. Evidence for a pre-cyclic AMP V_2 receptor defective mechanism. *Kidney Int.* 36:859(1989).

D.G. Bichet, N. Ruel, M.F. Arthus, and M. Lonergan, Rolipram, a phosphodiesterase inhibitor, in the treatment of two male patients with congenital nephrogenic diabetes insipidus (letter). *Nephron* 56:449(1990a).

D.G. Bichet, G.N. Hendy, D.J. Hirsch, M. Lonergan, M.F. Arthus, and J.L. Mandel, Congenital nephrogenic diabetes insipidus: from the ship Hopewell to restriction fragment length polymorphism studies. *Kidney Int.* 37:246A(1990b)

D.G. Bichet, M.F. Arthus, and M. Lonergan, Platelet vasopressin receptors in patients with congenital nephrogenic diabetes insipidus. *Kidney Int.*, 39:693(1991).

F.M. Booyse, G. Osikowicz, and S. Feder, Effects of various agents on ristocetin-Willebrand factor activity in long-term cultures of von Willebrand and normal human umbilical vein endothelial cells (letter). *Thromb. Haemost.* 46:668(1981).

E.J.P. Brommer, H. Brink, F.H.M. Derkx, M.A.H. Schalekamp, and J. Stibbe, Normal homeostasis of fibrinolysis in nephrogenic diabetes insipidus in spite of defective V_2-receptor-mediated responses of tissue plasminogen activator release. *Eur. J. Clin. Invest.* 20:72(1990).

S. Budiansky, False data confessed. *Nature* 301:101(1983).

A.K. Coffey, D.J. O'Sullivan, S. Homma, T.P. Dousa, and H. Valtin, Induction of intramembranous particle clusters in inner medullary collecting ducts of mice with nephrogenic diabetes insipidus (abstract). *Clin. Res.* 36:593A(1988).

A.K. Coffey, D.J. O'Sullivan, S. Homma, T.P. Dousa, and H. Valtin, Successful, specific treatment of nephrogenic diabetes insipidus (NDI) in mice (abstract). *Kidney Int.* 35:494(1989).

J.H. Cort, A.J. Fischman, W. Jean Dodds, J.H. Rand, and I.L. Schwartz, New category of vasopressin receptor in the central nervous system. *Int. J. Pept. Protein Res.* 17:14(1981).

J.D. Crawford and H.H. Bode, Disorders of the posterior pituitary in children. *in*: "Endocrine and Genetic Diseases of Childhood and Adolescence", (2nd edn), L.I. Gardner,ed., W.B. Saunders, Philadelphia (1975).

V. du Vigneaud, *The Harvey Lectures*, 49:1(1954-1955).

R.M. Hanley and A.L. Steiner, The second-messenger system for peptide hormones. *Hosp. Pract.* 24:59(1989).

S. Hashemi, E.S. Tackaberry, D.S. Palmer, G. Rock, and P.R. Ganz, dDAVP-induced release of von Willebrand factor from endothelial cells in vitro: The effect of plasma and blood cells. *Biochim. Biophys. Acta* 1052:63(1990).

A.T. Hirsch, V.J. Dzau, J.A. Majzoub, M.A. Creager, Vasopressin-mediated forearm vasodilation in normal humans. Evidence for a vascular vasopressin V_2 receptor. *J. Clin. Invest.* 84:418(1989).

R. Holemans, L.S. Mann, E.J. Mlynarczyk, and B.J. Polesz, Drug-induced plasminogen activator release. *Thromb. Diather. Haemorrhagica*, 18:298(1967).

D.A. Jans, B.A. van Oost, H.H. Ropers, and F. Fahrenholz, Derivatives of somatic cell hybrids which carry the human gene locus for nephrogenic diabetes insipidus (NDI) express functional vasopressin renal V_2-type receptors. *J. Biol. Chem.* 265:15379(1990).

S. Jard, : Vasopressin receptors, *in* "Frontiers in Hormone Research", Vol. 13: Diabetes insipidus in man, P. Czernichow and A.G. Robinson, eds, S. Karger, Basel (1985).

Z.S. Katusic, J.T. Shepherd, and P.M. Vanhoutte, Vasopressin causes endothelium-dependent relaxations of the canine basilar artery. *Circ. Res.* 55:575(1984).

L.B. Kinter, I. McConnell, B.G. Goodwin, S. Campbell, W.F. Huffman, M.F. Arthus, M. Lonergan, and D.G. Bichet, Vasopressin antagonist inhibition of clotting factor release in the rhesus monkey (*Macaca mulatta*). *J. Pharmacol. Exp. Ther.*, in press 1992.

L.B. Kinter, B.E. Ilson, S. Caltabianol, S., D.K. Jordasky, D.J. Murphy, H.A. Solloveld, G.R. Rhodes D.P. Brooks, C.R. Albrightson-Winslow, R.M. Stote and W.F. Huffman, Antidiuretic hormone antagonism in humans: Are there predictors? *in*: "Vasopressin" Vol. 208, S. Jard, and R. Jamison, eds. Colloque INSERM/John Libbey Eurotext Ltd, Paris, Londres (1991). pp. 321-329.

C.J. Kirk and D.A. Hems, Hepatic action of vasopressin: Lack of a role for adenosine-3',5'-cyclic monophosphate. *FEBS Lett.* 47:128(1974).

R. Kluge, M.F. Arthus, M. Lonergan, and D.G. Bichet, The stimulation of plasma cyclic GMP (cGMP) by dDAVP is an extrarenal V_2 specific response. *J. Am. Soc. Nephrol.* 2:723(1991).

L. Kovacs and B. Lichardus, Chapter 11. Vasopressin and anterior pituitary function. *in*: "Vasopressin. Disturbed Secretion and Its Effects". Kluwer Academic Publ, Dordrecht. Vol. 25. (1989a).

L. Kovacs and B. Lichardus, Chapter 12. Vasopressin and brain function. *in*: "Vasopressin. Disturbed Secretion and Its Effects". Kluwer Academic Publ, Dordrecht. Vol. 25. (1989b).

E. Kusano, A.N.K. Yusufi, N. Murayama, J. Braun-Werness, and P. Dousa, Dynamics of nucleotides in distal nephron of mice with nephrogenic diabetes insipidus. *Am. J. Physiol.* 260:F151(1986).

R.J. Lefkowitz, Variations on a theme. *Nature*, 351:353(1991).

J.F. Liard, Characterization of acute hemodynamic effects of antidiuretic agonists in conscious dogs. *J. Cardiovasc. Pharmacol.* 11:174(1988a).

J.F. Liard, Effects of a specific antidiuretic agonist on cardiac output and its distribution in intact and anephric dogs. *Clin. Sci.* 74:293(1988b).

J.F. Liard, Peripheral vasodilatation induced by a vasopressin analogue with selective V_2-agonism in dogs. *Am. J. Physiol.* 256:H1621(1989).

M.D. Lumpkin, W.K. Samson, and S.M. McCann, Arginine vasopressin as a thyrotropin-releasing hormone. *Science*, 235:1070(1987).

P.M. Mannucci, M. Aberg, I.M. Nilsson, and B. Robertson, Mechanism of plasminogen activator and factor VIII increase after vasoactive drugs. *Br. J. Haematol.* 30:81(1975).

P.M. Mannucci, G. Remuzzi, F. Pusineri, R. Lombardi, C. Valsecchi, G. Mecca, and T.S. Zimmerman, Deamino-8-D-arginine vasopressin shortens the bleeding time in uremia. *N. Engl. J. Med.* 308:8(1983).

P.M. Mannucci, Desmopressin: a nontransfusional form of treatment for congenital and acquired bleeding disorders. *Blood* 72:1449(1988).

R.H. Michell, C.J. Kirk, and M.M. Billah, Hormonal stimulation of phosphatidylinositol breakdown with particular reference to the hepatic effects of vasopressin. *Biochem. Soc. Trans.* 7:861(1979).

A.M. Moses and B.B. Coulson, Absence of overlapping resistance to vasopressin and parathyroid hormone in patients with nephrogenic diabetes insipidus and pseudohypoparathyroidism. *J. Clin. Endocrinol. Metab.* 55:699(1982).

A.M. Moses, R.S. Weinstock, M.A. Levine, and N.A. Breslau, Evidence for normal antidiuretic responses to endogenous and exogenous arginine vasopressin in patients withguaninenucleotide-bindingstimulatoryprotein-deficientpseudohypoparathyroidism. *J. Clin. Endocrinol. Metab.* 62:221(1986).

P. Niaudet, M. Dechaux, D. Leroy, and M. Broyer, Nephrogenic diabetes insipidus in children, *in* "Frontiers in Hormone Research", Vol. 13: Diabetes insipidus in man, P. Czernichow, and A.G. Robinson, eds, S. Karger, Basel (1985).

S. Ohno, "Monographs on Endocrinology. Sex Chromosomes and Sex-Linked Genes", Springer-Verlag, New York (1967).

G. Oliver and E.A. Schäffer, On the physiological action of extract of pituitary body and certain other glandular organs. *J. Physiol.* 18:277(1895).

V. Pliska, Pharmacology of deamino-d-arginine vasopressin. *in*: "Frontiers of hormone research". Vol. 13. Diabetes insipidus in man. P. Czernichow and A.G. Robinson eds. S. Karger, Basel (1985).

W.B. Reeves and T.E. Andreoli, Nephrogenic diabetes insipidus. *in* "The Metabolic Basis of Inherited Disease", C.R. Scriver, A.L. Beaudet, W.S. Sly, and D. Valle, eds. McGraw-Hill, New York (1989).

J. Schwartz, J.F. Liard, C. Ott, and A.W.J. Cowley, Hemodynamic effects of neurohypophyseal peptides with antidiuretic activity in dogs. *Am. J. Physiol.* 249:H1001(1985).

M.I. Simon, M.P. Strathmann, and N. Gautam, Diversity of G proteins in signal transduction. *Science* 252:802(1991).

A.M. Spiegel, Pseudohypoparathyroidism. *in*: "The Metabolic Basis of Inherited Disease", C.R. Scriver, A.L. Beaudet, W.S. Sly, and D. Valle, eds, McGraw-Hill, New York (1989).

E.H. Starling and E.B. Verney, The secretion of urine as studied on the isolated kidney. *Proc. Roy. Soc. London Ser. B*, 97:321(1924).

C. Van Dop, Pseudohypoparathyroidism: clinical and molecular aspects. *Sem. Nephrol.* 9:168(1989).

P.M. Vanhoutte, Endothelium and responsiveness of vascular smooth muscle. *J. Hypertens.* 5 (Suppl. 5):S115(1987).

T.D.M. Williams, S.L. Lightman, and M.J. Leadbeater, Hormonal and cardiovascular responses to dDAVP in man. *Clin. Endocrinol. (Oxf.)* 24:89(1986).

DISCUSSION

Kobrinski: My question concerns another experiment of nature, Bartter's syndrome, which has complete pressor resistance to V1 agonists, and is therefore a model for V1 receptor study. Is this so?

Bichet: In Bartter's syndrome there is also resistance to angiotensin infusion, and very high levels of prostaglandins. Apart from the first report, in 2 related boys, it is not as well defined a disease as nephrogenic diabetes insipidus. However, it has potential for research.

Brommer: Was there a time difference between the CGMP and the CAMP responses? Is this a secondary reaction?

Bichet: No, they were almost concomitant when sampling at 10 and 20 minute intervals.

THE VASOPRESSIN ANTAGONIST SK&F 105494 INHIBITS DESMOPRESSIN-STIMULATED CLOTTING FACTOR RELEASE IN VIVO

Lewis B. Kinter, B. Thomas Goodwin, Irving McConnell, Sarah Campbell, William F. Huffman, Marie-Francoise Arthus, Michele Lonergan, and Daniel G. Bichet

Departments of, Toxicology - U.S.(LBK), Laboratory Animal Science (IM, BTG, SC), and Peptidomimetic Research (WFH) SmithKline Beecham Pharmaceuticals, King of Prussia, PA, and Nephrology Research Service Hospital du Sacre-Coeur and University of Montreal (M-FA, ML, DGB), Montreal, PQ, Canada

SUMMARY

The antidiuretic (V_2) agonist, desmopressin (dDAVP), stimulates release of the clotting factors von Willebrand factor (vWF) and factor VIIIc (FVIIIc) in humans. dDAVP (3.0 µg/kg) stimulated release of vWF and FVIIIc, and was associated with hypotension and tachycardia in the pentobarbital-anesthetized rhesus monkeys (Macaca mulatta). The V_2 receptor antagonist, SK&F 105494 (30 µg/kg), had no effect on clotting factor release, blood pressure or heart rate, but prevented dDAVP stimulation of clotting factor release, hypotension, and tachycardia. The results support the hypothesis that dDAVP stimulation of clotting factor release and vasodilation are mediated by low-affinity, V_2-like receptor mechanisms.

INTRODUCTION

The mechanism of dDAVP-stimulation of circulating clotting factor concentrations is poorly understood (Mannucci et al., 1975). Because the vasopressin agonists AVP, LVP, and dDAVP share clotting factor-releasing activity and V_2, but not V_1 receptor affinity, it has been assumed that the vasopressin-clotting factor mechanism involved a V_2-like receptor (Bichet et al., 1988). In contrast to the renal V_2 receptor pathway, this extra-renal V_2-like mechanism requires circulating agonist concentrations in the ng/ml range, may have relatively low affinity for dDAVP, and may be linked to cyclic GMP metabolism (Bichet et al., 1988, 1992). The mechanism may also share pharmacological characteristics with other secondary actions associated with large doses of dDAVP, including flushing, hypotension, and stimulation of renin release (Williams et al., 1986; Bichet et al.,

Desmopressin in Bleeding Disorders, Edited by G. Mariani *et al.*
Plenum Press, New York, 1993

1988; Schwartz, 1989). The objective of this study was to identify and characterize dDAVP stimulation of clotting factor release in pentobarbital-anesthetized rhesus monkeys using dDAVP and a V_2 receptor antagonist (SK&F 105494).

MATERIALS AND METHODS

Drug: Desmopressin (1-deamino-8-D-arginine vasopressin, dDAVP) and SK&F 105494 (O-ethyl-D-tyrosyl-L-phenylalanyl-L-valyl-L-asparaginyl-5-[1-(carboxymethyl)cyclohexyl]-L-norvalyl-L-arginyl-D-argininamide, cyclic (5→1) peptide, Moore et al., 1988) were prepared by SB Peptidomimetic Chemists. The activity constant (K_{act}) for dDAVP for stimulation of human renal V_2-dependent adenylate cyclase is 24 nM; the inhibition constants (K_i) for SK&F 105494 for human and rhesus monkey renal V_2-dependent adenylate cyclase are 3.9 and 4.6 nM, respectively (Brooks et al., 1988a). DDAVP is an antidiuretic agonist and SK&F 105494 is an antidiuretic antagonist in the rhesus monkey (Brooks et al., 1988b and unpublished results). Both peptides were administered as solutions in 0.9% NaCl, infused intravenously over 20 minutes at a rate of 0.017 ml/minute per kg body weight. In order to avoid drug-induced hypotension that might compromise the study and/or the health of the monkeys, an upward dose titration was conducted with dDAVP (0.1 to 10 µg/kg). The dose of SK&F 105494 (30 µg/kg), was selected as that previously associated with maximal aquaretic (renal V_2 antagonist activity) in vivo in these monkeys (Brooks et al., 1988a).

Animals: Fourteen wild-caught female rhesus monkeys (Macaca mulatta, Hazelton Research Animals) were used in this study. The monkeys weighed between 3.8 and 8.0 kilograms and were of undetermined age at the start of the study. Monkeys were housed individually in stainless steel cages in environmentally controlled rooms (72°F ± 4°F; 50% ± 10% relative humidity) with a 12-hour light/dark cycle. Tap water was available ad libitum from an automatic watering system. The monkeys were fed a standard laboratory primate chow. The monkeys were fasted for approximately 16-20 hours prior to study, tranquilized (ketamine hydrochloride, 100 mg, i.m.), then lightly anesthetized with pentobarbital sodium (15 mg/kg, i.v.). Pentobarbital anesthesia has been shown not to interfere with V_2 agonist stimulation of plasma concentrations of vWF and FVIIIc (Johnstone and Crane, 1988). Anesthesia was maintained with supplemental doses of pentobarbital, to effect as necessary. Once a stable anesthesia was achieved, monkeys were placed in lateral recumbency on a thermo-controlled heating blanket and a thermocouple temperature probe inserted in the rectum. Catheters were placed in a radial (20g) and saphenous (22g) for administration of fluids and drugs and removal of blood samples, respectively. A slow intravenous drip (~0.2 ml/min) of 0.9% NaCl was started via the radial vein to maintain catheter patency. As a precaution against drug-induced hypotension mean arterial blood pressure and heart rate were monitored non-invasively at 5-10 min intervals using automated pneumatic blood pressure cuff placed around the uncatheterized forelimb.

The protocol used was modeled upon that described by Bichet and colleagues (1988). A blood sample (10 ml) was withdrawn into a chilled syringe (T=-30 min) and the monkey allowed to stabilize for 30 minutes. Following stabilization, another blood sample was withdrawn (T=0 min) and drug or vehicle infused intravenously over 20 minutes via the radial vein. Additional blood samples were withdrawn at 30, 60, 90, and 120 minutes following initiation of the drug or vehicle infusion. All monkeys were recovered from anesthesia and returned to their cages at the end of the study. Some monkeys repeated the protocol, no monkey received the same treatment twice. The minimum interval between studies in the same monkey was 41 days.

Analytical methodologies: Blood samples for determination of vWF and FVIIIc concentrations were transferred into pre-labeled citrate-buffered chilled evacuated tubes and centrifuged ($4^{o}C$, 650 x g). The plasma was transferred to prelabeled plastic cryogenic tubes and rapidly frozen and stored in a $-80^{o}C$ freezer until analyzed for vWF and FVIIIc. Von Willebrand factor was measured as previously described (Bichet et al., 1988, 1989) according to an enzyme-linked immunosorbent assay described by Cejka (1982); FVIIIc was measured with a chromogenic method (Lethagen et al., 1986). Values for the -30 and 0 min time points were averaged to define pretreatment (baseline) values. Data are expressed as percent change from baseline values and presented as means ± standard error of the mean (SEM). A one-factor repeated measures ANOVA was performed using SAS-based models (SAS Institute, NC). Tukey's multiple comparison procedure was used to determine statistically significant differences from vehicle- and dDAVP-treated responses. Statistical significance was defined as $p<.05$.

RESULTS

In 39 individual studies baseline (prior to drug treatment) plasma vWF concentrations ranged from 0.47 to 1.73 U/ml. In vehicle-treated monkeys plasma concentrations of vWF was stable for the duration of the study. dDAVP (3.0 μg/kg) caused a sustained and statistically significant increase (~40%) in plasma vWF concentrations (Figure 1); a higher dose (10 μg/kg) produced no further increase in vWF above those observed with the 3 μg/kg dosage. dDAVP (0.1 to 10 μg/kg) caused a transient, dose-dependent hypotension and reflex tachycardia. dDAVP (3.0 μg/kg) produced variable but sustained increases in plasma FVIIIc concentrations, similar to the increases in plasma vWF concentrations (data not shown).

The V_2 receptor antagonist SK&F 105494 (30 μg/kg) produced no changes in vWF, blood pressure, or heart rate in rhesus monkeys. However, pretreatment of monkeys with SK&F 105494 (30 μg/kg infused over T = 0 to 20 minutes) followed by dDAVP (3 μg/kg infused over T = 20 to 40 minutes) prevented the increases in vWF and the decrease in blood pressure and tachycardia associated with this dose of dDAVP.

DISCUSSION

Intravenous administration of the selective V_2 agonist, dDAVP, stimulated plasma concentrations of vWF and FVIIIc in pentobarbital-anesthetized female rhesus monkeys. The effect of dDAVP on vWF was prevented by prior administration of a vasopressin antagonist having high affinity for rhesus monkey renal V_2 receptors. The vasopressin antagonist was also effective in preventing the tachycardia and hypotensive effects of these dosages of dDAVP. The results are consistent with the existence of extra-renal V_2-like receptors that participate in the regulation of clotting factor release and cardiovascular dynamics in the rhesus monkey.

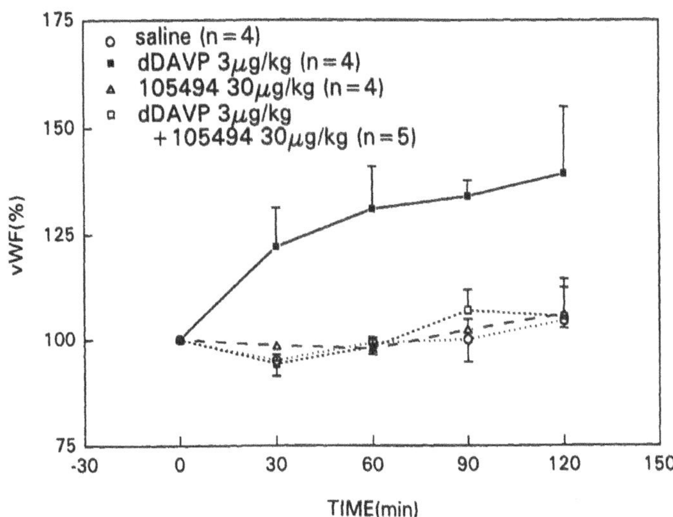

FIGURE 1: Effect of dDAVP (3.0 μg/kg) and SK&F 105494 (30 μg/kg) on plasma concentrations of von Willebrand factor (vWF) in anesthetized female rhesus monkeys. Values are means and are presented as % change from baseline (pre-treatment). Circles are vehicle-treated controls; filled squares are dDAVP (3.0 μg/kg); triangles are SK&F 105494 (30 μg/kg); and squares are dDAVP (3.0 μg/kg) plus SK&F 105494 (30 μg/kg); n=4-5.

Two general classes of vasopressin receptors have been characterized. V_1 receptors are linked to phosphatidyl inositol metabolism and mediate contraction of smooth muscle in peripheral vasculature and glucose turnover in hepatocytes. V_2 receptors are linked to adenylate cyclase and regulate water reabsorption in renal epithelia. DDAVP is a V_2 agonist which has little or no activity at V_1 receptors (Harris, 1989). In the rhesus monkey, SK&F 105494 is an antidiuretic hormone antagonist (Brooks et al., 1988a). In the rhesus monkey, SK&F 105494 blocked dDAVP stimulation of vWF, but did no stimulate vWF release when given alone. The effect of dDAVP to stimulate release of clotting factors appears appears to be mediated thru an extra-renal V_2-like receptor mechanism, perhaps linked to guanylate cyclase activity (Bichet et al., 1988, 1992). SK&F 105494 blockade of dDAVP-stimulation of clotting factor release is the first demonstration of inhibition of vWF release with a V_2 receptor antagonist and supports the existence of a specific extra-renal, V_2-like receptor mechanism mediating clotting factor release. Vilhardt and Barth (1991) have described dDAVP stimulation of FVIII release in dogs. Using the selective V_2 antagonist $d(CH_2)_5D\text{-}Ile^2Ile^4AVP$ these authors reported failure to block dDAVP-stimulation of FVIII and concluded that dDAVP stimulation of FVIII did not occur via an extrarenal V_2-like receptor. However, we have previously shown that V_2 receptor antagonists with branched side-chain amino acid substitutions at position 2 show substantial interspecies heterogeneity in affinity/activity for renal V_2 receptors and are effectively inactive in dogs (Kinter et al., 1988, 1990). Hence, we believe that the conclusions of Vilhardt and Barth regarding the mechanism of dDAVP-stimulation of FVIII release in dogs are premature.

Further evidence linking the vasopressin-clotting factor mechanism and V_2 receptors is the observation that most, if not all male patients with congenital X-linked nephrogenic diabetes insipidus (NDI) known to have a hereditary defect in their renal V_2 receptor-effector pathway (Jans et al., 1990) lack the dDAVP-clotting factor response (Kobrinsky et al., 1985; Bichet et al., 1988, 1989; Knoers et al., 1990). Other rare NDI patients with non-X-linked inheritance appear to have normal dDAVP-clotting factor responsiveness (Brenner et al., 1988; Ohzeki et al., 1988). NDI is a heterologous disorder (most cases being X-linked) and responsiveness to dDAVP appears to be consistent within family groups, and consistent with a genetic linkage between the renal V_2 receptor-effector mechanism and the dDAVP-clotting factor mechanism (Kobrinsky, 1988).

Large doses of dDAVP are reported to cause vasodilation, flushing, and hypotension (with reflex tachycardia) in humans (Harris, 1989). Direct vasodilator effects of both AVP and dDAVP have been reported in human forearm vasculature in vivo (Suzuki et al., 1989; Hirsch et al., 1989) and in rat and rabbit vascular tissues in vitro (Johns, 1990). These vasodilator effects are distinct from the well known vasoconstrictor (V_1) effect of AVP and are not apparent in X-linked NDI patients (Bichet et al., 1988), suggesting that they also are mediated by an extra-renal, V_2-like receptor. In the rhesus monkey, SK&F 105494 blocked the hypotension and tachycardia associated with dDAVP administration, but did not cause hypotension or tachycardia when given alone. This is the first demonstration of inhibition of the cardiovascular effects of dDAVP with a V_2 receptor antagonist and supports the existence of a specific extra-renal, V_2-like receptor mechanism mediating these responses.

The locations of the vasopressin receptor mechanism(s) responsible for the clotting factor and vasodilator/hypotensive effects of dDAVP are not precisely known. Proposed sites of dDAVP's actions include vascular endothelial cells, megakaryocytes, peripheral blood monocytes and mast cells (Schwartz, 1989; Hashemi et al., 1990; Macia et al., 1990; Johns, 1990; Murphy and Joran, 1992) The hemodynamic effects of dDAVP may be mediated or modulated by prostaglandins, serotonin, or other autocoids (Macia et al., 1990; Johns, 1990; Murphy and Joran, 1992) It is tempting to speculate that both clotting factors and vasodilatory autocoids are co-released from target cells by the same V_2 receptor mechanism in the rhesus monkey.

In summary, the V_2 receptor agonist, dDAVP (3.0 μg/kg) given intravenously, stimulated release of the clotting factors, von Willebrand's factor and factor VIIIc, and was associated with hypotension and tachycardia in pentobarbital-anesthetized female rhesus monkeys. The V_2 receptor antagonist, SK&F 105494 (30 μg/kg) given intravenously, had no effect on clotting factor release, blood pressure or heart rate, but prevented dDAVP stimulation of clotting factor release, hypotension and tachycardia. The results 1.) identify the rhesus monkey as a non-human species in which dDAVP stimulation of Factor VIIIc and von Willebrand factor occurs, and 2.) support the hypothesis that dDAVP stimulation of clotting factor release is mediated by a low-affinity, extra-renal, V_2-like receptor mechanism. The tachycardia associated with dDAVP administration are most likely secondary to vasodilation, also mediated by an extra-renal, V_2-like mechanism.

ACKNOWLEDGEMENTS

We acknowledge K. Schofield, K Morasco, J. Kissinger, S. Caltabiano, and D. Forman for expert technical assistance. We thank M. Landi and W. Matthews for their generous support of this work. A detailed description of these and other studies has previously been published (Kinter et al., 1992).

REFERENCES

Bichet, D.G., Razi, M., Arthus, M-F., Lonergan, M., Tittley, P., Smiley, R.K., Rock, G., and Hirsch, D.J.: Epinephrine and dDAVP administration on patients with congenital nephrogenic diabetes insipidus. Kidney Int. 36:859-866, 1989.

Bichet, D.G., Razi, M., Lonergan, M., Arthus, M-F., Papukna, V., Kortas, C., and Barjon, J-N.: Hemodynamic and coagulation responses to 1-desamino[8-D-arginine] vasopressin in patients with congenital nephrogenic diabetes insipidus. N. Engl. J. Med. 318:881-887, 1988.

Bichet, D.G., Arthus, M-F., and Lonergan, M., 1992, The hemodynamic and coagulant effects of dDAVP are specific extrarenal V_2-receptor responses. (this volume).

Brenner, B., Seligsohn, U., and Hochberg, Z.: Normal response of factor VIII and von Willebrand factor to 1-deamino-8-D-arginine vasopressin in nephrogenic diabetes insipidus. J. Clin. Endocrinol. Metab. 67:191-193, 1988.

Brooks, D.P., Caldwell, N.C., Koster, P.F., Albrightson-Winslow, C.R., and Kinter, L.B.: Effect of cyclo-oxygenase blockade on the renal actions of vasopressin and SK&F 105494 in the rhesus monkey. Br. J. Pharmacol. 99:750-752, 1990.

Brooks, D.P., Koster, P.F., Albrightson, C.R., Huffman, W.F., Moore, M.L., Stassen, F.L., Schmidt, D.B., and Kinter, L.B.: Vasopressin receptor antagonism in rhesus monkey and man: stereochemical requirements. European J. Pharmacol 160:159-162, 1989.

Brooks, D.P., Koster, P.F., Albrightson-Winslow, C.R., Stassen, F.L., Huffman, W.F., and Kinter, L.B.: SK&F 105494 is a potent antidiuretic hormone antagonist in the rhesus monkey (Macaca mulatta). J. Pharmacol. Expl. Ther. 245:211-215, 1988a.

Brooks, D.P., Koster, P.F., Stassen, F.L., Albrightson, C.R., Huffman, W.F., Wasserman, M.A., and Kinter, L.B.: Flushing and haemodynamic responses to vasopressin peptides in the rhesus monkey. Br. J. Pharmacol. 94:759-764, 1988b.

Cejka, J.: Enzyme immunoassay for factor VIII related antigen. Clin. Chem. 62:706-712, 1982.

Harris, A.S.: Clinical experience with desmopressin: efficacy and safety in central diabetes insipidus and other conditions. J. Pediatrics 114:711-718, 1989.

Hashemi, S., Tackaberry, E.S., Palmer, D.S., Rock, G., and Ganz, P.R.: DDAVP-induced release of von Willebrand factor from endothelial cells in vitro: the effect of plasma and blood cells. Biochemica et Biophysica Acta 1052:63-70, 1990.

Hirsch, A.T., Dzau, V.J., Majzoub, J.A., and Creager, M.A.: Vasopressin-mediated forearm vasodilation in normal humans: evidence for a vascular vasopressin V2 receptor. J. Clin. Invest. 84:418-426, 1989.

Jans, D.A., van Oost, B.A., Roper, H.H., and Fahrenholz, F.: Derivatives of somatic cell hybrids which carry the human gene locus for nephrogenic diabetes insipidus (NDI) express functional vasopressin renal V_2-type receptors. J. Biol. Chem. 265:15379-15382, 1990.

Johns, R.A.: Desmopressin is a potent vasorelaxant of aorta and pulmonary artery isolated from rabbit and rat. Anesthesiology 72:858-864, 1990.

Johnstone, I.B., and Crane, S.: Failure of sodium pentobarbital anesthesia to alter 1-desamino-8-D-arginine vasopressin-induced elevations of plasma factor VIII/von Willebrand factor in normal dogs. Can J. Vet. Res. 52:416-418, 1988.

Kinter, L.B., Caldwell, N., Caltabiano, S., Winslow, C., Brooks, D.P., and Huffman, W.F.: Physiological regulation of the renal vasopressin receptor-effector pathway in dogs. Am. J. Physiol. 258:R763-R769, 1990a.

Kinter, L.B., Huffman, L.B., and Stassen, F.L.: Antagonists of the antidiuretic activity of vasopressin. Am. J. Physiol. 254:F165-F177, 1988a.

Kinter, L.B., McConnell, I., Goodwin, B.I., Campbell, S., Huffman, W., Arthus, M-F., Lonergan, M. and Bichet, D.G.: Vasopresin antagonist inhibition of clotting factor release in the rhesus monkey (Macaca mulatta). J. Pharmacol. Expl. Ther. 261:462-469, 1992.

Knoers, N., Brommer, E.J.P., Willems, H., van Oost, B.A., and Monnens, L.A.H.: Fibrinolytic responses to 1-deamino-8-D-arginine vasopressin in patients with congenital nephrogenic diabetes insipidus. Nephron 54:322-326, 1990.

Kobrinsky, N.L.: Coagulation factor responsiveness in nephrogenic diabetes insipidus. J. Pediatrics 113:791, 1988.

Kobrinsky, N.L., Doyle, J.J., Israels, E.D., et al.: Absent factor VIII response to synthetic vasopressin analogue (DDAVP) in nephrogenic diabetes insipidus. Lancet 1:1293-1294, 1985.

Lethagen, S., Ostergaard, H., and Nilsson I.M.: Clinical application of the chromogenic assay of factor VIII in haemophilia A, and different variants of von Willebrand's disease. Scand. J. Haematol. 37:448-453, 1986.

Macia, R.A., Silver, A.C., Gabel, R.A., Campbell, G.K., Hanna, N., and DiMartino, M.J.: Hypotension induced by vasopressin antagonists in rats: role of mast cell degranulation. Toxicol. Appl. Pharmacol. 102:117-127, 1990.

Mannucci, P.M., Aberg, M., Nilsson, I.M., and Robertson, B.: Mechanism of plasminogen activator and factor VIII increase after vasoactive drugs. Brit. J. Haematol 30:81-93, 1975.

Moore, M.L., Albrightson, C., Brickson, B., Bryan, H.G., Caldwell, N., Callahan, J.F., Foster, J., Kinter, L.B., Newlander, K.A., Schmidt, D.B., Sorenson, E., Stassen, F.L., Yim, N.C.F., and Huffman, W.F.: Dicarbavasopressin antagonist analogues exhibit reduced in vivo agonist activity. J. Med Chem 31:1487-1489, 1988.

Murphy, D.J. and Joran, M.E., 1992, Respiratory and cardiovascular changes associated with toxic doses of a peptide antagonist of vasopressin in the rat. Fundamental Appl. Toxicol. 18:307-313.

Ohzeki, T., Sunaguchi, M., Tsunei, M., Shinzawa, T., Hanaki, K., Shiraki, K., and Shishido, H.: Coagulation factor responsiveness in nephrogenic diabetes insipidus. J. Pediatrics 113:790, 1988.

Schwartz, J.: Vasodilation associated with V_2-type vasopressin activity: findings and implications. Mol. Cell. Endocrinol. 64:133-136, 1989.

Suzuki, S., Tsutomu, T., Hirooka, Y., Yoshida, M., Ando, S., and Nakamura, M.: Biphasic forearm vascular responses to intraarterial arginine vasopressin. J. Clin. Invest. 84:427-434, 1989.

Vilhardt, H. and Barth, T.: The release of Factor VIII and tissue plasminogen activator can not be blocked by specific antagonists to vasopressin. J. Receptor Res. 11:239-245, 1991b.

Williams, T.D.M., Lightman, S.L., and Leadbeater, M.J.: Hormonal and cardiovascular responses to DDAVP in man. Clin. Endocrinol. 24:89-96, 1986.

DISCUSSION

Bichet: Does ELISA using human material work in dogs?
Nilsson: Human antibodies cannot be used in dogs.
Kinter: We did get a response. Perhaps the reason there was only a 50% increase in the monkey, as opposed to the 200 to 300% rise in humans was due to species difference. There was a consistent rise in vWf, but a tenfold increase in dose was needed than would be used in humans, and the rise was maximal. There was also a dose-related fall in blood pressure in monkeys at lower doses (around 1 mcg/kg).

The time course of the rise in vWf matched that in humans. The receptor antagonist had no effect on vWf even at a dose of 30 mcg/kg (ten times the DDAVP dose). However, pre-treatment with a receptor antagonist, then DDAVP, completely abolished all changes in vWf. The antagonist did not produce hypertension, and prevented tachycardia due to DDAVP. On the basis of these results we believe we have shown that in the rhesus monkey we can prevent DDAVP stimulation of vWf release by blocking the V2 receptor. This is consistent with the hypothesis that an extrarenal V2 receptor is responsible for this effect.

Kobrinsky: What insight does this give about the structure of DDAVP?
Kinter: SKF 105494 has a dicarba bridge, rather than a sulfur-sulfur bond, so it is permanently closed, and does not hydrolyse. There are two extra arginine molecules at the "tail" of the molecule giving an extra positive charge. This enhances the molecule's affinity for the receptor and reduces its partial agonist activity.

Mariani: Is this definitive abolition of the V2 receptor, or is it temporary?
Kinter: In vitro it is a pure V2 receptor antagonist. It blocks V1 receptors competitively, and once bound is very slow to dissociate. In vivo in animals it selectively increases the renal excretion of water, but in humans it is an antidiuretic agonist. It does not affect blood pressure in humans.

NON-RESPONSIVENESS OF t-PA, u-PA AND vWF TO DDAVP

E.J.P. Brommer[1], F.H.M. Derkx[2], M. Levi[3], G. Dooijewaard[1]

[1]Gaubius Laboratory, IVVO.TNO, Leiden, The Netherlands
[2]Univ. Hospital Dijkzigt, Rotterdam, The Netherlands
[3]Academic Medical Centre, Amsterdam, The Netherlands

HAEMOPHILIA / THROMBOPHILIA

What we should like to learn during this symposium is whether one can use desmopressin, or an analog, for the enhancement of fibrinolysis without affecting coagulation. What we will contribute are a number of observations with which we hope to help to answer this question. We realize that most of this audience are working towards the opposite: the possibility of achieving an elevation of factor VIII parameters in view of the haemostatic effects. Perhaps these observations will be useful to both these aims.

Apart from its use as an antidiuretic in patients with diabetes insipidus, our main experience with desmopressin is in the stimulation of the fibrinolytic system. Desmopressin has been proposed as a means of detecting thrombophilia, just as it is used by others for the detection of carriers of haemophilia. The "DDAVP-test" promised to be more specific and more convenient than the venous occlusion test. The side effects are minimal, most subjects only experience flushing of the face. However, despite a host of publications on the subject, it

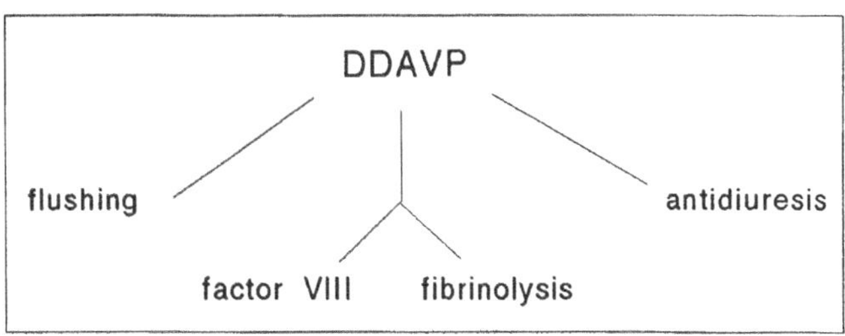

Figure 1. Principle actions of desmopressin

Desmopressin in Bleeding Disorders, Edited by G. Mariani *et al.*
Plenum Press, New York, 1993

is still an open question whether the DDAVP-test has any relevance for the detection of a tendency to thrombosis or a familial predisposition to thromboembolic disorders. In this regard our own interest has waned. Nevertheless, the fact that desmopressin can enhance fibrinolysis by the release of tissue-type and urokinase-type plasminogen activators, t-PA and u-PA, and does so in the vast majority of the subjects tested (Levi et al., 1989, 1991), indicates that it may be appealing for the prophylaxis or treatment of thrombotic disorders. In all the experiments I will refer to, a dose of 0.3 or 0.4 µg/kg body weight was injected or infused intravenously over 10 to 30 minutes, and blood was taken before, and within 30 minutes after the start of the infusion.

DISSOCIATION OF THE PA AND vWF RESPONSE?

The rise in factor VIII and Von Willebrand factor (vWF) by desmopressin infusion is usually accompanied by a rise in the fibrinolytic activity of the blood. There are, however, circumstances where the two effects seem to dissociate.

Many years ago we measured both vWF antigen and fibrinolytic activity of euglobulin fractions (on fibrin plates) in a series of patients with hyperlipoproteinaemia. We found (Brommer et al., 1982) that many of them failed to show a change in lytic activity after desmopressin infusion. We booked these patients out as non-responders and speculated that this might help explain the cardiovascular complications in hyperlipoproteinaemia. The fact that practically all patients responded with a rise in vWF:Ag only strengthened that hypothesis. In later years, when Dr Rijken had set up an assay for tissue plasminogen activator antigen (t-PA:Ag) in our laboratory, we re-analyzed the same plasma samples and found out that the response of t-PA:Ag was normal in the majority of the patients. The t-PA activity in their plasma did not parallel the change in t-PA:Ag because of the high level of the plasminogen activator inhibitor, PAI-1 in their plasma (Brommer et al., 1984c). After all, the release of vWF:Ag and t-PA:Ag after desmopressin injection appeared to be closely related.

In the meantime, Ludlam and coworkers (1980), and others in Austria and Scandinavia reported that in patients with severe forms of Von Willebrand disease, neither vWF nor the fibrinolytic activity rose after desmopressin. This particular disease is probably characterized by an endothelial defect, affecting both PA and vWF release.

Is it fortunate that a rise in vWF:Ag is most often accompanied by a rise in t-PA and u-PA? We should perhaps see this as a physiological defense mechanism: the enhancement of coagulation might give rise to thromboembolism if not counteracted by the enhancement of fibrinolysis. However, the increase in t-PA and u-PA is short-lived, and experience has taught that the danger of a thrombotic event after desmopressin infusion, even of acute myocardial infarction, is not imaginary (Van Dantzig et al., 1989). After an hour or two, only the levels of VIII:C and vWF remain elevated.

There seems to be little need for the isolated suppression of fibrinolytic enhancement. The opposite, the suppression of the rise of vWF without influencing fibrinolytic response, seems urgent in view of its multiple applications in thrombotic disease. In whichever direction we want to steer the system, we need to know something about the pathways of the stimulus. Animal experiments have proven that a dichotomy of t-PA and vWF response is possible (Tranquille & Emeis, 1991,1992). As we shall see, experience in humans also hints at this possibility.

MECHANISM OF ACTION OF DESMOPRESSIN

The rise in the plasma levels of t-PA, u-PA, vWF and other factors as a reaction to the infusion of desmopressin is not necessarily the result of an increased cellular production rate, but can also be the consequence of changes in blood flow.

One option is the interference of desmopressin with the clearance rate, especially hepatic clearance. A transient decrease in liver blood flow would increase the blood level of substances with a rapid hepatic clearance, such as t-PA, but would hardly influence the level of vWF. Since both parameters change after desmopressin infusion, the role of hepatic blood flow is improbable on theoretical grounds. Besides, we have shown that desmopressin does not diminish the liver blood flow (1982). Moreover, in another set of experiments we demonstrated that the clearance rate of t-PA in the liver did not change during infusion of desmopressin (1988), so that the rise in blood levels cannot be explained by this mechanism.

A second possibility is the rise in plasminogen activator and vWF levels as a consequence of its opening previously closed, resting, vascular beds, rather than of enhanced release. Desmopressin causes an increase in forearm blood flow (Hirsch et al., 1989) and induces peripheral vasodilatation, indicated by facial flushing (Mannucci & Rota, 1980) and hypotension (Brommer et al., 1982). After opening the vascular beds, the contact of the circulating blood with a larger endothelial surface will raise the level of any compound produced by the endothelium, among which t-PA, u-PA, and vWF. In addition, as a secondary reaction to the hypotension, secretion of catecholamines, which are known to stimulate the release of t-PA and vWF, will occur. However, the contribution of catecholamines is negligible, as beta-blockade does not diminish response to desmopressin (Brommer et al. 1984a). Up to now we have found no substantial evidence, either against, or in favour of the opening of blood vessels as an important contributor to the response to desmopressin.

The alternative is the effect of desmopressin on the production and release of t-PA, u-PA, and vWF in some or all organs in the body. Since most efforts to study the direct effect of desmopressin on endothelial cells have failed, the idea of at humoral messenger induced by desmopressin has received much attention. In order to explore this, we have subjected patients with severe organ failure or missing organs to a DDAVP-test: patients with terminal renal failure, autonomic dysfunction, congenital and acquired hypophysial defects, and patients who had undergone nephrectomy, adrenalectomy, or complete hypophysectomy. It was remarkable that despite their defective or missing organs most of our patients responded normally. Thus the whole pathway mediating the stimulus can be intact in the absence of kidneys, adrenals or pituitary gland. Interestingly, haemodialysis restored the previously absent response in patients with terminal renal failure, suggesting the presence of a low-molecular-weight inhibitor before dialysis (Brommer et al. 1984b).

Another approach to the elucidation of the nature of the humoral messenger is the administration of drugs before performing the DDAVP-test. No effort to suppress the response attained any success: high dosages of aspirin or beta-blockers (Brommer et al., 1984a), antihistaminics, and naloxone failed to influence the rise of fibrinolytic activity or vWF after desmopressin infusion. Of course this does not exclude the possibility that histamine, endorphins, prostaglandins or catecholamines may have an (inhibitory) effect on the response, but none of them appears to be the sole mediator or even an essential step in the final common pathway. Neither were we able to dissociate t-PA and vWF.

ROLE OF SPECIFIC RECEPTOR

Desmopressin is a selective V2-receptor agonist, which accounts for its antidiuretic action. Until a few years ago, V2-receptors were supposed to be present exclusively in renal tubule cells. We were the first to draw attention to the potent, fast, and reversible, hypotensive effect of desmopressin (1982, 1985), presumably mediated through an extrarenal site of action. V2-receptors have been postulated to be present in post-capillary venules (Adamski et al,

1985), and in forearm blood vessels (Hirsch, l.c.). In some areas of the vascular tree they are absent or play no measurable role, e.g. in digital arteries. An influence of desmopressin on V1 receptors has been postulated by Derkx et al. (1983). They surmised an antagonistic action of DDAVP on the V1-receptors, as inferred from the inhibition of vasopressin-induced platelet aggregation and renin secretion by kidney slices. In principle, desmopressin could suspend in this way the V1-receptor mediated vasoconstriction caused by vasopressin. This idea has been abandoned since the effects were achieved with unphysiologically high concentrations of desmopressin (Derkx et al., 1987). Moreover, cardiovascular effects of desmopressin have also been found in individuals with undetectable plasma vasopressin levels (Williams et al., 1986).

Kobrinsky et al. (1985), Brink et al. (1987), Bichet et al. (1989) and the authors of this paper (1990) reported on the non-responsiveness to desmopressin of patients with congenital nephrogenic diabetes insipidus, not only with regard to diuresis, but also to the rise in t-PA, vWF, active renin and to changes in blood pressure and flushing. The basal secretion of t-PA and vWF, however, seems to be normal, and venous occlusion as well as physical exercise can modulate the production or release of both substances. Apparently, physiological stimuli reach their target and induce release in this congenital disease. The question of whether these patients lack V2-receptors, or V2-like receptors, not only in the kidney, but also at extrarenal sites, viz. on endothelial cells, or whether the transmission of the signal between receptor and effector is blocked, has not yet been unequivocally answered. Vilhardt & Barth (1991) postulate a new class of vasopressin-receptors, different from V1- and V2-receptors.

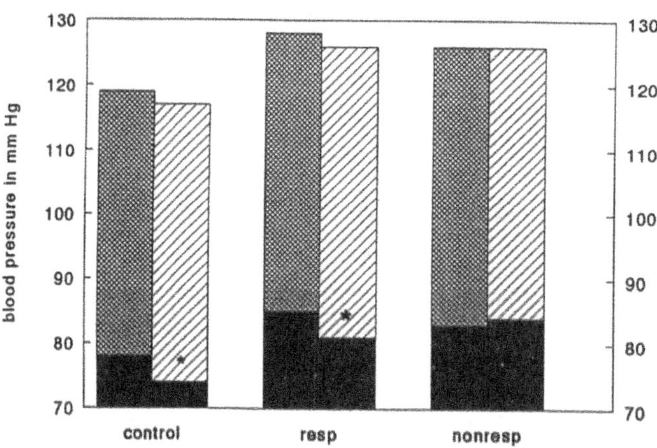

Figure 2. Blood pressure changes (diastolic in black) before (left bars) and after (right bars) infusion of desmopressin in patients treated with cyclosporin for renal transplantation. Patients who did respond (resp) or who did not respond (non-resp) with an increase in t-PA:Ag are represented separately. * = $p < 0.02$.

The next point to make in this context is the non-responsiveness to desmopressin in a group of patients treated with cyclosporin for immunosuppression after kidney transplantation, performed in Amsterdam. Among the 16 patients tested, 8 were non-responders in terms of the level of t-PA:Ag. Five of these patients did not respond with a rise in u-PA:Ag either. The other 8 patients responded with both parameters. The rise in vWF:Ag appeared to parallel the fibrinolytic parameters. In a control group of patients who received azathioprine for immunosuppression, all 9 patients responded with a rise in t-PA:Ag, u-PA and vWF. When the cyclosporin-treated patients were fed fish oil for four months, the response to desmopressin returned to normal. Control feeding with corn-oil failed to restore the response (Levi et al., 1992). The inference of this observation was that fish oil, e.g. by influencing the arachidonic acid and prostaglandin metabolism, re-established plasminogen activator production or release in response to desmopressin. To corroborate the hypothesis that cyclosporin and fish oil, directly or indirectly, exerted their effect on the transmission of the stimulus instead of the production and release of endothelial constituents, we have looked at responses other than release reactions in the same experiment. Interestingly, in the non-responsive phase after cyclosporin treatment, blood pressure did not drop during desmopressin infusion, whereas it did significantly fall in the control patients.

We conclude that cyclosporin interferes somewhere with the transfer of the stimulus induced by desmopressin, both to the effectors mediating vasodilatation and to those regulating the release of plasminogen activators and vWF. The failure to inhibit the response to desmopressin with aspirin in healthy volunteers, does not exclude a possible inhibitory role for prostaglandins in the regulation of the release reaction, as explained before.

MODULATION OF INTRACELLULAR PATHWAYS

The entire sequence of events from the occupation of the V2- or V2-like receptor to the release of t-PA, u-PA and vWF is far from clear at the moment. The main enzymes activated by the V2-receptor are those of the adenylate cyclase pathway with cyclic AMP (cAMP) as a crucial step. Concomitant activation of the pathway leading to the formation of arachidonate and PAF (platelet activating factor) via phospholipase A2 is a theoretical possibility.

vWF is stored in the Weibel-Palade bodies, a characteristic of endothelial cells, but the intracellular storage site of t-PA has escaped demonstration up to now. Nevertheless, Tranquille & Emeis (1990) have confirmed in animal experiments that the release of t-PA and vWF were tightly coupled under virtually every condition. Only recently have a few interesting exceptions been discovered.

After pretreatment with a xanthine derivative, a metabolite of pentoxifylline, a dissociation was observed in response to platelet activating factor (PAF). The experiments were performed in rat hindleg preparations. The pentoxifylline metabolite enhanced the PAF-induced release of t-PA, but decreased the release of vWF. The opposite effects were induced by forskolin. Both compounds are known to induce an increase in cAMP, so these experiments do not reveal the mechanism of the dissociation of t-PA and vWF.

Interference with the phospholipase pathway by a diacylglycerol analogue, the phorbolester PMA, also revealed a dichotomy of the t-PA and vWF release induced by PAF: the t-PA release was reduced by approximately 40%, and the release of vWF enhanced by almost 100%. Comparable effects were seen after induction of the release by the calcium ionophore, A 23187 (Tranquille & Emeis, 1992). The influx of extracellular calcium appears to be essential for the release of t-PA and vWF, as it is for the production of EDRF, the main mediator of hypotension induced by a variety of effectors. The fact that PMA differentiates between the responses of t-PA or vWF indicates a complex, probably post-receptor, regulating system. PAF itself is in the opinion of Hanss & Dechavanne (1988) not an obligatory intermediate in the induction of fibrinolytic activity: inhibition of PAF by 48740 RP did not decrease the baseline level of t-PA and vWF, and it failed to suppress their rise after venous occlusion. However, the effect of the inhibitor on the response to desmopressin has not yet been studied.

NON-RESPONSIVENESS IN DISEASE, THE ROLE OF THE KIDNEY?

In order to find out something about the principles of the regulation of t-PA and vWF release, we have carried out the DDAVP test in an array of diseases. The only patient groups with an exceptionally large percentage of non-responders were those with renal disease, not merely patients with terminal renal insufficiency, whether before or after nephrectomy, but also patients with glomerulonephritis or haemolytic uraemic syndrome (HUS).

Among 19 patients with terminal renal insufficiency we counted 6 with a poor or absent response of fibrinolytic activity (< 30% increase) and vWF:Ag (< 20% increase) to desmopressin, one patient with a poor response of fibrinolytic activity alone, and 6 with a poor response of vWF:Ag. This was the first hint that vWF and t-PA are not of necessity released together.

Recently, we studied the changes in t-PA (activity, antigen and drop in PAI-1 activity), u-PA:Ag and vWF:Ag after DDAVP infusion in 22 patients admitted with glomerulonephritis of various origins. Here also we noted a dissociation of the responses of t-PA, u-PA, and vWF to desmopressin: only 6 patients responded normally with all parameters; 8 showed a rise in two of the three parameters, 5 responded with one parameter, and three showed no response at all. The responses of t-PA:Ag and vWF were the most closely linked. The bleeding time was normal in all patients, so we have no data on the response of platelet function. In order to exclude a direct effect of uraemia, we compared the patients admitted for glomerulonephritis, with a group of patients with a similar impairment of renal function caused by adult-type polycystic kidney disease. The conclusion was that the abnormalities depended on the acute stage of the disease, probably the inflammatory component, rather than renal failure per se.

We have also analyzed plasma samples from 10 children with haemolytic uraemic syndrome (HUS) sent to us by Prof Monnens (Nijmegen). We found a poor t-PA response to desmopressin in 4 of them (Monnens et al., 1988), but the u-PA response was defective in all ten. A similar observation has been reported by the group of Prof. ten Cate in Amsterdam. They tested the patients not only in the acute stage of the disease, but also in the subacute stage and in remission. A dissociation was noted between the various responses: the u-PA response remained impaired during the whole observation period, whereas the responses of t-PA and vWF normalized (Menzel et al., 1991). This is another example of a dissociation of the responses to desmopressin.

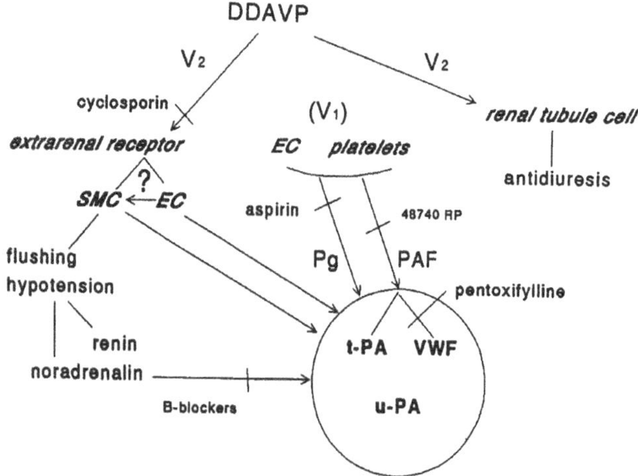

Figure 3. Major pathways leading to release of t-PA, u-PA, and VWF. Pg = prostaglandins; PAF = platelet activating factor; SMC = smooth muscle cells; EC = endothelial cells.

CONCLUDING REMARKS

It can be inferred from the segregation of responses in renal disease as well as from animal experiments, that the release of vWF and fibrinolytic enzymes is not necessarily coupled. Three possibilities have not yet been fully explored: the involvement of different anatomical or histological areas, the modulation of the response by secondary factors or drugs, and the difference between acute and chronic responses. The most important, presently known mechanisms involved in the action of desmopressin are summarized in the diagram (Figure 3), which also indicates some pharmacological interactions. The negative results of the numerous efforts to inhibit the response to DDAVP with single drugs elicits the idea that the induction of the release of t-PA, u-PA, and vWF by desmopressin involves more than a single pathway. Recent years have seen a dramatic evolution in the knowledge of intracellular processes regulating the production of receptors, enzymes, eicosanoids and regulating proteins within the cell, some of which are linked to the cell membrane. This knowledge should be used in our opinion to launch new efforts to unravel the regulation of vWF and plasminogen activator release.

The potent hypotensive capacity of desmopressin and its ability to stimulate fibrinolysis or haemostasis could be applied separately in the future, provided that we can manipulate and direct the various effects selectively. The investigation of the response to desmopressin applied alone, or in combination with certain drugs, in healthy volunteers or in disease remains an appealing approach to that goal.

REFERENCES

Adamski, S.W., Svensjö, E.S., and Grega, G.J., 1985, Effects of AVP and DDAVP on histamine-induced increases in macromolecular permeability in the hamster cheek pouch, Microcirc. Endothel. Lymphat. 2:41.

Bichet, D.G., Razi, M., Lonergan, M., Arthus, M.-F., Papukna, V., Kortas, C., and Barjon, J.-N., 1988, Hemodynamic and coagulation responses to 1-desamino[8-D-arginine] vasopressin in patients with congenital nephrogenic diabetes insipidus, N. Engl. J. Med. 318:881.

Bichet, D.G., Razi, M., Arthus, M.-F., Lonergan, M., Tittley, P., Smiley, R.K., Rock, G., and Hirsch,D.J., 1989, Epinephrine and dDAVP administration in patients with congenital nephrogenic diabetes insipidus. Evidence for a pre-cyclic AMP V2 receptor defective mechanism, Kidney Int. 36:859.

Brink, H., Derkx, F., Brommer, E., Stibbe, J., Kolstee, N., and Schalekamp, M., 1987, The fibrinolytic,factor VIII:C, von Willebrand factor and hemodynamic responses to DDAVP in patients with hereditary nephrogenic diabetes insipidus, Thromb. Haemostas. 58:517.

Brommer, E.J.P., Barrett-Bergshoeff, M.M., Allen, R.A., Schicht, I., Bertina, R.M., and Schalekamp, M.A.D.H., 1982, The use of desmopressin acetate (DDAVP) as a test of the fibrinolytic capacity of patients - analysis of responders and non-responders, Thromb. Haemostas. 48:156.

Brommer, E.J.P., Derkx, F.H.M., Barrett-Bergshoeff, M.M., and Schalekamp, M.A.D.H., 1984a, The inability of propranolol and aspirin to inhibit the response of fibrinolytic activity and factor VIII-antigen to infusion of DDAVP, Thromb. Haemostas. 51:42.

Brommer, E.J.P., Schicht, I., Wijngaards, G., Verheijen, J.H., and Rijken, D.C., 1984b,

Fibrinolytic activators and inhibitors in terminal renal insufficiency and in anephric patients, Thromb. Haemostas. 52:311.

Brommer, E.J.P., Verheijen, J.H., Chang, G.T.G., and Rijken, D.C., 1984c, Masking of fibrinolyticresponse to stimulation by an inhibitor of tissue-type plasminogen activator in plasma, Thromb. Haemostas. 52:154.

Brommer, E.J.P., Van Brummelen, P., and Derkx, F.H.M., 1985, Desmopressin and hypotension, Ann. Intern. Med. 103:962.

Brommer, E.J.P., Derkx, F.H.M., Schalekamp, M.A.D.H., Dooijewaard, G., and Van der Klaauw,M.M.,1988, Renal and hepatic handling of endogenous tissue-type plasminogen activator (t-PA) and its inhibitor in man, Thromb. Haemostas. 59:404.

Brommer, E.J.P., Brink, H., Derkx, F.H.M., Schalekamp, M.A.H., and Stibbe, J., 1990, Normal homeostasis of fibrinolysis in nephrogenic diabetes insipidus in spite of defective V2-receptor-mediated responses of tissue plasminogen activator release, Eur. J. Clin. Invest. 20:72.

Derkx, F.H.M., Man in 't Veld, A.J., Jones, R., Reid, J.L., and Schalekamp, M.A.D.H., 1983, DDAVP(1-desamino-8-D-arginine vasopressin): an antagonist of the pressor action of endogenous vasopressin?, J Hypertension 1(suppl 2):58.

Derkx, F.H.M., Brommer, E.J.P., Boomsma, F., and Schalekamp, M.A.D.H., 1984, Activation of plasma prorenin by plasminogen activators in vitro and increase in plasma renin after stimulation of fibrinolytic activity in vivo, Neth. J. Med. 27:124.

Derkx, F.H.M.,Brink, H.S., Merkus, P., Smits, J., Brommer, E.J.P., and Schalekamp, M., 1987,Vasopressin V2-receptor-mediated hypotensive response in man, J Hypertension, 5 (suppl 5):S107.

Emeis, J.J., and Kluft, C., 1985, PAF-acether-induced release of tissue-type plasminogen activator from vessel walls, Blood 66:86.

Grant, M.B., Guay, C., and Lottenberg, R., 1988, Desmopressin stimulates parallel norepinephrine and tissue plasminogen activator release in normal subjects and patients with diabetes mellitus, Thromb. Haemostas. 59:269.

Hanss, M., and Dechavanne, M., 1988, 48740 RP, an antagonist of PAF, does not affect human plasma fibrinolysis before and after venous occlusion, Thromb. Res. 49:129.

Hirsch, A.T., Dzau, V.J., Majzoub, J.A., and Creager, M.A., 1989, Vasopressin-mediated forearm vasodilation in normal humans. Evidence for a vascular vasopressin V2 receptor, J. Clin. Invest. 84:418.

Keber, D., 1988, Mechanism of tissue plasminogen activator release during venous occlusion, Fibrinolysis 2(suppl 2):96.

Kobrinsky, N.L., Doyle, J.J., Israels, E.D., Winter, J.S.D., Cheang, M.S., Walker, R.D., and Bishop,A.J.,1985, Absent factor VIII response to synthetic vasopressin analogue (DDAVP) in nephrogenic diabetes insipidus, Lancet June 8:1293.

Levi, M., Ten Cate, J.W., Dooijewaard, G., Sturk, A., Brommer, E.J.P., and Agnelli, G., 1989, DDAVP induces systemic release of urokinase-type plasminogen activator, Thromb. Haemostas. 62:686.

Levi, M., Lensing, W.A., Büller, H.R., Prandoni, P., Dooijewaard, G., Cuppini, S., and ten Cate, J.W.,1991, Deep vein thrombosis and fibrinolysis. Defective urokinase type plasminogen activator release, Thromb Haemostas. 66:426.

Levi, M., Wilmink, J., Büller, H., and ten Cate, J.W., 1992, Impaired fibrinolysis in cyclosporin-treatedrenal transplant patients: analysis of the defect and beneficial effect of fish-oil, Transplantation (in press).

Ludlam, C.A., Peake, I.R., Allen, N., Davies, B.L., Furlong, R.A., and Bloom, A.L., 1980,

Factor VIII and fibrinolytic response to deamino-8-D-arginine vasopressin in normal subjects and dissociate response in some patients with haemophilia and von Willebrand's disease, Br. J. Haematol. 45:499.
Mannucci, P.M., and Rota, L., 1980, Plasminogen activator response after DDAVP: a clinico-pharmacological study, Thromb Res 20:69.
Menzel, D., Levi, M., Peters, M., Dooijewaard, G., Monnens, L., and Ten Cate, J.W., 1991, Impaired fibrinolysis in haemolytic uremic syndrome of childhood, Blood 78:216a.
Monnens, L., Brommer, E., Van de Kar, N., and Knoers, N., 1990, The role of the fibrinolytic system in the epidemic form of hemolytic uremic syndrome, Ped. Nephrol. 4:C51.
Tranquille, N., and Emeis, J.J., 1990, The simultaneous acute release of tissue-type plasminogen activatorand von Wilebrand factor in the perfused rat hindleg region, Thromb Haemostas 63:454.
Tranquille, N., and Emeis, J.J., 1991, The effect of pentoxifylline (Trental) and two analogues, BL 194 and HWA 448, on the release of plasminogen activators and von Willebrand factor in rats, J. Cardiovasc. Pharmacol. 18:35.
Tranquille, N., Emeis, J.J., 1992, The involvement of products of the phospholipase pathway in the acuterelease of tissue-type plasminogen activator from perfused rat hidlegs, Eur. J. Pharmacol. (in press)
Van Dantzig, J.M., Düren, D.R., and Ten Cate, J.W., 1989, Desmopressin and myocardial infarction, Lancet March 25:664.
Vilhardt H. and Barth, T., 1991, The release of factor VIII and tisue plasminogen activator can not beblocked by specific antagonists to vasopressin, J Receptor Res 11:239
Williams, T.D.M., Lightman, S.L., and Leadbeater, M.J., 1986, Hormonal and cardiovascular responses to DDAVP in man, Clin. Endocrinol. 24:89.

DISCUSSION

Rao: How did you measure fibrinolytic activity?
Brommer: We used the fibrin plate method.
Rao; The tPAag rise is two or three times, and is modest, so that it would not cause significant fibrinolytic activity, and in any case, it is complexed. Also tPA has a half life of 4 minutes, so is there any evidence that an increase in fibrinolytic activity post-DDAVP is clinically significant?
Brommer: tPA activity rises considerably, and when we make clots of the plasma they show enhanced spontaneous clot lysis with a small increase in tPA antigen.

Rao: Is this enough to say that fibrinolytic activity diminishes clots and impairs haemostasis?
Brommer: Yes.

Mannucci: How do you explain good hemostasis in surgery?
Brommer: Because there is also a rise in Factor VIII which lasts much longer.
Mannucci: If a clot forms with a lot of tPA around, tPA is trapped, and lysis is prompt. If you give DDAVP before surgery, by the time the patient comes to theatre, the effect is washed out.
Brommer: Correct.

Kobrinski: Overall in a population of congenital nephrogenic diabetes insipidus patients there

is a Factor VIII response and a vWf response of around 50%, but one may occur without the other. It would be interesting to do the tPA responses in these heterozygotes, to see if there are separate endothelial cell sets or tPA disorders.
Brommer: We have seen parallel FVIII and vWf responses in the heterozygotes.
Kobrinski: This suggests they are the same endothelial cells, and not anatomically discordant.
Brommer: They are both V2 receptor related, but not necessarily at the same sites.

Mannucci: Is u-PA produced by endothelial cells only?
Brommer: No, it is produced by other cells, including kidney cells.

Mannucci: You saw rises of twice baseline levels. Are you convinced they are bona fide?
Brommer: For all these parameters we used a threshold of 1.2. For clinical medicine u-PA may be more important than we know, because pro-urokinase may be critical for lysis of fibrin deposits. It may start fibrinolysis.
Mannucci: In addition, there is no natural inhibitor.

CONTROL OF BLEEDING IN UREMIC PATIENTS

Y. Sultan

Centre des Hémophiles
Hopital Cochin
Paris, France

INTRODUCTION

Patients with acute or chronic renal failure exhibit an increased tendency to bleed. The severity of the hemorrhagic diathesis is not always correlated with the severity of uremia. Hemorrhagic episodes remain a major contributory factor to the morbidity and mortality associated with renal failure (1).

Mucosal bleeding particularly of the gastrointestinal tract is perhaps the most frequent manifestation of the hemorrhagic diathesis. Other manifestations include: ecchymoses, epistaxis, bleeding from the venipuncture site, hemorrhagic pericarditis and subdural hematoma. The incidence of gastrointestinal hemorrhage in patients with established acute renal failure is approximately 30 to 40% of the overall mortality (2). In the setting of chronic renal failure, hemorrhagic complications tend to be more frequent and rise from 60 to 75% in dialysed patients (3). Patients with renal failure bleed during surgical procedures, tooth extraction and renal biopsy necessary for diagnosis.

ETIOLOGY OF UREMIC BLEEDING

The etiology of uremic bleeding is unknown but is probably multifactorial and reflects a complex disorder of hemostasis. No abnormalities of the coagulation factors or the fibrinolytic system have been described.The primary hemostasis is the target abnormality, as the test that most closely correlates with clinical bleeding is the Bleeding Time. The Bleeding Time is a global measure of primary hemostasis and prolonged bleeding times reflect a defect of the platelet plug formation. Primary hemostasis itself is multifactorial resulting of the interaction of platelets with the vessel wall and von Willebrand factor (vWF). Many tests are available for assessing primary hemostasis and historically as each test was developed, abnormal values in uremic patients were soon reported.

Desmopressin in Bleeding Disorders, Edited by G. Mariani *et al.*
Plenum Press, New York, 1993

Anemia

Most patients with renal failure also have anemia and this contributes to the hemostatic defect. Platelet adhesion is influenced not only by platelet number, but also by red cell number. Red blood cells appear to promote platelet-vessel wall interaction by enhancing the radial diffusion of platelets within the lumen, thereby increasing the collision of platelets with vessel walls. In addition the mechanical effects of red cells release ADP, allowing further aggregation (4, 5).

Platelets in uremic patients

Thrombocytopenia is often detected but rarely severe enough to be the sole cause of bleeding.

Defective clot retraction was described as early as 1956 by Lewis et al (6) and confirmed by several others: Rath et al in 1957 (7) and O'Grady in 1957 (8). More recently Carr and Zekert, using a new device, a clot retractometer, allowed the measurement in dynes per square centimeters of platelet mediated force development during clot retraction. This force is decreased and altered in a standardized clot containing 72.10^9 platelets per liter measuring the force developed at 800 S. post thrombin addition. Improvement of clot retraction after infusion of DDAVP was reported in a test using platelet rich plasma adjusted at 72.10^9 platelets per liter with platelet poor plasma studies at 37°C. After DDAVP the patient retraction curve improved substantially. The reason for decreased clot retraction and improvement after DDAVP was still unclear after the study.

Defective platelet factor 3 (PF_3) was first described by Lewis et al in 1956 (6) and confirmed by Rabiner and Hrodek (10) twelve years later, showing that PF_3 activity improved following dialysis.

Platelet aggregation tests using various aggregation agents detected defects in uremic patients in a study published by Castaldi et al (11) and also showed by Rabiner and Drake in 1975 using ADP and collagen. Abnormal aggregation tests were shown to reverse following dialysis (12).

Decreased platelet adhesion on the subendothelium was shown by Castillo et al in 1986 (13). Since 1983, Mannucci et al (14) reported an increase in cyclic AMP levels in platelets of uremic patients which remained elevated after DDAVP.

More recently Soslau (15) and coworkers described a storage pool defect in the plateletsof renal failure patients. Content in 5HT was found significantly depressed while the ATP/ADP content was not. Even though the platelet ATP/ADP content is usually in the normal range, the release of ATP upon activation was significantly depressed relative to control values. The perturbation of 5HT storage and ATP release reflects disturbances in plasma factors that interact with the platelet membrane. The reduced serotonin content of plateletscontributes to the hemostatic process by inducing vasoconstriction.

Disturbed regulation of platelet calcium content has also been described as secondary to elevated parathyroid hormone levels.

Abnormal platelet linking to fibronectin following thrombin stimulation was described in uremic patients. It was suggested that a better linking to fibronectin following cryoprecipitate infusion was a possible mechanism in the reduction of the BT.

Vessel Walls

Remuzzi et al in 1980 (16) showed that veins taken from patients with renal failure exhibit strikingly greater prostacyclin (PGI_2) production than those from controls and that this increased production of PGI2 was not lessened by dialysis. These authors also showed that plasma from uremic patients suppressed thromboxane A_2 (TXA_2) production from platelet and that dialysis did not reverse the diminished TXA_2 production.

Factor VIII - von Willebrand factor activity

Von Willebrand factor (vWF) plays a crucial part in primary hemostasis: it induces platelet adhesion to the subendothelium through specific platelet receptors. For this reason, vWF has been intensively investigated and the possibility that an abnormal vWF accounts for the prolonged bleeding time and reduced platelet adhesiveness is not confirmed. As early as 1974, Ekberg and coworkers (17) described elevated levels of vWF antigen in glomerulonephritis. Kazatchkine et al (18) reported also elevated F VIII and vWF antigen but reduced vWF activity indicated by decreased ristocetin cofactor, suggesting a functional defect of vWF. Two other studies did not confirm abnormal activity of the elevated vWF antigen. However a Janson and coworkers study in 1980 demonstrated lower ristocetin cofactor activity than vWF antigen in these patients (19).

Abnormalities of the multimeric structure of the molecule have not been detected after being carefully examined in three different studies. Therefore the overall data do not suggest a structural or functional abnormality of vWF even though two patients with an abnormal multimeric pattern were described by Rodighiero in 1988 (20). One of them had a vWF multimeric pattern resembling the IB variant of vW disease and the other had a larger than normal multimer resembling the one found in thrombotic thrombocytopenic purpura.

THERAPEUTIC APPROACH

Dialysis

It was first noticed that dialysis improved the hemostatic defect in uremia in studies by Castaldi et al in 1966 (11) and Remuzzi et al in 1978 (21). Abnormal platelet functions may improved after dialysis suggesting that molecules present in the plasma of uremic patients might be responsible for impaired primary hemostasis. However dialysis does not eliminate the risk of bleeding and only some of the abnormal platelet functions were corrected. Moreover dialysis can contribute to bleeding because of platelet activation by artificial membranes and anticoagulation necessary to maintain patency of extracorporeal circuits.

Red blood cell transfusion and erythropoietin

Livio et al in 1982 (22) and Fernandez et al (23) in 1985 have indicated beneficial effects of red cell transfusion on the bleeding time.

More recently, Moia et al (1987) (24) showed that recombinant erythropoietin given to patients with chronic uremia improved hemostasis by correcting anemia. The progressive rise in hematocrit was paralleled by a pronounced shortening of the bleeding time. After 100 days of treatment, hematocrit below 22% in seven patients increased to 33% and above , coincident with the shortening of the bleeding time. In the 7 patients however only two of them were totally corrected. During the study platelet adhesion to the subendothelium, very low before the study, increased and became normal in 6 patients. The incomplete correction of the BT by erythropoietin was also noticed by Jacquot and coworkers (25) who mentioned in one patient that the BT although shortened from >45 to 22 minutes was only partially corrected by the improved hematocrit. Following DDAVP infusion the BT almost normalized indicating an additional beneficial effect of DDAVP and incomplete correction in presence of red cells alone.

Cryoprecipitate

In 1980 Janson et al (19) administered bags of cryoprecipitate to a uremic patient with a prolonged BT greater than 30 minutes and rectal bleeding. One hour later the BT was 4 minutes and the bleeding stopped. 6 additional similar uremic patients were treated and in 5, BT returned to normal. 5 patients underwent surgical or invasive procedures without bleeding abnormally.

Although this study suggested that the shortening of the BT was a specific effect of vWF the mechanism was not established.

Infusion of DDAVP

Watson (26) in 1982 suggested that DDAVP may exert a beneficial effect on the hemostatic abnormalities in chronic uremia. Mannucci and colleagues (14) in 1983 postulated that if the shortening of the BT were due to the infusion of the large von Willebrand multimers in cryoprecipitate, administration of DDAVP should also shorten the BT. In a prospective controlled study they gave DDAVP (0.3 µg/kg) to 12 uremic patients who had greatly prolonged BT. DDAVP infusion shortened the BT in all patients with the effect lasting at least four hours, however 6 of them did not normalize. This effect of DDAVP was confirmed in 9 additional patients in an uncontrolled study in which DDAVP was given in surgical condition for nephrectomy in two patients, hemorroidectomy and renal biopsy.

Appearance in plasma of larger multimers than had been present before DDAVP were changes that consistently accompanied the effects of DDAVP on BT.

Even though vWF antigen and activity were high in uremic patients before DDAVP infusion, vWF and F VIII increased from two to four times after infusion.

In 1984, beneficial effect of DDAVP on the BT of uremic patients was confirmed in two case reports by Watson et al (27) by showing efficacy in a patient with diffuse gastritis and active bleeding. One hour after DDAVP, BT was 6 minutes and coincident with the cure of hemorrhage. A second patient bleeding during reconstruction of an arteriovenous fistula was stopped after DDAVP while the BT shortened from 16 to 4 minutes. Watson and Koegh completed a study on 8 uremic patients showing efficacy on the BT (28).

More recently in 1990, Soslau (15) and colleagues published a study on 5 HT uptake by platelets in uremic patients before and after infusion of DDAVP. This study demonstrated correction of the BT in 16 renal failure patients coincident with an increased uptake of 5HT by platelets and higher ATP release.

It was also shown that other routes of administration than intravenous perfusion gave interesting results. Shapiro and Kelleher (29) showed that administration of desmopressin via the intranasal route in two uremic patients decreased the bleeding time and improved clinical bleeding.

In the first patient 2 hours after intranasal administration of DDAVP, the BT was 3 minutes and the upper gastrointestinal bleeding slowed.

The second patient had a BT greater than 20 minutes and suffered from oozing at the stump after amputation. 90 minutes after administration of 3 µg/Kg of DDAVP intranasally, BT was 9 minutes and a decrease in the amount of oozing was noted.

Vigano and colleagues (30) demonstrated the efficacy of the subcutaneous route in shortening the bleeding time of uremic patients. A controlled study in nine uremic patients was carried out to evaluate shortening of the BT after subcutaneous injections of DDAVP. One hour after, the BT was significantly shorter and became normal in 7 of the 9 patients. Köhler et al (31) carried out a trial on 8 patients with uremic bleeding and confirmed the efficacy of 0.4 µg/kg to shorten the bleeding time and increase platelet retention. Therefore subcutaneous injection is an alternative method with the possibility of self administration by patients at home,however with a less pronounced effect on hemostasis.

Side effects

Cerebral thrombosis in an elderly patient with evidence of atherosclerosis was described by Byrnes et al in 1988 (32) incriminating the release of unusually large vWF multimers induced by DDAVP infusion. DDAVP should be given with greater caution to patients with atherosclerosis.

Fistula thrombosis 24 hours after DDAVP intravenous infusion was observed in a 35 year old woman (33).

Finally a decrease in functional protein C was detected in uremic patients following the administration of DDAVP (34). Before DDAVP protein C antigen is elevated in uremic patients associated to lower functional protein C than in normals. If confirmed this abnormality may contribute to thromboembolic complications.

CONCLUSION

Causes of clinical bleeding and prolonged bleeding time in uremic patients are not yet clearly defined. However two major hypotheses seem likely. The first in chronological order, assumes that the presence in uremic plasma of substances influences blood cell functions, mainly platelets and endothelial cells. This hypothesis is supported by the improvement of hemorrhagic diathesis following dialysis, which is more likely to be related to plasmatic abnormalities. In this group of causes, anemia, i.e. decrease number of circulating red blood cells can cause a mechanical disorder in platelet - vessel wall interaction. However neither dialysis nor correction of anemia by red cell transfusion or erythropoietin in most of the cases totally correct the bleeding tendency.

The hypothesis of abnormal von Willebrand factor, even though vWF antigen is usually higher than controls and even though the multimeric structure is identical to the one found in normal plasma, is appealing. This hypothesis is supported by the beneficial effect of cryoprecipitate and DDAVP infusion giving high molecular weight multimers of vWF in the patient's circulation. In addition DDAVP seems to have a more beneficial effect thatn cryoprecipitate: some patients who do not respond to cryoprecipitate do respond to DDAVP (35) and it might also have an effect on the platelet dysfunction described in uremia improving interaction of platelets with vessel subendothelium (36): increased serotonin uptake and ATP release indicating a platelet membrane modification after DDAVP, and improvement in clot retraction (15).

REFERENCES

1 Rabiner SF: Bleeding in uremia. Med Clin North Am 1972, 56: 221-233.

2 Anagnostou A, Fried W, Kurtzman NA: Hematological consequences of rena failure in Brenner B, Rector FC (eds)1981. The Kidney, Philadelphia, WB Saunders.

3 Kleinknecht D, Jungers P, Clianard J et al: Uremic and non-uremic complications in acute renal failure: evaluation or early and frequent dialysis in prognosis. Kidney Int 1972, 1: 190-196.

4 Small M, Lowe GDO, Cameron et al: Contribution of the haematocrit to the bleeding time. Haemostasis 1983, 13: 379-384.

5 Saniabadi AR, Lowe GDO, Barhenel JC et al: Haematocrit, bleeding time and platelet aggregation. Lancet 1983, 1: 1409-1411.

6 Lewis JH, Zucker MB, Ferguson JH: Bleeding tendency in uremia. Blood 1956, 11: 1073-1076.

7 Rath CE, Mailliard JA, Schreiner GE: Bleeding tendency in uremia. N Engl J Med 1957, 257: 808-811.

8 O'Grady JA: Bleeding tendency in uremia. JAMA 1959, 169: 1727-1732.

9 Carr ME Jr and Zekert SL: Force monitoring of clot retraction during DDAVP therapy for the qualitative platelet disorder or uraemia: report of a case. Blood Coagulation and Fibrinolysis 1991, 2: 303-308.

10 Rabiner SF, Hrodek O: Platelet factors in normal subjects and patients with renal failure. J Clin Invest 1968, 47: 901-912.

11 Castaldi PA, Rozenberg MC, Stewart JH: Bleeding disorder of uremia: a qualitative platelet defect. Lancet1968, 2: 66-69.

12 Rabner SF, Drake RF: Platelet function as an indicator of adequate dialysis. Kidney Int 1975, 7: S144-S146.

13 Castillo R, Lozano T, Escolar G et al: Defective platelet adhesion on vessel subendothelium in uremic patients. Blood 1986, 68: 337-342.

14 Mannucci PM, Remuzzi G, Pusineri F, Lombardi R et al: Deamino-8-D-arginine vasopressin shortens the bleeding time in uremia. The N Eng J of Med 1983, 6: 8-12.

15 Soslau G, Schwarts AB, Putatunda B, Conroy JD Parker J, Abel RF, Brodsky I:

Desmopressin-induced improvement in bleeding times in chronic renal failure patients correlates with platelet serotonin uptake and ATP release. Am J Med Sciences 1990, 300, 6: 372-379.

16 Remuzzi G, Marchesi D, Livio M, Schiepetti A, Mecca G, Donati MB, De Gaetano G: Prostaglandins, plasma factors and hemostasis in uremia. In Hemostasis, Prostaglandins and Renal Disease, edited by Remuzzi G., De Gaetano G., New York, Raven Press, 1980, 273-281.

17 Ekberg MR, Nilsson IM, Linell F: Significance of increased factor VIII in early glomerulonephritis. Ann Intern Med 1975, 83: 337-341.

18 Kazatchkine M, Sultan Y, Caen JP, Bariety J: Bleeding in uremia: a possible cause. Br Med J 1976, 2: 612-615.

19 Janson PA, Jubelirer SJ, Weinstein MJ, Deykin D,: Treatment of the bleeding tendency in uremia with cryoprecipitate. N Engl J Med 1980, 303:1318-1322.

20 Rodeghiero F, Castaman G, Lombardi R, Mannucci PM: von Willebrand factor abnormalities in two patients with uraemia. The Lancet 1988, 29: 1016-1017.

21 Remuzzi G, Livio M, Marchiaro G, Mecca G, de Gaetano G: Bleeding in renal failure: altered platelet function in chronic uraemia only partially corrected by haemodialysis. Nephron 1978, 22: 347-353.

22 Livio M, Marchesi D, Remuzzi G, Gotti E, Mecca G, de Gaetano G: Uraemic bleeding: role of anaemia and beneficial effect or red cell transfusions. Lancet 1982, ii: 1013-1015.

23 Fernandez F, Goudable C, Sie P et al: Low hematocrit and prolonged bleeding time in uraemic patients: effect of red cell transfusions. Br J Haematol 1985, 59: 139-148.

24 Moia M, Mannucci PM, Vizzotto L, Casati S, Cattaneo M, Ponticelli C: Improvement in the haemostatic defection uraemia after treatment with recombinant human erythropoietin. Lancet 1987, ii: 1227-1229.

25 Jacquot Ch, Masselot JP, Berthelot JM et al: Addition of desmopressin to recombinant human erythropoietin in treatment of haemostatic defect of uraemia. The Lancet, 1988, 20: 420.

26 Watson AJS, Koegh JAB: Effect of 1-deamino-8-D-arginine vasopressin on the prolonged bleeding time in chronic renal failure. Nephron 1982, 32: 49-52.

27 Watson AJ, Koegh JAB: 1-deamino-8-D-arginine vasopressin as a therapy for the bleeding diathesis of renal failure. Am J Nephrol 1984, 4: 49-51.

28 Watson AJ and Koegh AB: 1-deamino-8-D-arginine vasopressin (DDAVP): a potential new treatment for the bleeding diathesis of acute renal failure. Pharmatherapeutica 1984,3,9: 618-622.

29 Shapiro MD, Kelleher SP: Intranasal deamino-8-D-arginine vasopressin shortens the bleeding time in uremia. Am J Nephrol 1984, 4: 260-261.

30 Vigano GL, Mannucci PM, Lattuada A et al: Subcutaneous desmopressin (DDAVP) shortens the bleeding time in uremia. Am J Hematol 1989, 31: 32-35.

31 Köhler M, Hellstern P, Tarrach H, Bambauer R, Wenzel E, Jutzler GA: Subcutaneous injection of desmopressin (DDAVP): evaluation of a new, more concentrated preparation.Haemostasis 1989, 1: 38-44.

32 Byrnes JJ, Larcada A, Moake JL: Tgrombisis following desmopressin for uremic bleeding. Am J Hematol 1988, 28: 63-65.

33 Viron B, Michel C, Serrato T, Verdy E: Risque thrombogene du DDAVP dans l'insuffisance rénale chronique. Néphrologie 1987, 8: 225.

34 Aunsholt NA, Schmidt EB, Stoffersen E: 1-deamino-8-D-arginine vasopressin lowers protein C activity in uremics. Nephron 1989, 53: 6-8.

35 Triulzi DJ, Blumberg N: Variability in response to cryoprecipitate treatment for hemostatic defects in uremia. The Yale J of Biol and Med 1990, 63: 1-7.

36 Escolar G,Cases A, Monteagudo J, Garrido M, Lopez J, Ordinas A, Revert L and Castillo R: Uremic plasma after infusion of desmopressin (DDAVP) improves the interaction of normal platelets with vessel subendothelium. J Lab Clin Med 1989, 114: 36-42.

HEMOSTATIC EFFECTIVENESS OF DESMOPRESSIN IN THE BLEEDING DISORDERS OF UREMIA

Gianluigi Viganò[1] and Giuseppe Remuzzi1 [2]

[1]Istituto di Ricerche Farmacologiche Mario Negri
Laboratori Negri Bergamo
Bergamo
Italy

[2]Divisione di Nefrologia e Dialisi
Ospedali Riuniti di Bergamo
Bergamo
Italy

Bleeding is a common complication of uremia[1]. The modern management of renal failure has reduced the incidence of severe hemorrhages, but bleeding still presents a problem for uremic patients, particularly during surgery or invasive procedures.

CLINICAL MANIFESTATION

The most common hemorrhagic complications of uremia are ecchymoses, purpura, epistaxis and bleeding from venipuncture sites[1]. Severe bleeding, such as intracranial or gastrointestinal hemorrhage is less frequent. Though more common in acute renal failure, gastrointestinal bleeding can be found in chronic renal insufficiency, often associated with telangiectasias[2]. Cardiac tamponade following hemorrhagic pericarditis, and hemorrhagic pleural effusion were frequently described in the early days of dialysis but are now rare. Spontaneous retroperitoneal bleeding has occurred in patients with hydronephrosis, periarteritis nodosa, hypertension, or spontaneous rupture of the kidney. A recognized complication of chronic hemodialysis is subdural hematoma, which occurs in 5 to 15% of cases[3]. Prognosis is variable and death may ensue in 90% of cases.

Despite major advances in understanding the cause of the bleeding disorders associated with chronic renal failure, relatively few studies are available that allow the identification of laboratory markers of clinical bleeding. In this context, the most important study is that of

Desmopressin in Bleeding Disorders, Edited by G. Mariani *et al.*
Plenum Press, New York, 1993

Steiner and coworkers[4] who investigated 26 uremic patients to find correlations between the degree of uremia, bleeding and abnormal laboratory tests. They found that platelet aggregation was impaired and of little value in predicting bleeding, but a correlation was shown between bleeding time, blood urea nitrogen and clinical bleeding, suggesting that the skin bleeding time is the most useful platelet function test in predicting uremic bleeding.

PATHOGENESIS

Although the pathogenesis has still not been fully elucidated, a defect in primary hemostatis appears to be the main cause[1].

The etiology is certainly multifactorial. An acquired platelet dysfunction plays a major a role including reductions in platelet serotonin and adenosine diphosphate, the elevation of cyclic adenosine monophosphate, a defective cyclooxygenase activity with a reduced thromboxane A_2 generation as well as an abnormal mobilization of platelet Ca^{++} content with the consequent impairment of calcium-dependent platelet functions.

Studies that have focused on platelet-vessel wall interactions have disclosed several abnormalities, especially the abnormally high synthesis of vascular prostacyclin (a prostaglandin that potently inhibits platelet aggregation) and quantitative and/or qualitative defects of plasma and platelet von Willebrand Factor (vWF). The hemorrhagic tendency in uremia is also influenced by low hematocrit. Red blood cells play a pivotal role in primary hemostasis, and anemia may have a negative effect on the rheological component of the platelet-vessel wall interaction.

Since bleeding time is a global test of primary hemostasis which is influenced simultaneously by the platelet number and function and by integrity of vascular endothelium as well as by the hematocrit, it is not surprising that in patients with multifactorial impairment of hemostasis, abnormal bleeding time is a good marker of clinical bleeding[4].

CRYOPRECIPITATE AND DESMOPRESSIN

In recent years, several pharmacological approaches have been proposed for the treatment of uremic patients with active bleeding.

Studies on vWF in uremia produced a rationale for the use of cryoprecipitate. This is a precipitate enriched in vWF containing fibrinogen and fibronectin in addition to smaller amounts of all plasma proteins (including viruses such as hepatitis B and C, or human immunodeficiency virus). Cryoprecipitate has been reported to decrease bleeding time and reduce the complications of bleeding in uremic patients undergoing major surgery[5]. The effect is apparent within a few hours from the time of the infusions, but the maximal effect is obtained between 4 and 12 hours and by 24 hours post-infusion, the effect is no longer detectable. An increase in levels of fibrinogen and vWF properties was the only change noted after the infusion. Like blood transfusion, cryoprecipitate unfortunately carries the risk of transmitting blood-borne diseases including hepatitis and AIDS, so alternatives have been sought.

The possibility that the beneficial effect of cryoprecipitate may be related to the increase in vWF related properties suggested that desmopressin - a synthetic derivative of the antidiuretic hormone that induces release of autologous vWF from storage sites in healthy subjects and patients with vWF deficiency[6] - might be considered an alternative to cryoprecipitate. Desmopressin was also employed in the prevention of hemorrhages in mild hemophilia and vWF disease during and after surgical procedures[6].

In an open study[7] involving 12 patients on choronic hemodialysis, continuous peritoneal dialysis or with severe renal failure, and in a double-blind, placebo-controlled, cross-over study[8] including 12 hemodialysis patients, 0.4 µg/kg or 0.3 µg/kg of desmopressin respectively, were intravenously administered in patients who had a history of bleeding episodes and a prolonged bleeding time (greater than 15 min). Watson and Keogh[7] in the open study found that 1 and 2 hours after infusion of desmopressin the bleeding times significantly shortened to 6.7 ±1.7 and 7.2 ± 1.8 minutes, respectively. The differences in these values were statistically significant in comparison with the basal ones. In 5 of these patients, bleeding time was also measured 24 hours after desmopressin and it had returned to approximate the baseline values, suggesting that the effect of desmopressin is a temporary one.

Our group gave desmopressin or placebo in a double-blind study[8] at a dose of 0.3 µg/kg intravenously, added to 50 ml saline to avoid possible side effects. We found that desmopressin but not placebo shortened bleeding times 1 to 4 hours after infusion. The magnitude and duration of the responses varied: the bleeding time was still shorter in 10 patients at 4 hours in 7 patients at 8 hours. 24 hours after, bleeding time returned to basal values in all patients. Platelet count, platelet cAMP levels, platelet retention on glass beads, plasma fibronectin serum TxB_2 and residual prothrombin, hematocrit and plasma osmolarity were unchanged after desmopressin. A consistent post-infusion increase in FVIII coagulant activity, related antigen, and ristocetin cofactor was associated with the shortening of bleeding time. Before desmopressin, the multimeric structure of vWF in uremic plasma was no different from that observed in normal plasma. After desmopressin, larger vWF multimers than those present in pre-treatment plasma appeared, reaching a maximum at 1 to 4 hours. No change in multimeric structure was observed when the patients were treated with placebo. The shortening of bleeding time parallels the appearance of larger vWF multimers in plasma[8]. Two explanations may be hypothesized: the larger vWF multimers may be more effective in promoting platelet adhesion to subendothelium or, alternatively, the vWF released by desmopressin from storage sites may correct an abnormality of vWF present in uremia.

A further study was aimed at improving hemostasis in patients with uremia due to acute renal failure and with prolonged bleeding time, in order to allow a diagnostic percutaneous renal biopsy9. All patients admitted to the study had prolonged bleeding times (more than 10 minutes). Patients were given washed red cell transfusions, when hematocrit was less than 30%, or desmopressin, when hematocrit was more than 30%, with the aim of normalizing the patient's bleeding time before biopsy. Red blood cell transfusions normalized bleeding time in all patients except one. Four patients with hematocrit greater than 30% received desmopressin alone, and bleeding time performed one hour after the end of the infusion became normal in 3. Computerized tomography revealed an incidence of perirenal hematomas comparable to that usually reported in patients with normal or slightly depressed renal function who undergo renal biopsy. This study indicated that desmopressin, as well as red blood cell transfusions, can temporarily restore hemostasis, allowing a diagnostic percutaneous renal biopsy in patients with acute renal failure.

A more recent study[10] documented that desmopressin can be also given subcutaneously. In this placebo controlled cross-over trial, 9 patients on chronic hemodialysis and prolonged bleeding time received 0.3 µg/kg intravenous or subcutaneous desmopressin or subcutaneous placebo. The bleeding time returned to normal range 1 to 4 hours after the administration of desmopressin but not after placebo. vWF antigen levels increased significantly 1 hour after desmopressin infusion. When values obtained before and 1 hour after desmopressin were pooled together, a significant negative correlation was found between bleeding time and vWF antigen levels. This finding suggests that although baseline vWF levels are normal or elevated in patients with uremia, further elevation induced by desmopressin might induce platelet adhesion and contribute to bleeding time shortening.

An alternative means of administering the drug to uremics is via the intranasal route[11], as is done in patients with hemophilia or vWF disease[6]. Intranasal administration is well tolerated and appears to be safe. A dose ten to twenty times the amount given intravenously is required. Intranasal desmopressin administered in a dose of 3 µg/kg has been shown to decrease prolonged bleeding time and to reduce upper gastrointestinal bleeding in two patients with uremia[11]. No adverse effects on serum sodium or systemic blood pressure were observed.

There have been publications of uncontrolled cases of desmopressin treatment of patients with acute or chronic renal failure to prevent bleeding before invasive procedure or to stop spontaneous bleeding[6]. However, the evidence that desmopressin stops spontaneous bleeding or prevents excessive blood loos after surgery is still lacking because no controlled double blind clinical trial has been performed thus far.

In some patients desmopressin loses efficacy after repeated administration[12]. This has been attributed to a progressive depletion of the storage sites from which vWF is released by the drug. The development of tachyphylaxis would limit the usefulness of desmopressin in clinical management of these patients. However, the prevalence extent and pattern of development of tachyphylaxis are not known and proper studies are needed to clarify this issue.

SIDE EFFECTS

The side effects of desmopressin are generally of mild degree ranging from mild facial flushing to headache, a 10-20% increase in pulse rate, and minor falls in blood pressure[6].

Recently, some thrombotic events have been reported during desmopressin treatment[13-15], one of these in an old patient with uremia[16]. These thrombotic events are probably related to the release of the multimeric forms of vWF found in normal plasma and of large forms not normally present in the circulation.

A recent review of all cases[17], however, has concluded that desmopressin does not significantly increase the incidence of thrombosis when the increasing number of patients who use the drug is considered. Even so, close surveillance is warranted, especially in patients with clinical and laboratory evidence of coronary or cerebral atherosclerosis. To gain additional insight, Mannucci and Lusher[17] also perused the clinical trials (published and unpublished) evaluating the hemostatic efficacy of desmopressin in reducing blood loss and transfusion requirements in patients undergoing cardiac surgery with cardiopulmonary bypass. They analyzed nine trials on 763 patients. Twenty six clinical adverse events could be ascribed to thrombosis (myocardial infarction, stroke, venous thromboembolism), 15 in 382 desmopressin-treated patients (3.9%) and 11 in the 381 untreated patients (2.9%). All these trials were carried out on patients undergoing cardiac surgery, a condition associated with a risk of coronary and cerebral thrombosis, thus the data support the view that desmopressin does not significantly increase the incidence of thrombosis.

THERAPEUTIC STRATEGIES FOR UREMIC BLEEDING

New therapeutic tools for the prevention and the treatment of uremic bleeding have been recently developed. The therapeutic strategy one should choose depends on the urgency of the situation, the severity of uremia, and the previous treatment employed.

Acute bleeding episodes may be treated with desmopressin in a dose of 0.3 µg/kg given intravenously or subcutaneously[8,10].

We suggest that desmopressin be used as an alternative to cryoprecipitate[5] because of the difficulty of obtaining reproducible results with the latter and to avoid the risk of transmitting viral hepatitis. The effect of desmopressin, however, lasts only a few hours and desmopressin appears to lose its efficacy when administered repeatedly.

Conjugated estrogens given intravenously at a dose of 3 mg/kg divided into daily dose are ideal for the treatment of dramatic bleeding because of their long-lasting effect[18]. The effect does not become evident for several hours, but lasts for 14 days.

Severely anemic patients should receive red blood cell transfusion[19] or recombinant human erythropoietin[20] to increase the hematocrit to more than 30%. A recent controlled study was designed to establish the minimum level of hematocrit achieved with erythropoietin that corrects the prolonged bleeding time of uremic patients[21]. The results indicated that a threshold of hematocrit between 27% and 32% had to be reached for bleeding time to become normal, indicating that a partial correction of renal anemia is enough to normalize bleeding time. The initial dose should be 50 U/kg IV thrice weekly and the single doses should be increased by 25 U/kg to reach hematocrit of 30-32%.

REFERENCES

1. G. Remuzzi, Bleeding in renal failure, Lancet 1:1205(1988).
2. J.T. Cunningham, Gastric telangiectasias in chronic hemodialysis patient: a report of six cases, Gastroenterology 81:1131 (1981).
3. A.Pan, A.G.Rogers, and D.Pearlman, Subdural hematoma complicating anticoagulant therapy, Canadian Medical Association Journal 82:1162 (1960).
4. R.W.Steiner, C.Coggins, and A.C.A. Carvalho, Bleeding in uremia: a useful test to assess clinical bleeding, Am J Hematol 7:107 (1979).
5. P.A.Janson, S.J.Jubiler, M.J. Weinstein, and D.Deykin, Treatment of the bleeding tendency of uremia with cryoprecipitate N Engl J Med 303:1318 (1980).
6. P.M.Mannucci, Desmopressin: a non-transfusional form of treatment for congenital and acquired bleeding disorders, Blood 72:1449 (1988).
7. A.J.S. Watson, and J.A.B. Keogh, Effect of 1-deamino-8-D-arginine vasopressin on the prolonged bleeding time in chronic renal failure , Nephron 32:49 (1982).

8. P.M. Mannucci, G.Remuzzi, F.Pusineri, R.Lombardi, C.Valsecchi G.Mecca, and T.S.Zimmerman, Deamino-8-D-arginine vasopressin shortens the bleeding time in uremia ,N Engl J Med 308:8 (1983).
9. E.Gotti, G.Mecca, C.Valentino, E.Cortinovis, T.Bertani, and G.Remuzzi, Renal biopsy in patients with acute renal failure and prolonged bleeding time: a preliminary report, Am J Kidney Dis 6:397 (1985).
10. G.Viganò, P.M.Mannucci, A.Lattuada, A.Harris, and G.Remuzzi, subcutaneous desmopressin (DDAVP) shortens the bleeding time in uremia Am J Hematol 31:32 (1989).
11. M.D.Shapiro, and S.P.Kelleher, Intranasal deamino-8-D-arginine vasopressin shortens the bleeding time in uremia, Am J Nephrol 4:260 (1984).
12. C.Canavese, M.Salomone, A.Pacitti, G.Magiarotti, and V.Calitri,Reduced response of uraemic bleeding time to repeated doses of desmopressin , Lancet 1:867 (1985).
13. J.R.O'Brien, P.J.Green, G.Salmon, et al, Desmopressin and myocardial infarction, Lancet 1:664 (1989).
14. L.Bond, and D.Bevan, Myocardial infarction in a patient with hemophilia treated with DDAVP, N Engl J Med 318:121 (1988).
15. Editorial, Desmopressin and arterial thrombosis, Lancet 1:938 (1989).
16. J.J.Byrnes, A.Larcada, and J.L.Moake, Thrombosis following desmopressin for uremic bleeding, Am J Hematol 28:63 (1988).
17. P.M.Mannucci, and J.M.Lusher,Desmopressin and Thrombosis, Lancet 2:675 (1989).
18. M.Livio, P.M.Mannucci, G.Viganò, G.Mingardi, R.Lombardi, G.Mecca, and G.Remuzzi, Conjugated estrogens for the management of bleeding associated with renal failure, N Engl J Med 315:731 (1986).
19. M.Livio, D.Marchesi, G.Remuzzi, E.Gotti, G.Mecca, and G. de Gaetano, Uraemic bleeding:role of anemia and beneficial effect of red cell transfusion, Lancet 2:1013 (1982).
20. Ad hoc Committee for the National Kidney foundation, Statement on the clinical use of recombinant erythropoietin in anemia of end-stage renal disease, Am J Kidney Dis 14:163 (1989).
21. G.Viganò, A.Benigni, D.Mendogni, G.Mingardi, G.Mecca, and G.Remuzzi, Recombinant human erythropoietin to correct uremic bleeding, Am J Kidney Dis 18:44 (1991).

DISCUSSION

Kobrinski: Recently Montgomery, and we ourselves, have seen in children with congenital heart disease an increase in bleeding times due to turbulent flow through the shunts. The discordant results of ristocetin co-factor may be due to the different venous access technologies, such as shunts.

Weinstein (United States): VWf may not be abnormal itself in uraemia; instead toxins may bind to vWf binding sites for platelets. Perhaps infusions of cryoprecipitate or vWf introduces fresh amounts into the circulation that can interact with platelets. Maybe vWf is more effective

than cryoprecipitate because cryoprecipitate does not contain the higher molecular weight multimers of vWf.
Sultan: If there is an abnormality of vWf it is acquired. It happens after its release into the circulation, perhaps it is interfering with platelet function.
Vigano: The large multimers appear in all patients. However the issue is open to speculation.

Mannucci: Dr Weinstein, I think that your hypothesis that fresh unimpeded vWf is being released and is used before it can be effective is the most reasonable, but it is difficult to prove. We work with washed platelets, so the toxins may not be there. Do you have evidence of such toxins?
Weinstein: We have looked for them, but have not found them. It IS difficult. Dr Sultan, how did you do the ristocetin co-factor study?
Sultan: We used washed platelets prepared the same day from blood donors.

Lusher: You recommended i.v. or s.c. DDAVP for acute, but not longer term bleeding. Is this because of tachyphylaxis? How do conjugated estrogens compare in efficacy with DDAVP?
Vigano: I suggest subcutaneous treatment at home and for acute treatment in hospital. The oestrogen effect starts after a few hours and have maximum effect after 24 hours. They are better in severe traumatic bleeding where the patient requires major surgery.
Mannucci: Tachyphylaxis has never been demonstrated in the DDAVP treatment of uraemia.

Stuart (United States): Have the speakers used methylprednisolone intravenously for severe bleeding? We used it successfully over 4 days in a woman with severe haemorrhage.
Vigano: We have no experience with it. However, I agree that it has a rationale, in that methylprednisolone, as shown for estrogens, at least in uraemia, can stop bleeding by a general hormone receptor mechanism. Indeed , the treatment with glucocorticoid or estrogen receptor antagonist blocked the effect of shortening the prolonged bleeding time of uraemic rats. The protein involved is not yet known.

Bichet: Since we have been using high efficiency dialysis and erythropoietin we rarely have haemostatic complications. We maintain hemoglobin between 12 and 14, and the hematocrit above 30.

Nilsson (Sweden): In the 1970's we took part in an international exchange study and looked at methods of measuring Factor VIII, vWf and ristocetin co-factor. The first two were easily standardized, but the third was subject to very wide variations. I suggest the ristocetin co-factor studies are repeated using the much more reliable modern methods.

Kessler (United States): We do not have uniform responses in our renal failure patients after cryoprecipitate, DDAVP or estrogens. I'd like to know the statistics from colleagues on correcting bleeding times. DOes correcting bleeding times matter? Do you see increased bleeding after surgery? Are there differences of quality of cryoprecipitate between institutions. We have noticed that many bags of cryoprecipitate before cooling have no active vWf. The multimers are degraded.
Sultan: We have no data for correction of bleeding time after DDAVP. We can operate on patients without correction, as they do not bleed excessively at surgery. If vWf is important, it is not the only factor causing platelet problems: other vessel wall factors are responsible.
Vigano: I agree. Patients have multifactorial problems and it is difficult to correct them all.

Kohler: We changed from cryoprecipitate to Factor VIII concentrates, which contains high levels of vWf multimers. This works for uremics.

RENAL FUNCTION AND THROMBOEMBOLISM IN HIGH DOSE DESMOPRESSIN TREATMENT

Per Anders Flordal

Department of Surgery
Danderyd Hospital
S-182 88 Danderyd, Sweden

INTRODUCTION

When desmopressin is used in relation with surgery some possible side effects have to be taken into consideration. A risk of arterial thrombosis has been proposed, but seems to be minimal (Mannucci and Lusher, 1989)*. A proposed risk of postoperative venous thromboembolism (Melissari et al., 1986) is contradicted by two pilot studies indicating beneficial effects in the prophylaxis (Nilsen et al., 1984) and treatment (Törnebohm et al., 1987) of deep vein thrombosis. This paper will account for the first data available on the effect of desmopressin on phlebographically verified postoperative deep vein thrombosis (Flordal et al., 1991b; Flordal et al., 1991a).

But first it addresses the question of renal effects of high dose desmopressin treatment (Flordal and Ljungström, 1991). Anecdotic data indicate that the antidiuretic effect is no problem, despite the potent antidiuretic effect of desmopressin in doses considerably lower than those used to reach hemostatic effects. Desmopressin and dextran were studied together, since this combination seems to be favorable with regard to both transfusion requirements and postoperative thromboembolism.

METHODS TO ASSESS RENAL FUNCTION

Volunteers

Two men aged 20 and 28 years and two women aged 33 and 37 participated as volunteers. They were all healthy and taking no medication. They abstained from physical exercise, heavy meals and alcohol from 12 hours before up to the end of each experiment.

Each volunteer participated in four experiments, with an interval of at least one week between experiments, receiving all combinations of desmopressin, dextran and placebo (saline / saline, saline / dextran, desmopressin / saline and desmopressin / dextran).

On arrival at 8.00 a venous blood sample was drawn and then a venous cannula was put into a vein on the dorsal aspect of the left forearm. In a single blind manner 50 ml saline or desmopressin (Ferring AB, Sweden) 0.3 µg/kg body weight diluted in 50 ml saline was infused over 20 minutes, starting at 8.30. Then 500 ml 6% dextran 70 in saline (Pharmacia AB, Sweden) or 500 ml saline was infused between 9.00 and 10.00, single-blindedly. To prevent allergic reactions, 20 ml 15% dextran 1 (Pharmacia AB, Sweden) was injected before dextran 70.

Further venous samples were taken from an antecubital vein in the right arm 2, 3, 5, 7 and 24 hours after the 8 o'clock start. On each occasion the hemoglobin concentration (Hb) was determined.

Desmopressin in Bleeding Disorders, Edited by G. Mariani *et al.*
Plenum Press, New York, 1993

Urine was collected in four fractions: from 07.00 to 11.00, from 11.00 to 15.00, from 15.00 to 21.00 and from 21.00 to the following morning at 07.00. After measuring the volume of each sample it was analysed for osmolality and creatinine.

Surgical Patients

Eight women, mean age 63 (range 43–72) years, and four men, mean age 67 (range 55–73) years, scheduled for total hip replacement were also studied. The indication for surgery was primary arthrosis in eight, sequelae to hip fractures in two patients, repeated hip prosthesis dislocations in one and prosthesis loosening in one patient. Methyl-metacrylate cement was used in all patients.

In a double-blind fashion each patient received an infusion of placebo or desmopressin (Ferring AB, Sweden) 0.3 μg/kg body weight diluted in 50 ml saline at the start of surgery. The same infusion was repeated 6 hours later, on both occasions at an infusion rate of 20–30 minutes.

Venous samples were taken at 8.00 (before anesthesia and surgery), at 12.00 (1 hour after the end of the operation), at 15.00 and on the following day at 8.00. Analyses were made for Hb, Na^+, K^+, creatinine and albumin.

Operations started at 9.15–9.30. Ringer acetate 500 ml was infused before induction of spinal anesthesia with plain bupivacaine 0.5% (Astra AB, Sweden). All but one patient also had an epidural catheter for postoperative pain relief with bupivacaine and morphine. Ephedrine was administered pre- or intraoperatively to prevent the systolic blood pressure from falling below 100 mmHg.

During surgery all patients received an intravenous infusion of 6% dextran 70 (Pharmacia AB, Sweden) 500–1000 ml for thrombosis prophylaxis and plasma expansion, the volume infused depending on the amount of blood loss. In addition, a balanced isotonic crystalloid solution (2.5% glucose in Na^+ 70 mmol, Cl^- 45 mmol, Ac^- 25 mmol/l) was infused at the rate of 2 ml/kg per hour intra- and postoperatively for the first 24 hours.

The mean operation time was 101 (range 75–135) minutes, blood loss during surgery 640 (range 225–1750) ml and drainage loss up to the following morning 560 (range 150–1400) ml. Erythrocyte concentrate corresponding to a mean of 560 (range 0–1800) ml donor blood and balanced crystalloid solutions at a mean of 4070 (range 3200–5300) ml were infused during surgery and postoperatively. One patient received 300 ml plasma and 200 ml 20 % albumin. There where no significant differences betwen the groups in these variables.

All patients had an indwelling bladder catheter and urine production was measured hourly. Urine was pooled in three fractions: from 09.00 to 12.00, from 12.00 to 15.00 and from 15.00 to 06.00 and analysed for osmolality (first four patients in each group only) and creatinine. Furosemide was administered intravenously to maintain urine flow at about 100 ml/hour.

Urine production and creatinine clearance

For each interval of urine collection urine production was expressed as the volume collected over the duration of the interval. Glomerular filtration rate was estimated with the clearance of endogenous creatinine, using the standard formula

$$\frac{\text{Urinary creatinine} * \text{Urinary volume}}{\text{Serum creatinine} * \Delta\text{Time}}$$

Serum creatinine was determined at both ends of all urine collection intervals and the mean values were used.

Analysis of variance with a repeated measures design (Winer, 1971; Brain Power, 1986) was used to compare differences between groups when repeated measurements had been done over time.

RENAL FUNCTION IN VOLUNTEERS

Baseline urine osmolalities before the start of experiments did not vary significantly. Dextran did not affect urine osmolality, urine volumes or clearance of endogenous creatinine.

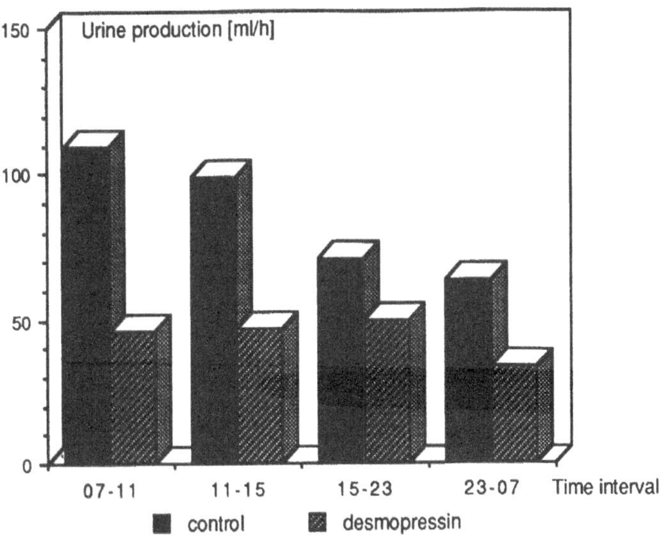

Fig. 1. Mean urine production in four healthy volunteers, each studied twice with and twice without desmopressin. Significant (p=0.02) antidiuretic effect of desmopressin, administered in the middle of the first time interval.

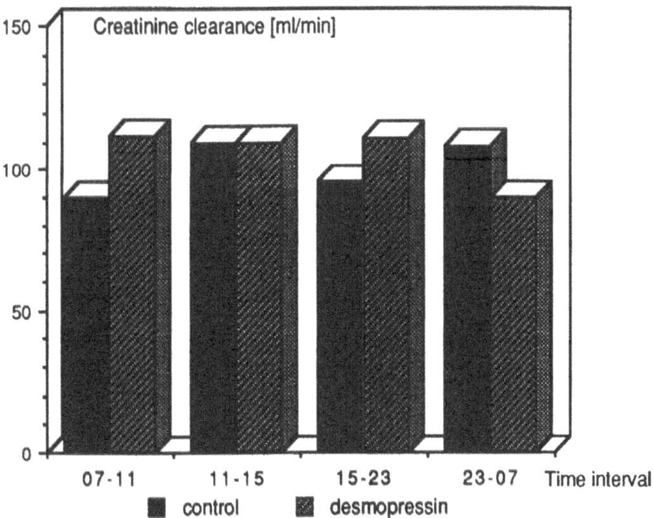

Fig. 2. Mean clearance of endogenous creatinine in four healthy volunteers, each studied twice with and twice without desmopressin. No significant effect of desmopressin, administered in the middle of the first time interval.

Desmopressin caused marked reduction in urine production (*p*=0.02, Fig. 1). The antidiuretic effect persisted over the whole 24-hour period and urine flow was approximately halved even 14–22 hours after the end of the infusion (*p*=0.01). The mean 24-hour urine volume was 890 ml less (*p*=0.001) in periods with desmopressin than in periods without desmopressin. The mean clearance of endogenous creatinine (as an estimate of the glomerular filtration rate) was not significantly affected by desmopressin (Fig. 2). All Na^+, K^+ and creatinine determinations were within normal limits and desmopressin had no significant effect on these variables.

RENAL FUNCTION IN TOTAL HIP REPLACEMENT PATIENTS

Renal function was also studied in 12 patients undergoing total hip replacement. Mean urine volume was 50% lower in those who received desmopressin than in the untreated control patients in the 3-hour period including surgery and 26% higher in the postoperative period (Fig. 3), but the differences between groups did not reach statistical significance. The total 21-hour urine volume was similar in both groups.

Mean urine osmolalities before anaesthesia and surgery were similar (484 and 489 mOsm/kg in the the placebo and desmopressin groups, respectively). Osmolality had an inverse relation to urine production, both during and after surgery.

The creatinine clearance was constant in the placebo group, but it increased in the desmopressin group in the postoperative period (*p*=0.001, Fig. 4).

The mean amount of furosemide administered was 17 mg in the desmopressin group (range 0–40 mg) and 15 mg in the controls (0–35 mg). The mean total volume of liquids infused was 5020 ml in the desmopressin group and 5250 ml in the control group. Mean fluid losses (urine volume plus blood loss) were 3710 and 3570 ml, respectively. Thus, the excess of liquids infused over liquids lost was a mean of 1310 ml in the desmopressin group and 1680 ml in the controls. Blood loss, transfusion rate and Hb before and after surgery did not differ significantly between the groups.

Desmopressin had no statistically significant effect on Na^+, K^+ or creatinine concentrations, which were within normal limits; only a marginal hyponatraemia and hypokalaemia was seen in one patient on one occasion in each group.

DIFFERENT EFFECTS ON URINE PRODUCTION IN VOLUNTEERS AND SURGICAL PATIENTS

The antidiuretic effect of desmopressin lasted for at least 24 hours after a single dose in healthy volunteers. Nonetheless, several investigators have found no untoward effects of desmopressin on renal function when given in the context of surgery (Mannucci et al., 1977; Salzman et al., 1986; Czer et al., 1987; Kobrinsky et al., 1987; Rocha et al., 1988). In the present study the control patients had the expected pattern of urine production (Fig. 3). No antidiuretic effect of desmopressin was ascertained in the surgical patients, although there was a trend to decreased urine volumes during surgery (Fig. 3).

The fact that the 21-hour urine output was the same in the desmopressin-treated patients as in the controls does not in itself prove that urine production was unaffected by desmopressin. These patients were monitored in the recovery room and their urine output was checked by the anesthesiologist to be about 100 ml/h. However, since the patient groups did not differ in body weight, preoperative hydration, blood loss, or urine volume, any significant antidiuretic activity should have been reflected in an increased requirement for diuretic drugs and/or fluid infusions. These were similar in both groups, and therefore it can be said that desmopressin had a very transient antidiuretic effect, if any, in the surgical patients, in contrast to what was seen in the volunteers.

Increased secretion of ADH is a normal response to surgery (Kehlet, 1984). This response is of a smaller magnitude under epidural than under general anaesthesia (Bonnet et al., 1982; Punnonen and Viinamäki, 1983). Still, Bonnet et al. (1982), studying total hip replacement performed with epidural anaesthesia, found plasma ADH to increase from 1 pg/ml before, to 3 pg/ml during and 20 pg/ml early after surgery.

The apparent distribution volume of desmopressin is 0.21 l/kg and the plasma half-life is 55 minutes (Vilhardt et al., 1986). The plasma concentration of desmopressin in our

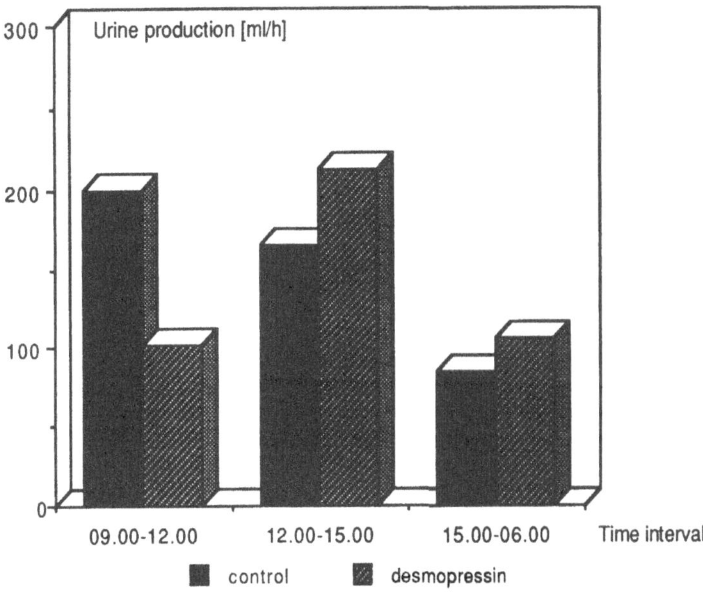

Fig. 3. Mean urine volumes, six total hip replacement patients in each group. Desmopressin infusions were started at 9.00 and 15.00. No significant effect of desmopressin.

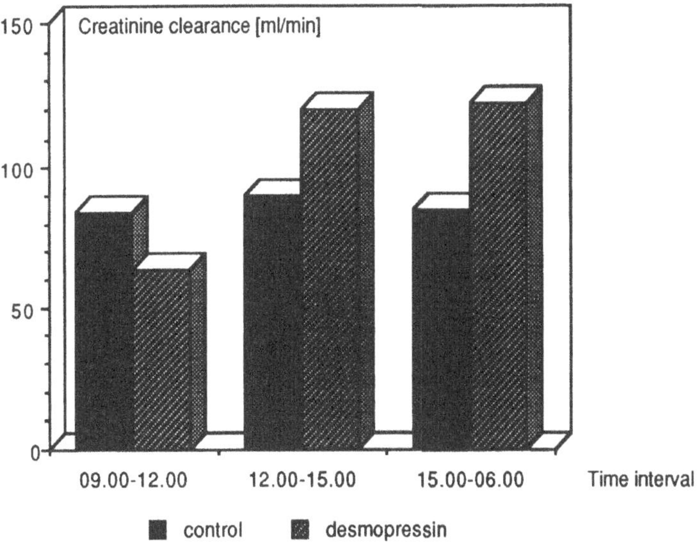

Fig. 4. Mean values for clearance of endogenous creatinine, six total hip replacement patients in each group. Desmopressin infusions were started at 9.00 and 15.00. Desmopressin increased creatinine clearance in the postoperative period (p=0.001).

patients, who received 0.3 μg/kg in a 20–30 minute infusion, would then have been at a peak of about 1300 pg/ml at the end of the infusion and have declined exponentially to reach about 20 pg/ml just before the second dose. Desmopressin has a 60% higher affinity than ADH for the V_2 receptor (Richardson and Robinson, 1985).

Even if the ADH increase in response to surgery were in some way inhibited by desmopressin, this would not influence urine production much, since ADH consequently accounts for only a minor part of the V_2 receptor activity during the early postoperative period. Moreover, it is unlikely that desmopressin could inhibit the increase in ADH, since this response depends on nociceptive inflow and not on plasma volume or Na^+ concentration changes (Bonnet et al., 1982), and it is reasonable to think that only the latter two may have been affected by desmopressin.

Ephedrine is known to affect blood pressure as well as glomerular filtration rate and urine production (Westman et al., 1988). In the present study ephedrine was used to treat postanesthetic hypotension. A mean of 32 (0–85) mg being given in the desmopressin group and 23 (15–35) mg in the placebo group (n.s.). There was no correlation between ephedrine dose and creatinine clearance and since ephedrine was administered in similar doses to both groups it cannot be held responsible for any differences observed.

Regional anesthesia does not modify water or electrolyte homeostasis (Kehlet, 1984) and it was used uniformly in both groups.

DIFFERENT EFFECTS ON CREATININE CLEARANCE IN VOLUNTEERS AND IN SURGICAL PATIENTS

In connection with orthopedic surgery under regional anesthesia the antidiuretic effect of desmopressin seemed to be nil, or very transient. An increased glomerular filtration rate (evaluated as creatinine clearance, Fig. 4) and a consequent rise in primary urine flow may be a compensatory mechanism. In the volunteers, the antidiuretic effect of desmopressin was longlasting, and creatinine clearance did not increase (Fig. 2).

The increase in creatinine clearance after desmopressin was not explained by a higher systemic arterial blood pressure, but reduced resistance in renal afferent arterioles or an increased resistance in efferent arterioles cannot be ruled out.

Prostacyclin secretion is stimulated by ADH. In turn, prostacyclin is known to inhibit ADH activity (Goodman-Gilman et al., 1990). Prostacyclin might very well be a link in another compensatory mechanism moderating the antidiuretic effect of desmopressin.

There seems at present to be no explanation of why there was a compensatory creatinine clearance response or why a prostacyclin-mediated regulation should be in effect in the surgical patients but not in the volunteers. However, the neuroendocrine and metabolic systems are profoundly affected by anesthesia and surgery (Kehlet, 1984), so a different mode of reaction may very well be expected.

A plausible explanation for the different effects of desmopressin in healthy volunteers and in surgical patients is based on the fact that desmopressin is actually an antagonist to ADH on the V_1 receptor (Derkx et al., 1983). The surgical trauma induces increased secretion of ADH (Bonnet et al., 1982). Stimulating the V_1 receptor, ADH is a vasoconstrictor and can markedly reduce renal blood flow and glomerular filtration rate (West, 1985). Apparently, since the glomerular filtration rate does not decrease despite the ADH increase (Kehlet, 1984), there are also mechanisms *stimulating* glomerular filtration. By antagonism on the V_1 receptor, desmopressin may abolish the depressing effect of ADH on the glomerular filtration rate, allowing it to increase in response to these stimulating mechanisms.

In conclusion, these data agree with and offer an explanation of the lack of cases of water retention and renal failure from desmopressin in other studies.

METHODS TO ASSESS THROMBOEMBOLIC RISK

The twelve patients studied with respect to coagulation parameters (see "Desmopressin corrects the hemostatic disorder induced by dextran ..." in this volume) were also studied with respect to fibrinolysis and coagulation inhibition (Flordal et al., 1991b). The fifty patients studied with respect to blood loss (see same article) were also studied with respect to postoperative thromboembolism (Flordal et al., 1991a).

All patients were mobilized from the first postoperative day with the aid of a physiotherapist. Compressive stockings were not used. On the third and eighth postoperative days patients were clinically assessed for signs of venous thrombosis or pulmonary embolism. On the eighth postoperative day all but six patients in the blood loss study underwent ascending phlebography (Rabinov and Paulin, 1972) on the operated leg. Two patients were lost due to intercurrent complications, three due to technical difficulties in inserting the venous cannula on the dorsum of the foot, and one patient refused cooperation. The anterior and posterior tibial, peroneal, popliteal, femoral and external and common iliac veins were evaluable in all 44 patients and the muscle veins of the calf in 43 patients. All phlebography was performed and assessed by the same senior radiologist.

ANTICOAGULANT ACTIVITIES

In six placebo-treated control patients undergoing total hip replacement, the mean tPA activity did not change significantly, but it increased twofold in the six desmopressin treated patients (Table 1). The tPA increase after desmopressin is known to be of short duration (Mannucci et al., 1975) and may have mainly disappeared by the time of the first postoperative venous sampling, which was 2.5 hours after administration of the first dose of desmopressin.

PAI-1 activities did not change significantly in the control group (Table 1), but it decreased significantly in the desmopressin group, returning to the preoperative level on the morning after surgery. The difference between groups before surgery was not statistically significant. High PAI-1 levels have been shown to correlate to postoperative deep venous thrombosis (Eriksson et al., 1989; Eriksson et al., 1991). An early stimulation of fibrinolysis, indicated by a rise in tPA and a fall in PAI-1, may be beneficial in regard to the risk for thromboembolism, since most thrombi already form during surgery (Modig et al., 1980; Westermann et al., 1981; Ogston, 1987).

Protein C decreased similarly during surgery in both groups (Table 1), in each individual very closely related to hemodilution. Low protein C levels are known to carry a risk for venous thrombosis (Felez, 1990). It was not confirmed in this study that protein C is decreased by desmopressin, as was found by Melissari et al. (1986).

Antithrombin III was decreased in the postoperative period in both groups (Fig. 5), but significantly less in the desmopressin group ($p<0.05$). All placebo-treated patients had antithrombin III concentrations below the normal level on all sampling occasions in the postoperative period (45–83%, normal range 85–125%), except for one patient who returned to a normal value at the last sampling point. Four of the six control patients, but none of the desmopressin patients, had a mean postoperative antithrombin III concentration below 80% (range: placebo 60–81%, desmopressin 80–85%).

Table 1. tPA, PAI-1 and protein C in total hip replacement patients (n=6 in each group) and statistical significance of change within treatment (over time) and of difference between treatments.

	Time of day 08.00	12.00	15.00	08.00	Within treatment	Between treatments
tPA [IU/ml]						
placebo	0.42 ±0.11	0.34 ±0.07	0.54 ±0.10		n.s.	p=0.005
desmopressin	0.66 ±0.17	1.39 ±0.28	1.41 ±0.28		p<0.05	
PAI-1 [U/ml]						
placebo	33 ±10	35 ±10	27 ±5	44 ±11	n.s.	p=0.01
desmopressin	16 ±4	9 ±3	8 ±2	19 ±5	p<0.05	
Protein C [percentage of population mean]						
placebo	133 ±12	88 ±8	91 ±13	92 ±12	p<0.001	n.s.
desmopressin	122 ±11	95 ±8	90 ±5	93 ±10	p<0.001	

Means ±SEM.

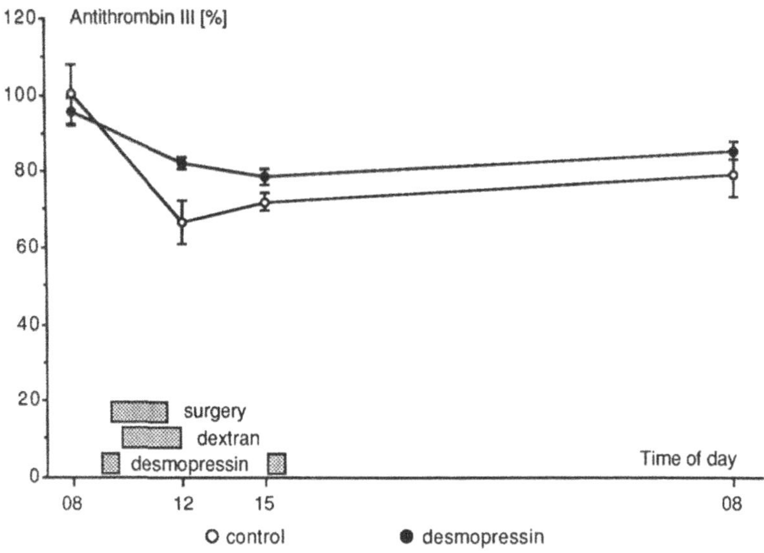

Fig. 5. Antithrombin III concentrations as percentages of mean of a healthy reference population. Mean and SEM for six patients in each group. Decreases were significant in both groups ($p<0.01$), but levels were significantly higher in the desmopressin group in the postoperative period ($p<0.05$).

The mean antithrombin III concentration of 67% directly after surgery is a level known to be in the risk zone (Reeve, 1980; Welin-Berger et al., 1982; Francis et al., 1989). This pronounced drop in antithrombin III in the control patients is in accord with the findings of other authors (Francis et al., 1989). There is no effective compensatory mechanism for antithrombin III loss as there is for several other factors (Myllylä, 1988).

The drop was found to be partly prevented by desmopressin, which kept antithrombin III levels within the normal range. Lack of antithrombin III may make heparin ineffective (Gitel et al., 1979). Antithrombin III infusion, in combination with heparin, has been shown to prevent postoperative venous thrombosis in total hip replacement (Francis et al., 1989). Desmopressin could possibly replace antithrombin III infusions, which are extremely expensive.

THROMBOEMBOLISM

Deep venous thrombi were found in six out of 44 patients, examined by phlebography on day 8 ±1 after total hip replacement (Table 2). All thrombi were short (5–30 mm) and non-occluding and none produced clinical signs or needed medical treatment.

Table 2. Thromboembolic complications in 50 total hip replacement patients.

	Control	Desmopressin	Difference
Deep venous thrombi	4/22	2/22	n.s.
- distal	2/22	2/22	n.s.
- proximal	2/22	0/22	n.s.
Pulmonary embolism	1/25	1/25	n.s.
Deep venous thrombosis or pulmonary embolism	5/25	2/25	n.s.

One patient in each group developed pulmonary embolism, confirmed by pulmonary ventilation and perfusion scintigraphy on clinical suspicion. The placebo patient had sudden dyspnoea on the 13th postoperative day. Phlebography had been unsuccessful in his case because of difficulties inserting the venous cannula in the foot. The desmopressin-treated patient had light coughing from the fifth postoperative day and pulmonary embolism was not confirmed until the 42nd postoperative day. On phlebography he was seen to have a 30-mm thrombus in the peroneal vein. Both patients were treated with heparin and warfarin and recovered completely.

Two patients in the placebo group had proximal thrombosis; none did in the desmopressin group. Five patients in the placebo group had thromboembolic events, compared with two in the desmopressin group. The differences were not statistically significant, so one cannot conclude that desmopressin reduces the risk of thromboembolic events, but no evidence was found of an increase, as speculated by some authors (Melissari et al., 1986).

Previously reported fears that a FVIII complex increase induces a risk of venous thrombosis (Bonnar et al., 1973; Bredbacka et al., 1986; Melissari et al., 1986; Petäjä et al., 1989) were contradicted by this study. Platelet function is of minor importance to the risk of formation of venous thrombi (Ogston, 1987). The vWF increase should therefore be without risks, and the increase in FVIII seems to be balanced by the simultaneous stimulation of fibrinolysis.

REFERENCES

Bonnar, J., Walsh, J.J., Haddon, M., Fairweather, J., and Denson, K.W.E., 1973, Coagulation system changes induced by pelvic surgery and the effect of dextran 70, *Bibl Anat.* 12:351–5.

Bonnet, F., Harari, A., Thibonnier, M., and Viars, P., 1982, Suppression of antidiuretic hormone hypersecretion during surgery by extradural anaesthesia, *Br J Anaesth.* 54:29–35.

Brain Power, Inc., 1986, "StatView 512+", Abacus Concepts Inc, Calabasas.

Bredbacka, S., Blombäck, M., Hägnevik, K., Irestedt, L., and Raabe, N., 1986, Per- and postoperative changes in coagulation and fibrinolytic variables during abdominal hysterectomy under epidural or general anaesthesia, *Acta Anaesthesiol Scand.* 30:204–10.

Czer, L.S.C., Bateman, T.M., Gray, R.J., Raymond, M., Stewart, M.E., Lee, S., Goldfinger, D., Chaux, A., and Matloff, J.M., 1987, Treatment of severe platelet dysfunction and hemorrhage after cardiopulmonary bypass: reduction in blood product usage with desmopressin, *J Am Coll Cardiol.* 9:1139–47.

Derkx, F.H., Man in't Veld, A.J., Jones, R., Reid, J.L., and Schalekamp, M.A.D.H., 1983, DDAVP (1-desamino-8-D-arginine vasopressin): an antagonist of the pressor action of endogenous vasopressin? *J Hypertens.* 1(suppl 2):58–61.

Eriksson, B.I., Eriksson, E., Gyzander, E., Teger-Nilsson, A.C., and Risberg, B., 1989, Thrombosis after hip replacement. Relationship to the fibrinolytic system, *Acta Orthop Scand.* 60:159–63.

Eriksson, B.I., Eriksson, E., and Risberg, B., 1991, Impaired fibrinolysis and postoperative thromboembolism in orthopedic patients, *Thromb Res.* in press.

Felez, J., 1990, Biochemical aspects of the pathogenesis of venous thrombosis, *Acta Chir Scand.* suppl 556:9–17.

Flordal, P.A., and Ljungström, K.-G., 1991, Renal effects of high dose desmopressin and dextran, *Acta Anaesthesiol Scand.* in press.

Flordal, P.A., Ljungström, K.-G., Fehrm, A., Ekman, B., and Neander, G., 1991a, Desmopressin in total hip replacement – effects on blood loss and thromboembolism, submitted for publication.

Flordal, P.A., Ljungström, K.-G., Svensson, J., Ekman, B., and Neander G., 1991b, Effects on coagulation and fibrinolysis of desmopressin in patients undergoing total hip replacement, *Thromb Haemost.* 66:562–6.

Francis, C.W., Pellegrini, V.D., Marder, V.J., Harris, C.M., Totterman, S., Gabriel, K.R., Baughman, D.J., Roemer, S., Burke, J., Goodman, T.L., and Evarts, C.M.C., 1989, Prevention of venous thrombosis after total hip arthroplasty. Antithrombin III and low-dose heparin compared with dextran 40, *J Bone Joint Surg. [Am]* 71-A:327–35.

Gitel, S.N., Salvati, E.A., Wessler, S., Robinson, H.J., and Worth, M.H., 1979, The effect of total hip replacement and general surgery on antithrombin III in relation to venous thrombosis, *J Bone Joint Surg. [Am]* 61-A:653–6.

Goodman-Gilman, A., Rall, T.W., Nies, A.S., and Taylor, P., eds., 1990, "Goodman and Gilman's The Pharmacological Basis of Therapeutics", 8th ed., Pergamon Press, Inc., New York.

Kehlet, H., 1984, The stress response to anaesthesia and surgery: release mechanisms and modifying factors, *Clin Anaesthesiol.* 2:315–39.

Kobrinsky, N.L., Letts, R.M., Patel, L.R., Israels, E.D., Monson, R.C., Schwetz, N., and Cheang, M.S., 1987, 1-desamino-8-D-arginine vasopressin (desmopressin) decreases operative blood loss in patients having Harrington rod spinal fusion surgery. A randomized, double-blinded, controlled trial, *Ann Intern Med.* 107:446–50.

Mannucci, P.M., Åberg, M., Nilsson, I.M., and Robertson, B., 1975, Mechanism of plasminogen activator and factor VIII increase after vasoactive drugs, *Br J Haematol.* 30:81–93.

Mannucci, P.M., and Lusher, J.M., 1989, Desmopressin and thrombosis, *Lancet* ii:675–6.

Mannucci, P.M., Ruggeri, Z.M., Pareti, F.I., and Capitano, A., 1977, 1-deamino-8-D-arginine vasopressin: a new pharmacological approach to the management of haemophilia and von Willebrand's disease, *Lancet* i:869–72.

Melissari, E., Scully, M.F., Paes, T., Ellis, V., and Kakkar, V.V., 1986, The influence of DDAVP infusion on the coagulation and fibrinolytic response to surgery, *Thromb Haemost.* 55:54–7.

Modig, J., Malmberg, P., and Karlström, G., 1980, Effect of epidural versus general anaesthesia on calf blood flow, *Acta Anaesthesiol Scand.* 24:305–9.

Myllylä, G., 1988, New transfusion practice and haemostasis, *Acta Anaesthesiol Scand.* 32(suppl 89):76–80.

Nilsen, D.W.T., Haerem, J., Westheim, A., Skjennald, A., Grendahl, H., and Godal, H.C., 1984, Venous thrombosis following diagnostic transvenous catheterization by percutaneous catheter insertion: an evaluation of desmopressin as a thromboprophylactic agent, *Thromb Haemost.* 52:121–3.

Ogston, D., 1987, "Venous Thrombosis. Causation and Prediction", Wiley, Chichester.

Petäjä, J., Myllynen, P., Rokkanen, P., and Nokelainen, M., 1989, Fibrinolysis and spinal injury. Relationship to post-traumatic deep vein thrombosis, *Acta Chir Scand.* 155:241–6.

Punnonen, R., and Viinamäki, O., 1983, Vasopressin release following operation upon the vagina performed under general anesthesia or epidural analgesis, *Surg Gynecol Obstet.* 156:781–4.

Rabinov, K., and Paulin, S., 1972, Roentgen diagnosis of venous thrombosis in the leg, *Arch Surg.* 104:134–44.

Reeve, E.B., 1980, Steady state relations between factors X, Xa, II, IIa, antithrombin III and alpha-2 macroglobulin in thrombosis, *Thromb Res.* 18:19–31.

Richardson, D.W., and Robinson, A.G., 1985, Desmopressin, *Ann Intern Med.* 103:228–39.

Rocha, E., Llorens, R., Páramo, J.A., Arcas, R., Cuesta, B., and Martín Trenor, A., 1988, Does desmopressin acetate reduce blood loss after surgery in patients on cardiopulmonary bypass? *Circulation* 77:1319–23.

Salzman, E.W., Weinstein, M.J., Weintraub, R.M., Ware, J.A., Thurer, R.L., Robertson, L., Donovan, A., Gaffney, T., Bertele, V., Troll, J., Smith, M., and Chute, L.E., 1986, Treatment with desmopressin acetate to reduce blood loss after cardiac surgery. A double-blind randomized trial, *N Engl J Med.* 314:1402–6.

Törnebohm, E., Bratt, G., Granqvist, S., Lockner, D., and Egberg, N., 1987, A pilot study: desmopressin (DDAVP) in the treatment of deep venous thrombosis, *Thromb Res.* 45:635–43.

Vilhardt, H., Lundin, S., and Falch, J., 1986, Plasma kinetics of DDAVP in man, *Acta Pharmacol et Toxicol.* 58:379–81.

Welin-Berger, T., Bygdeman, S., and Mebius, C., 1982, Deep vein thrombosis following hip surgery. Relation to activated factor X inhibitor activity: effect of heparin and dextran, *Acta Orthop Scand.* 53:937–45.

West, B.J., ed., 1985, "Best and Taylor's Physiological Basis of Medical Practice", 11th ed., Williams & Wilkins, Baltimore, p 467.

Westermann, K., Trentz, O., Pretschner, P., and Mellmann, J., 1981, Thromboembolism after hip surgery, *Int Orthop.* 4:253–7.

Westman, L., Hamberger, B., and Järnberg, P.O., 1988, Effects of ephedrine on renal function in patients after major vascular surgery, *Acta Anaesthesiol Scand.* 32:271–7.

Winer, B.J., 1971, "Statistical Principles in Experimental Design", Mc Graw-Hill, New York, pp 514–603.

DISCUSSION

Bichet: What were the glomerular filtration rates of the controls and the surgical patients? Could the rise in GFR be due to osmotic diuresis? Did you measure the urinary osmolarity in the patients?

Flordal: Urinary output in both groups was the same. They had the same pre-operative hydration and osmolarity. The excretion of osmoles was the same, with the same fluids, the same blood loss, and no difference in the administration of anaesthetics.

Bichet: The volunteers had no blood loss! In the surgical patients the rise in GFR may have been due to the additional blood and fluids over and above the controls. The total osmolar excretion in the surgical patients must be higher than in the controls, so that there must be some osmotic diuresis. This could explain the results.
Flordal: The mean total osmolar excretion was exactly the same in the surgical patients as in the volunteers, and in both groups exactly the same with as without desmopressin. We did not measure free water clearance or natriuresis.

Kinter: Did you measure endogenous vasopressin?
Flordal: No.
Kinter: The levels were probably between 10 and 100pg/ml. With no more than 1000 pg/ml DDAVP and let's say 100 pg/ml vasopressin, there was only a 10-fold excess of DDAVP. Given the published affinities of these peptides for the V1 receptor, DDAVP would not be expected to displace AVP. I would look for other explanations, such as the osmotic hypothesis, or the role of other autocoids.
Flordal: Our hypothesis is that DDAVP binds to V1, but causes no activity.
Kinter: There is no evidence from the literature that this occurs.
Flordal: The antidiuretic effect, in any case, is not a problem in surgery.

DDAVP CORRECTS THE PLATELET DYSFUNCTION PRODUCED BY CARDIOPULMONARY BY-PASS, HEMODIALYSIS, AND PROLONGED STORAGE: RE-EXPRESSION OF GLYCOPROTEIN Ib ON THE PLATELET MEMBRANE

E.M. Sloand[1], C.M. Kessler[2], J. Sloand[3], and K. Prodouz[4]

[1]National Heart, Lung, and Blood Institute
Bethesda, Maryland
[2]The George Washington University Medical Center
Washington DC
[3]The University of Rochester, Rochester, New York
[4]Center for Biologics Evaluation and Research, FDA
Bethesda, Maryland

INTRODUCTION

Varying degrees of qualitative platelet dysfunction are observed in all patients who have undergone surgical procedures utilizing cardiopulmonary bypass (CPB), often resulting in severe hemorragic complications[1-8]and necessitating mediastinal reexploration to control excessive bleeding in up to 3% of patients[5]. Because similar platelet abnormalities have been described following hemodialysis (HD), the mechanism for defective hemostasis is believed to be related to activation and in vivo release of platelets circulating over oxygenation and dialysis membranes[4],perhaps creating an acquired storage pool defciency[7]. Platelet transfusions are often indicated in these patients to initiate hemostasis. The effectiveness of these platelets are influenced by conditions and duration of storage, which ironically may be conducive to the development of platelet defects resembling those produced by CPB and HD[9]. Desmopressin acetate (DDAVP) has been used succesfully to reverse the severe platelet dysfunction and hemorrhage produced by CPB[10,11]via a mechanism which involves von Willebrand factor protein interactions between the platelets and subendothelial connective tissue[10]. This study examines the alterations of platelet membrane glycoproteins induced by CPB, HD, and blood bank storage and demonstrates that DDAVP can stimulate the redistribution of cytosolic glycoprotein Ib, which can be translated into enhanced platelet function in vitro.

Desmopressin in Bleeding Disorders, Edited by G. Mariani *et al.*
Plenum Press, New York, 1993

METHODS AND MATERIALS

Patient Population

Nine patients undergoing cardiopulmonary bypass (CPB) for coronary artery bypass grafting or valve replacement, between the ages of 20 and 80, were recruited from George Washington University. All but patients denied ingestion of aspirin or other non-steroidal anti-inflammatory agents. Patients receiving platelet concentrates during or immediately after their surgery were excluded from the study. Amembrane oxygenator was used for all cases. One additional patient receiving chronic hemodilysis (HD) for renal failure secondary to hypertension was also recruited.

Platelet Preparation

Arterial blood was obtained through an indwelling arterial catheter in CPB patients or from a catheter placed in the arteriovenous fistula of a HD patient. Blood was drawn into polypropylene tubes containing citrate to a final concentration of 3.8% (v/v). Platelet-rich plasma (PRP) was prepared by centrifuging blood at 1600g for 3 minutes. PRP was diluted immediately by addition of phosphate buffered saline (PBS) pH 7.4, after which an equal volume of PBS with 2 percent formalin was added. Samples were incubated for 5 minutes at 37°C and refrigerated at 4°C until tests of antibody binding could be performed. Samples were stored less than three days before antibody binding was determined.

DDAVP: EFFECT OF PLATELET MEMBRANE GLYCOPROTEIN EXPRESSION

Effect in CPB and HD Patients

In order to assess the effect of DDAVP on platelets obtained from patients subjected to CPB and HD, DDAVP (Rorer Pharmaceutical Corp, Fort Washingto, Pa) (0.004 µg/ml) was added to one aliquot from a split sample of PRP obtained after CPB or HD and incubated for 1 hour at room temperature with intermittent agitation; the other aliquot of the sample was incubated in a similar manner but without the addition of DDAVP. Platelets were then prepared for flow cytometry as described below after staining with antibodies.

Effect on Stored Platelets

In a second set of experiments, nine 100 ml samples of plateletpheresis concentrates obtained from normal donors were stored for five days in PL732 platelet storage bags (Fenwal, Baxter Health Care, Deerfield, Ill) at 22°C with constant agitation. Samples were split into two 50 ml aliquots and DDAVP (0.004 µg/ml) was added to one of the bags. Both aliquots were stored under similar conditions for 24 hours. Samples were removed from the storage bags after 24 hours and prepared for platelet antibody staining as described below.

Measurement of Antibody Binding

Monoclonal antibodies to platelet glycoproteins were incubated with the platelet preparations for twenty minutes at room temperature. The monoclonal antibodies that were used were anti-CD42b-FITC (Gen Trak, Inc., Plymouth Meeting, Pa), an antibody to the vWF binding site of GPIb; anti GPIb/IX (Gen Trak, Inc.); and Plt-1-FITC (Coulter Immunology, Hialeah, Fl), an antibody directed against GPIIb/IIIa. Fluorescence intensity indicative of antibody binding

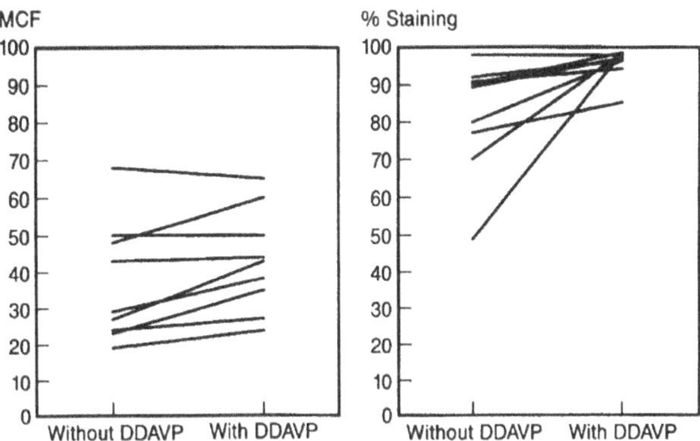

Figure 1. Samples of PRP obtained from patients undergoing CPB at the completion of surgery were incubated with DDAVP (0.004 µg/mL) for one hour at room temperature with intermittent agitation. Samples were stained with FITC-conjugated antibody to GPIb as previously described. Mean Channel Flourescence (MCF) and percent of platelet staining are shown above

was analized on a Becton Dickinson FACScan flow cytometer with Consort 30 Software (Becton Dickinson, San Jose, Ca).

Effect of DDAVP on Platelets Response to Ristocetin

We prepared formalin-fixed platelets for ristocetin agglutination by a method modified from Coller et al[12] using Gaintner's buffer (5 mM KH_2PO_4, 41 mM $NaH_2PO_4H_2O$, 0.1 M NaCl, 0.1% dextrose, pH 4.5). The platelet suspension (0.35 mL) was adjusted to a count of 3 X 10^5 per mm^3 and incubated at 37°C with 0.1 mL of pooled normal plasma (6 donors). We induced agglutination by adding 0.05 mL of ristocetin (1.5 mg/mL) and then measured the mean rate of agglutination.

DDAVP (0.004 µg/mL) was added to 20 mL aliquots of plateletpheresis concentrated previously stored for 5 days at 22°C with constant agitation. After an additional 24 hours, samples were formalinized and used for flow cytometry studies or ristocetin-induced agglutination.

Statistical Analysis

Mean channel fluorescence (MCF) measurements and percent of platelets binding antibody were compared for platelets incubated with DDAVP and platelets non incubated with DDAVP by using a one sample Wilcoxan test for non-parametric statistics.

RESULTS

Effect of DDAVP on Samples Obtained After CPB and HD

When platelet samples obtained immediately following CPB or HD were incubated with 0.004 µg/ml of DDAVP for one hour at room temperature, there was an increase in binding of anti-CD42b antibody in all ten samples from CPB patients and in the one HD patient as measured by increases in both mean channel fluorescence and percent of platelets staining. The differences in samples obtained form patients on CPB were statistically significant ($p = 0.02$ when both percent of platelets binding antibody and mean channel fluorescence were analyzed) (Figure 1). Similar changes were seen when anti-GPIb/IX antibody was used (Figure 2). There were no changes in binding of antibody to GPIIb/IIIa induced by DDAVP.

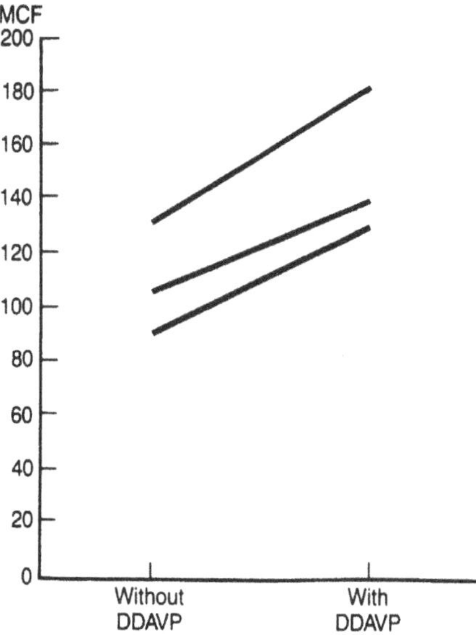

Figure 2. Samples of PRP obtained from CPB patients at the completion of surgery were incubated with DDAVP (0.004 µg/mL) for one hour with intermittent agitation and stained with antibody to GPIb/IX (Coulter Immunology) as previously described. MCF of platelet staining with antibody is shown above.

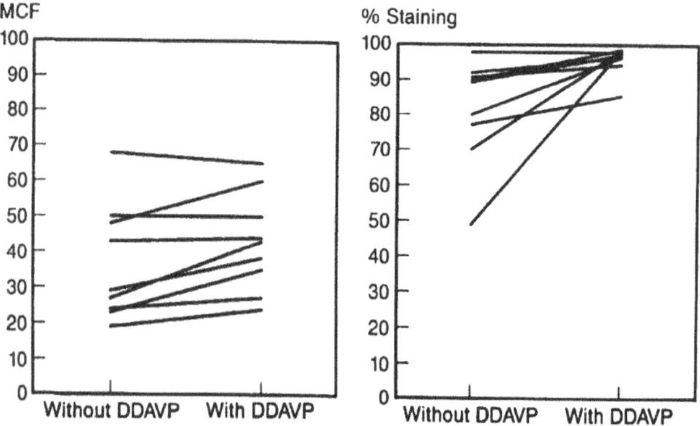

Figure 3. Nine plateletpheresis samples obtained from normal donors and stored for five days in PL732 platelet storage bags were split into two aliquots. DDAVP was added (0.004 µg/mL) to one of the split samples and both samples were stored at 22°C with constant agitation for 24 hours in PL732 platelet storage bags. Samples were then removed and stained with antibody to GPIb (Gen Trak Inc) as previously described. MCF and percent of platelet staining with

Effect of DDAVP on Stored Platelet Samples

When six sets of 5 day old platelets were incubated with DDAVP (0.004 µg/ml) for 24 hours with constant agitation at 22°C, all samples demonstrated a statistically significant increase in the percent of platelets binding anti-CD42b ($p = 0.032$) (Figure 3). There was no significant difference in the MCF between treated and non-treated samples ($p = 0.124$). Neither the platelet count, the mean platelet volume, nor the pH of the PRP were changed by DDAVP. There were no changes in binding of antibody to GPIIb/IIIa induced by DDAVP. The increase responsiveness to ristocetin induced platelet aggregation was correlated proportionally to increases in anti-GPIb antibody binding, as seen for four additional samples in Table 1.

CONCLUSION

Excessive bleeding is a fairly frequent phenomenon accompanying cardiopulmonary bypass[1-5]. There are multiple reasons for defective hemostasis. These include dilutional thrombocytopenia[3] and coagulation factor depletion[5], as well as acquired platelet disfunction. The latter is generally transient in nature and is characterized by prolongation of bleeding time[4], defective platelet adhesion to glass beads[6], abnormal congregation in response to agonists (adenosine diphosphate, epinephrine, collagen)[4,6,7] and decreased agglutination to ristocetin[6,8]. Platelet defects are more pronounced when a bubble oxygenator rather than a membrane oxygenator is used. Prior coating of the oxygenator with albumin or low molecular weight dextran helps minimize the adverse effects on platelets6,13. The structural composition of the large molecular weight multimers of von Willebrand factor protein have been reported to be abnormal by some investgators[1,14,15] but normal by others[16]. George et al[17] have demonstrated a loss of platelet membrane GPIb and GPIIb/IIIa in patients on CPB; loss of membrane glycoproteins is accompanied by appearance of microvesicles in the plasma which are capable of binding antibody to both GPIb and GPIIb/IIIa. These findings are distinctly different from those seen following platelet activation by thrombin, which results in decreased membrane GPIb and increases in membrane GPIIb/IIIa. Changes induced by thrombin are believed to result from internalization of GPIb and mobilization of intracytoplasmic GPIIb/IIIa. However, Michelson et al[18] did not demonstrate any changes in platelet GPIb during CPB. Differences in duration of bypass, sample preparation, and type of oxygenator could have accounted for these discrepancies. In a previous study[19] we demonstrated decreases in platelet membrane and total platelet GPIb which occured during surgery in the majority of patients; the most pronounced changes occured in those having the longest time on bypass. Samples obtained the day following surgery showed an increase in platelet membrane GPIb, while total platelet GPIb was unchanged; the increase in membrane expression following surgery may have resulted from mobilization of intracytoplasmic stores. Similar findings were also seen in one patient on HD (data non presented).

The changes observed in platelets incubated with DDAVP are of great interest. DDAVP infusion has been shown to decrease blood loss during and following CPB in some studies[10,11], although others have failed to demonstrate an effect[16,20-23]. In one study the only group of patients demonstrating benefit from DDAVP was the group with abnormal platelet response to ristocetin before surgery[22]. As ristocetin agglutination is GPIb-dependent, these findings are consistent with our observations that DDAVP influences GPIb expression. Studies showing a DDAVP-associated improvement in bleeding time in patients with platelets storage pool disease and Glanzman's thrombasthenia[23] but no effect on persons with Bernard Soulier Disease (who lack GPIb)[24] also suggest an association between DDAVP-induced changes in hemostasis and changes in GPIb expression.

In conclusion, DDAVP was able to increase platelet membrane expression of GPIb without changes in other membrane proteins in platelets obtained after CPB and HD, as well as in platelets stored five days under blood banking conditions. These observations may lead to increased understanding of the platelet dysfunction related to extra-corporeal procedures and may have clinical implications for patient management.

Table 1. Effect of DDAVP on the Staining and Functional Properties of Stored Platelets

Sample Number	DDAVP	MCF	% staining	Slope of Ristocetin Agglutination
1	yes	41.0	97	0.40
	no	42.1	98	0.52
2	yes	50.7	95	1.10
	no	36.7	96	0.0
3	yes	50.4	86	1.3
	no	44.1	77	0.4
4	yes	53.0	97	0.3
	no	41.0	98	0.0

Samples of plateletpheresis concentrates stored for 5 days in PL732 platelet storage bags (Fenwal) at 22°C with constant agitation were divided into two 20 mL aliquots. DDAVP (0.004 µg/mL) was added to one sample and an equal volume of saline was added to the other sample. Samples were stored for 24 hours at 22°C with constant agitation in PL732 storage bags for 24 hours. Samples were then fixed with formalin, prepared for flow cytometry and stained with anti-GPIb (GenTrak) as previously described. Samples to be prepared for ristocetin agglutination were washed in PBS as previously described. The mean slope of agglutination, MCF, and percent of platelet staining with antibody were recorded for samples stored with DDAVP and compared to those stored without.

REFERENCES

1. E.F. Mammen, M.H. Koets, B.C. Washington,et al: Hemostasis changes during cardiopulmonary bypass surgery. Sem Thromb Hemosta 11:281(1985).
2. R. McKenna, F. Bachmann, B. Whittaker, J.R. Gilson, M. Weinberg: The hemostatic mechanism after open-heart surgery. II. Frequency of abnormal platelet functions during and after extracorporeal circulation. Thorac Cardiovascu Surg 70:298(1975).
3. L.A. Harker, T.W. Malpass, H.E. Branson, E.A. Hessel,S.J. Slichter: Mechanism of abnormal bleeding in patients undergoing cardiopulmonary bypass: acquired transient platelet dysfunction associated with selected _-granule release. Blood 56:824 (1980).
4. R.L. Bick: Alterations of hemostasis associated with cardiopulmonary bypass: Pathophysiology, prevention, diagnosis,and management. Sem Thromb Hemosta 3:59 (1976).

5. F. Bachmann, R. Mc Kenna, E.R. Cole, H. Najafi: The hemostatic mechanism after open-heart surgery. I. Studies on plasma coagulation factors and fibrinolysis in 512 patients after extracorporeal circulation. J Thorac Cardiovasc Surg 70:76 (1975).
6. R.L. Bick: Hemostasis defects associated with cardiac surgery,prosthetic devices, and other extracorporeal circuits. Sem Thromb Hemostas 11:249 (1985).
7. W.R. Friedenberg, W.O. Myers, E.D. Plotke, J.N. Beathard, D.J. Kummer, P.F. Gatlin, D.L. Stoiber, J.F. Ray, R.D. Sautter: Platelet dysfunction associated with cardiopulmonary bypass. Ann Thorac Surg 25:298 (1978).
8. R. Mohr, M.Golan, U. Martinowitz, E. Rosner, D.A. Goor, B. Ramot: Effect of cardiac operation on platelets. J Thora Cardiovasc Surg 92:434 (1986).
9. A.D. Michelson, B. Adelman, M.R. Barnard, E. Carrol, R.I. Handin: Platelet storage results in a redistribution of glycoprotein Ib molecules. J. Clin Invest 81:1734 (1988).
10. E.W. Salzman, M.J. Weinstein, R.M. Weintraub, et al: Treatment with desmopressin acetate to reduce blood loss after cardiac surgery. A double-blind randomized trial. N Engl J Med 314:1402 (1986).
11. L.S. Czer, T.M. Batemen, R.J. Gray, et al: Treatment of severe platelet dysfunction and hemorrhage after cardiopulmonary bypass: reduction in blood product usage with desmopressin. JACC 9:1139 (1987).
12. B.S. Coller, B.R. Franza, Jr., H.R. Gralnick: The pH dependance of qualitative ristocetin-induced platelet aggregation: Theoretical and practical implications - a new device for maintenance of platelet rich plasma pH. Blood 47:841 (1975).
13. V.P. Addonizio, E.J. Macarak, K.C. Nicolaou, L.H. Edumunds, R.W. Colman: Effects of prostacyclin and albumin on platelet loss during in vitro simulation of extracorporeal circulation. Blood 53:1033 (1979).
14. E. Rocha, R. Llorens, J.A. Paramo, R. Arcas, B. Cuesta, A.M. Renor: Does desmopressin acetate reduce blood loss after surgery in patients on cardipulmonary bypass? Circulation 77:1319 (1988).
15. M. Weinstein, A.J. Ware, J. Troll, E. Salzman: Changes in von Willebrand factor during cardiac surgery : effect of desmopressin acetate. Blood 71:1648 (1988).
16. T.L.G. Anderson, J. Otto Solem, L. Tengborn, E. Vinge: Effects of Desmopressin acetate on platelet aggregation, von Willebrand factor, and blood loss after cardiac surgery with extracorporeal circulation. Circulation 81:872 (1990).
17.J.N. George, E.B. Pickett, S. Saucerman: Platelet membrane glycoproteins: Studies on resting and activated platelets and platelet membrane in normal subjects and observations in patients during Adult Respiratory Distress Syndrome and cardiac surgery. J Clin Invest 78:340 (1986b).
18. A.S. Kestin, C.R. Valeri, S.F. Khuri, et al: The platelet function defect of cardiopulmonary bypass surgery. Blood 78:144a (1991).
19. E.M. Sloand,J. Sloand, C. Kessler, K.Prodouz: Loss of glycoprotein Ib from platelets on hemodialysis (HD) or cardiopulmonary bypass (CABG) is followed by it reexpression on the platelet membrane. Blood 78:388a (1991).
20. M.D. Sear, L.D. Wadsworth, P.C. Rogers, S. Sheps, P.G. Ashmore: The effect of desmopressin acetate (DDAVP) on postoperative blood loss after cardiac operations in children. J Thorac Cardiovasc Surg 98:217 (1989).
21. G.S. Hedderich, D.J. Petsikas, B.A. Cooper, et al: Desmopressin acetate in uncomplicated coronary artery bypass surgery: a prospective randomized clinical trial. CJS 33:33 (1990).
22. W.D. Lazenby, I. Russo, J.A. Zadeh: Treatment with Desmopressin acetate in routine coronary artery bypass surgery to improve postoperative hemostasis. Circulation 82:IV-413 (1990).

23. J.M. Lusher: Pharmacology and pharmacokinetics of Desmopressin in haemostatic disorders. Drug Invest 2 (Suppl 5):25 (1990).
24. E. Waldenstrom, L. Holmberg, U. Axelsson, I. Wingvist, I.M. Nilsson: Bernard Soulier syndrome in two Swedish families: Effect of DDAVP on bleeding time. Eur J Haematol 46:182 (1991).

DISCUSSION

Cattaneo: Can you speculate how DDAVP may affect platelets?
Kessler: It may mediate calcium fluxes in platelets. we are now studying in vivo samples to see if the changes in surgery and hemodialysis can be prevented by DDAVP. We may be able to store platelets for 5 days, increase ristocetin co-factor and perhaps restore them to make them more functional.

Stuart: Have you correlated platelet function to your results?
Kessler: To give platelets that have been stored would need first an institutional review. We do not yet have this.
Rao: We found no effect of DDAVP on platelet calcium levels, ADP, thrombin, or PAF, so I do not feel that it enhances calcium distribution.

DESMOPRESSIN IN THE TREATMENT OF CONGENITAL AND ACQUIRED DEFECTS OF PLATELET FUNCTIONS

Marco Cattaneo and Pier Mannuccio Mannucci

Angelo Bianchi Bonomi Hemophilia and Thrombosis Centre
Institute of Internal Medicine
I.R.C.C.S. Maggiore Hospital and University of Milano
Milano, Italy

INTRODUCTION

Desmopressin (DDAVP) is mainly used in an autologous replacement therapy in patients with congenital or acquired deficiencies of factor VII and von Willebrand factor, which are raised in plasma by the drug. Its efficacy as hemostatic agent in these disorders has been clearly established[1] (see also corresponding chapters in this book).

There, however, several observations indicating that DDAVP may also be effective, through less specific mechanisms, in congenital and acquired defects of primary hemostasis not caused by defects of von Willebrand factor[1]. Most of the studies have evaluated the effects of DDAVP on the bleeding time, which is the most useful test to explore primary hemostasis, but may be an unsatisfactory predictor of post-surgical bleeding[2]. It must be emphasized, therefore, that, although there are anecdotal reports on the clinical efficacy of the drug, definite evidence that desmopressin reduces the risk of bleeding in patients with defects of primary hemostasis is still lacking, because no controlled, double-blind clinical study has been performed so far.

CONGENITAL DEFECTS OF PLATELET FUNCTION

Intravenous DDAVP, at a dose of 0.3 µg/Kg, shortens or normalizes the bleeding time of patients with congenital platelet dysfunctions[3-7]. There is usually a good response in patients with defects of the platelet release reaction, with platelet cyclooxygenase deficiency and in those with isolated and unexplained prolongations of the bleeding time. Some patients with congenital storage pool deficiency respond but others do not[4]. Since there is no established laboratory or clinical predictor of the effect of the drug in these patients, but the response tends to be consistent for each individual patient, responders should be identified by performing a test infusion of the drug at the time of diagnosis or before clinical use.

Clinical studies suggest that DDAVP can be used as an alternative to blood products

Desmopressin in Bleeding Disorders, Edited by G. Mariani *et al.*
Plenum Press, New York, 1993

do not respond[4], indicating that the integrity of the glycoprotein IIb/IIIa complex is essential for the drug to be efficacious.

ACQUIRED DEFECTS OF PLATELET FUNCTION

Uremia

Two indipendent groups of investigators[8,9] gave 0.3 or 0.4 µg/Kg of DDAVP intravenously to patients with chronic renal failure and found that the prolonged bleeding time became normal in 75% of these patients 1 hour after the infusion started. In one of the original studies, and in subsequent studies, DDAVP was also successfully employed to prevent bleeding after surgical procedures in patients with acute or chronic renal failure[9-11] (see corresponding chapters). Recently it has been shown subcutaneous desmopressin too (0.3 µg/Kg) markedly shortens the bleeding time in patients with uremia[12].

Liver cirrhosis

It is not completely understood why the bleeding time is prolonged in some patients with liver cirrhosis. There is usually mild or moderate thrombocytopenia, but counts are not correlated negatively with the bleeding time. Factor VIII and von Willebrand factor levels in cirrhosis are in the high normal range or even higher. Two double-blind, placebo-controlled crossover studies showed that intravenous DDAVP (0.3 µg/Kg) shortened the prolonged bleeding time of patients with liver cirrhosis[4,13]. More recently, it has been shown that also subcutaneous DDAVP is efficacious[14]. Hence DDAVP is a possible treatment for patients with liver cirrhosis and prolonged bleeding times who need invasive diagnostic procedures or with spontaneous mucosal bleedings; however, as already noticed, controlled clinical trials are needed to test this hypothesis and validate DDAVP treatment (see De Franchis et al in this book).

Thrombocytopenia

DDAVP is ineffective in patients with severe thrombocytopenia[4] indicating that there is a critical platelet number for the effect to be manifested (at approximately 50,000 platelets/µl). More recently, however, Kobrinski et al showed that DDAVP may be hemostatically effective in severe amegacaryocytic thrombocytopenia (see Kobrinski et al in this book).

Antiaggregating drugs

Desmopressin counteracts the antihemostatic effects of severaldrugs employed for treatment of thrombotic disorders. It does shorten the prolonged bleeding times of individuals who are taking the antiaggregating agents aspirin[3,4] and ticlopidine[4]; the prolonged bleeding time and activated partial thromboplastin times of patients treated with heparin[15]; the bleeding time of rabbits treated with aspirin and streptokinase[16], but human data are not available; finally, it counteracts the antihemostatic effects on dextran, with no apparent impairment of the antithrombotic properties of this product[17]. Even though there is no evidence yet that DDAVP can prevent or stop bleeding complications developing in association with the use of these products, it might give us an opportunity to control drug-induced bleeding without stopping treatment and perhaps avoiding recurrence or progression of thrombosis.

MECHANISMS INVOLVED IN DDAVP-INDUCED SHORTENING OF THE BLEEDING TIME

It is not completely understood why the compound shortens the bleeding time in clinical conditions with no associated defect or abnormalities of factor VIII and von Willebrand factor. It has been postulated that in these cases the favourable effects are mediated by the attainment of supranormal levels of von Willebrand factor in the circulation. As a matter of fact, the extent of platelet adhesion to the subendothelium appears to be correlated with the plasma levels of von Willebrand factor and is potentiated by the in vitro addition of purified von Willebrand factor[18]. Moreover, supralarge von Willebrand factor multimers, normally contained in endothelia cells but not in plasma, appear transiently in plasma after the infusion of DDAVP. Supra large multimers may be hemostatically more effective than "normal" multimers.

More recent data have demonstrated that DDAVP potentiates shear-induced platelet aggregation[19]. Shear-induced platelet aggregation requires von Willebrand factor and ADP, whereas it is completely independent of plasma and platelet fibrinogen[20-24]. Under conditions of blood flow characterized by high shear stress, which can be found in the microcirculation or at sites of severe arterial stenosis, plasma von Willebrand factor directly interacts with the platelet glycoprotein Ib/IX complex, leading to platelet activation, exposure of receptor function for adhesive glycoproteins on the platelet membrane glycoprotein complex IIb/IIIa, to which plasma and/or platelet von Willebrand factor bind, supporting platelet aggregation[24]. Therefore, different adhesive proteins and platelet membrane glycoproteins are involved in aggregation depending on the shear stress conditions. Fibrogen interaction with glycoprotein IIb/IIIa appears necessary at low shear[24], while von Willebrand factor interaction with both glycoprotein Ib/IX and IIb/IIIa is required at high shear.

The intravenous infusion of DDAVP (0.3 µg/Kg body weight) in normal volunteers significantly increases shear-induced platelet aggregation both under basal conditions and after its partial inhibition by oral ticlopidine[19]. The increase in shear-induced platelet aggregation is correlated with the plasma levels of von Willebrand factor. In contrast to shear-induced platelet aggregation, DDAVP does not affest the fibrogen-dependent platelet aggregation induced by exogenous agonists such as ADP, collagen or the thromboxane A_2 analogue U46619. Hence, the potentiation of shear-induced platelet aggregation by DDAVP is likely due to the induced increase in plasma von Willebrand factor levels and the appearance in the circulation of supralarge von Willebrand factor multimers, which support shear-induced platelet aggregation more effectively than "normal" multimers[20].

In summary, since supranormal levels of plasma von Willebrand factor increase platelet adhesion to the subendothelium and potentiate platelet aggregation at high shear, it is biologically plausible that the shortening of the bleeding time caused by DDAVP in patients with normal plasma von Willebrand factor levels is mediated, at least in part, by released von Willebrand factor.

Mechanisms independent of released von Willebrand factor have also been advocated[4,9], but only recently have they been demostrated to operate in vitro.

In 1989 a double blind randomized crossover study showed that the infusion of DDAVP in patients with severe von Willebrand desease (who are usually completely deficient in von Willebrand factor in plasma, endothelial cells and platelets) shortens their bleeding times, which had previously been partially corrected but not normalized by the infusion of cryoprecipitate[25]. Plasma von Willebrand factor levels, which had been normalized by the infusion of cryoprecipitate, did not change after the infusion of DDAVP and supralarge von Willebrand factor multimers did not appear in the circulation, since patients with severe von during or after surgery, assuring satisfactory hemostasis. Patients with Glanzmann Thrombasthenia

Willebrand desease lack von Willebrand factor in tissue stores. These findings must be taken as evidence that DDAVP shortens the prolonged bleeding time independently of released von Willebrand factor.

A second demonstration that DDAVP acts through a mechanism that is independent of released von Willebrand factor was given by Johnstone et al[16], who showed that DDAVP shortened the prolonged bleeding times of rabbits treated with streptokinase and aspirin without causing an increase in their plasma von Willebrand factor levels.

The nature of the mechanism independent of released von Willebrand factor is unknown. The hypothesis that the DDAVP-induced decrease in prostacylin production plays a major role in shortening the bleeding time[26] is unlikely, since the drug is efficacious in subjects treated with doses of aspirin high enough to abolish completely prostacylin production[3,4]. In an in vitro study, Barnhart et al[27] showed that desmopressin exerts its hemostatic effects by enhancing platelet adhesion onto damaged vessel wall through a mechanism not necessarily involving the release of von Willebrand factor. Recent data suggest that this effect might be mediated by the inhibition by DDAVP of 13-HODE, a lypooxygenase metabolite of linoleic acid which inhibits platelet adhesion (see corresponding chapter in thes book).

In conclusion, DDAVP shortens the prolonged bleeding times in a variety of congenital and acquired defects of primary hemostasis not caused by decreased and/or dysfunctional von Willebrand factor. Although case reports indicate that DDAVP might be clinically useful in such conditions, carefully designed controlled clinical trials should be performed to test its hemostatic effect. There are demonstrations that the effect of DDAVP is mediated by a mechanism that is independent of released von Willebrand factor, although its nature its not completely understood. On the other hand, it is biologically plausible that the effect of DDAVP is also partly mediated by released von Willebrand factor.

REFERENCES

1. P.M. Mannucci, Desmopressin: a nontransfusional form of treatment for congenital and acquired bleeding disorders, Blood 72:1449 (1988).
2. S.E. Lind, The bleeding time does not predict surgical bleeding, Blood 77:2547 (1991).
3. N.L. Kobrinsky, E.D. Israel, J.M. Gerrard, et al, Shortening of bleeding time by 1-deamino-8-D-arginine vasopressin in various bleeding disorders, Lancet 1:1145 (1984).
4. P.M. Mannucci, V. Vicente, L. Vianello, et al, Controlled trial of desmopressin (DDAVP) in liver cirrhosis and other conditions associated with a prolonged bleeding time, Blood 67:1148 (1986).
5. S. Schulman, H. Johnson, N. Edberg, et al, DDAVP-induced correction of prolonged bleeding time in patients with congenital platelet function defects, Thromb Res 45:165 (1987).
6. H.K. Nieuwenhuis and J.J. Sixma, 1-deamino-8-D-arginine vasopressin (desmopressin) shortens the bleeding time in storage pool deficiency, Ann Inern Med 108:65 (1988).
7. T.B. Kentro, R. Lottenberg, C.S. Kitchens, Clinical efficacy of desmopressing acetate for hemostatic control in patients with primary platelet disorders undergoing surgery, Am H Hematol 24:215 (1987).
8. A.J.S. Watson and J.A.B. Koegh, Effect of 1-deamino-8-D-arginine vasopressing on the prolonged bleeding time in chronic renal failure, Nephron 32:49 (1982).
9. P.M. Mannucci, G. Remuzzi, F. Pusineri, et al, Deamino-8-D-arginine vasopressing shortens the bleeding time in uremia, N Engl J Med 308:8 (1983).

10. E. Gotti, G. Mecca, C. Valentino, et al, Renal biopsy in patients with acute renal failure and prolonged mbleeding time, Lancet 2:978 (1984).
11. C. Canavese, M. Salomone, A. Paciti, et al, Reduced response of uremic bleeding time to repeated doses of desmopressin, Lancet 1:967 (1985).
12. G.L. Viganò, P.M. Mannucci, A. Lattuada, et al, Subcutaneous desmopressin (DDAVP) shortens the bleeding time in uremia, Am J Hematol 31:32 (1989).
13. A.K. Burroughs, K. Matthews, M. Qadiri, et al, Desmopressing and bleeding time in patients with cirrhosis, Br Med J 291:1377 (1985).
14. M. Cattaneo, P.M. Tenconi, I. Alberca, et al, Subcutaneous desmopressin (DDAVP) shortens the prolonged bleeding time in patients with liver cirrhosis, Thromb Haemostas 64:358 (1990).
15. S. Schulman, H. Johnsson, Heparin, DDAVP and the bleeding time, Thromb Haemostas 65:242 (1991).
16. M.T. Johnstone, T. Andrews, J.A. Ware, et al, Bleeding time prolongation with streptokinase and its reduction with 1-deamino-8-D-arginine vasopressin, Circulation 82:2142 (1990).
17. P.A. Flordal, K.-G. Ljungstrom, J. Svensson, Desmopressin reverses effects of dextram on von Willebrand factor, Thromb Haemostas 61:541 (1989).
18. K.S. Sakariassen, M. Cattaneo, A.V.D. Berg, et al, DDAVP enhances platelet adherence and platelet aggregate growth on human artery subendothelium, Blood 64:229 (1984).
19. M. Cattaneo, R. Lombardi, A. Lecchi, et al, Shear-induced platelet aggregation: potentiation by DDAVP and inhibition by ticlopidine, Thromb Haemostas 65:976 (abs.) (1991).
20. J.L. Moake, N.A. Turner, N.A. Stathopoulos, et al, Involvement of large plasma von Willebrand factor (vWF) multimers and usually large vWF forms derived from endotheial cells in shear stress-induced platelet aggregation, J Clin Invest 78:1456 (1986).
21. D.M. Peterson, N.A. Stathopoulos, T.D. Giorgio, et al, Shear-induced platelet aggregation requires von Willebrand factor and platelet membrane glycoproteins Ib and IIb-IIIa, Blood 69:625 (1987).
22. J.L. Moake, N.A. Turner, N.A. Stathopoulos, et al, Shear-induced platelet aggregation can be mediated by vWF released from platelets, as well as by exogenous large or unusually large vWF multimers, requires adenosine diphosphate, and is resistant to aspirin, Blood 71:1366 (1988).
23. M.W. Moritz, R.C. Reimers, R.K. Baker, et al, Role of the cytoplasmic and releasable ADP in platelet aggregation induced by laminar shear stress, J Lab Clin Med 101:537 (1983).
24. Y. Ikeda, M: Handa, K. Kawano, et al, The role of von Willebrand factor and fibrogen in platelet aggregation under varying shear stress, J Clin Invest 87:1234 (1991).
25. M. Cattaneo, m: Moia, P. Della Valle, et al, DDAVP shortens the prolonged bleeding times of patients with severe von Willebrand desease treated with cryoprecipitate. Evidence for a mechanism of action independent of released von Willebrand factor, Blood 74:1972 (1989).
26. M.J. Stuart, C. Ganley, M. Reed, et al, DDAVP inhibits prostacyclin formation: a potential mechanism for bleeding time correction in hemostatic disorders. Thromb Haemostas 54:151 (1985).
27. M.I. Barnhart, Shan-te Chen, M. Lusher, DDAVP: does the drug have a direct effect on the vessel wall? Thromb Res 31239 (1983).

DISCUSSION

Mayadas-Norton: Could the DDAVP be causing retraction of endothelial cells to expose the subendothelium which could allow more vWF to bind to the subendothelium?
Cattaneo: This mechanism is independent of vWf release, but it may be so.

Schulman: We did the same with human plasma concentrates and added DDAVP in patients with prolonged bleeding times before surgery. We can confirm your findings.

THE EFFECTIVENESS OF DESMOPRESSIN IN PATIENTS WITH DISORDERS OF PRIMARY HAEMOSTASIS

Sam Schulman

Department of Internal Medicine
Karolinska Hospital
S-104 01 Stockholm
Sweden

INTRODUCTION

Already in 1973 it was demonstrated by Gader et al that the vasopressin analog 1-deamino-8-D-arginine vasopressin (desmopressin) elevates the plasma concentration of coagulation factor VIII (F VIII), and one year later Ruggeri et al (1974) reported a similar effect on the von Willebrand factor (vWf). Subsequently, Mannucci et al (1977) demonstrated the clinical applicability of desmopressin in patients with mild forms of hemophilia A and von Willebrand's disease (vWD). A few years later it became obvious that desmopressin could shorten the bleeding time in uremia (Mannucci et al ., 1983), congenital or aspirin-induced platelet defects (Kobrinsky et al., 1984) as well as liver cirrhosis (Burroughs et al., 1985), in spite of the fact that the level of F VIII and vWf was normal or often high in these patients. We could show that most of the patients (27 of 37) with congenital platelet function disorders had a normalisation of the bleeding time after injection with desmopressin 0.2 µg/kg, and that 8 of those patients, undergoing surgery or vaginal delivery, did not experience bleeding complications when prophylaxis with desmopressin was given (Schulman et al., 1987).

It has been hard to prove the effectiveness of desmopressin in a placebo-controlled randomized study in these patients. Firstly, many of the patients have experienced bleeding complications in connection with previous surgical procedures, when no prophylaxis against hemorrhage was provided, leading to the diagnosis of the coagulopathy. It would be unethical to risk another hemorrhage giving them placebo. Secondly, it would be a difficult task to find a sufficient number of patients with the same type and severity of the coagulopathy, undergoing the same surgical procedure, with the possible exception of tooth extractions.

Since 1985, when we consistently started testing patients with disorders of primary hemostasis with desmopressin and thereafter using it instead of blood products in the responders in connection with surgery or bleeding episodes, we have gathered considerable patient material. Among those cases there are several who have undergone identical or at least similar procedures without as well as with desmopressin. This allowed us to perform a comparison, using the patients as their own controls.

METHODS

During a period of five years (1985-1989) we tested the effect of desmopressin in 370 consecutive patients with disorders of primary hemostasis, referred to the unit of blood coagulation disorders at the Department of Internal Medicine, Karolinska Hospital, due to a

Desmopressin in Bleeding Disorders, Edited by G. Mariani *et al.*
Plenum Press, New York, 1993

hemorrhagic tendency, abnormal findings in a preoperative hemostatic screening or a positive family history. The routine was to give 0.2μg/kg of desmopressin (Minirin®, Ferring AB, Malmö, Sweden) in 100 ml saline intravenously over 30 minutes and measure the bleeding time before and 30 minutes after the end of the infusion. However, in some cases where the patient needed emergency surgery, or the referring physician was unwilling to postpone the procedure, we gave 0.3 μg/kg as above and if the bleeding time was shortened, the patient went straight to surgery. The rationale for this routine was, that most of the patients responded very well to 0.2 μg/kg of desmopressin, thus obviating the need for a higher dose, and in those who had a partial reduction but no normalisation of the bleeding time, we could expect an improved effect by giving 0.3 μg/kg for surgery.

A responder was defined as a patient who obtained a normalisation or a reduction by at least 20% of the bleeding time. In those cases with vWD and a minimally prolonged bleeding time at baseline, we also required a more than twofold increase of the level of vWf.

At the end of the five year period mention above, we reviewed all the episodes for which these patients had obtained desmopressin as prophylaxis against hemorrhage or as therapy against manifest bleeding. We had initially, after the desmopressin test, informed the patient and referring physician to contact us whenever desmopressin could be used, so that we would have notes about the dose and procedure. We also retrospectively checked with the patients and physicians if there had been any other treatment occasions, of which we did not know.

The first dose of desmopressin was given not more than one hour before the start of surgery, except for vaginal delivery, where it was given immediately post partum in order to avoid any, albeit unlikely, effects on the labour. In total 3-5 doses with an interval of 8-24 hours were given. After the first six months we reduced the number of doses to 1-3 in order to avoid excessive retention of water. Since it is well known that the fibrinolytic activity is high in mucous membranes, we always added the fibrinolytic inhibitor tranexamic acid (Cyklokapron®, KabiPharmacia AB, Stockholm, Sweden) for procedures in such organs and sometimes also for other types of surgery. Furosemide 20 mg was given, in cases where there was a positive fluid balance.

Whenever possible we obtained data on the amount of blood loss or duration of bleeding from all available sources (anesthetist, surgeon, dentist, patient etc).

Bleeding time was measured with a Simplate-II device (General Diagnostics, Morris Plains, USA) and our normal range was 140-570 s (Mielke et al., 1969). Platelet aggregation was studied on a Payton dual channel aggregometer (Scarborough, Ont, Canada), using ADP, adrenalin, arachidonic acid, collagen and ristocetin as aggregating agents.

RESULTS

Of the 370 patients with a disorder of the primary hemostasis, tested with desmopressin 0.2 - 0.3 μg/kg, 322 (87%) fulfilled the criteria for responders. The distribution thereof is presented in Table 1.

Table 1. Positive response rate to test with desmopressin according to diagnosis

Diagnosis	Number of patients	Responders (%)
vWD	133	90
type I (mild)	113	97
type I (moderate)	10	60
type IIA	3	100
type IIB	4	25
type III (severe)	3	0
Platelet disorder	237	85
Congenital	77	83
Hepatopathy	16	88
Myeloproliferative disease	7	71
Acetylsalicylic acid	4	75
Isolated prolonged bleeding time	123	89
Other	10	70

Desmopressin was used clinically on 173 occasions (as prophylaxis against hemorrhage in 159 and for active bleeding in 14 cases) in 127 patients. In 13 of the 173 episodes (7.5%) hemostasis was not completely satisfactory. This should be compared with the fact that 56 of these 127 patients (44%) had experienced hemorrhagic complications previously, when desmopressin was not used.

Description of Adverse Events

The 13 "unsatisfactory" cases will be described here.

Four of the patients had vWD and underwent tooth extractions. One of those had a moderate form of vWD, got only one dose of desmopressin and started bleeding two days after the extraction. After that we always gave at least two doses to this type of patient. The second, third and fourth patients had mild forms of vWD. One developed a submucous hematoma, another patient bled more than normally for one hour after the extraction but afterwards there was no further hemorrhage and two subsequent extractions were uneventful. The last patient did not take tranexamic acid and bled for several hours, but when he at three subsequent extractions followed our instructions and took the medicine, no complications occurred.

Two patients with platelet function disorders underwent tonsillectomy and were considered to bleed more than normally during surgery, but postoperative hemostasis was excellent.

One patient with vWD underwent cholecystectomy, and the surgeon remarked that blood was oozing during surgery. There was, however, no bleeding postoperatively.

One patient with platelet dysfunction and multiple myeloma underwent implantation of Harrington rods. Peroperative blood loss was 1500 ml, mainly from tumor tissue, but after surgery there were no problems.

One patient with isolated prolonged bleeding time had a tumor in the scull. During the resection she bled profusely from the tumor, total blood loss amounting to 1000 ml, but at the end of surgery hemostasis was excellent.

One patient with liver cirrhosis and platelet function defect underwent sclerotherapy of esophageal varices and bled intensively afterwards, necessitating insertion of a Sengstaken tube. She also received desmopressin for liver biopsy, resection of a benign skin tumor and middle ear surgery without bleeding complications.

One patient with a congenital platelet function disorder received one dose of desmopressin for active vaginal bleeding, which then ceased, but restarted the following day. She unfortunately did not tell us until several weeks later.

Finally, two patients with congenital platelet function defects (release defect in both) received desmopressin immediately after delivery, which was complicated by retention of the placenta in one case and threatening asphyxia of the baby, necessitating rapid delivery with a vacuum bell in the other. Blood loss was 1200 and 1070 ml, respectively, but most of it actually before all of the desmopressin infusion had been administered, and thereafter there was no abnormal bleeding.

Excessive fluid retention was only observed in two patients, receiving multiple doses of desmopressin, and it was rapidly alleviated with furosemide. In one patient with vaginal delivery, desmopressin was given by mistake during labour, which thereafter ceased for six hours and had to be induced again.

Patients as Matched Controls

Among the 127 patients who received desmopressin in clinical situations, we were able to identify 18, who had undergone an identical or similar procedure previously without desmopressin. Most of those had, however, been treated with tranexamic acid then. Six of the patients had vWD, four had a congenital platelet function disorder, one had liver cirrhosis and seven had isolated prolonged bleeding time. The types of matched events and outcome are shown in Table 2.

In these comparisons treatment with desmopressin turns out favourably in every single case, and if a statistical comparison of the blood losses in matched pairs, wherever available, were to be performed, it would of course be significant. The patient described above with retention of the placenta and a blood loss of 1200 ml during delivery, after which she received desmopressin, had a previous delivery without desmopressin and without such obstetric complications with a blood loss of 1400 ml.

Table 2. Types of matched events without and with desmopressin and the outcome.

Operation etc	Patients	Without desmopressin	With desmopressin
Tooth extractions	4	Prolonged or late bleeding (up to six days) (n=5)	No bleeding (n=7)
Tongue tie	1	Excessive blood loss	No blood loss
Resection of parotid adenoma	1	Blood loss 500 ml	Blood loss 300 ml
Adenoid-/tonsillectomy	1	Excessive blood loss	Blood loss 300 ml
Breast surgery	1	Four separate operations, Excessive bleeding, evacuation, transfusion	One operation – almost no bleeding
Cesarian section	1	Blood loss 600 ml	Blood loss 500 ml
Vaginal delivery / vacuum extraction / uterine curettage / cervical surgery	9	Transfusions. Bleeding for two months. Mean blood loss 1057 ml (n=7)	Bleeding was none or normal. Mean blood loss 507 ml (n=7)

Active Bleeding

Another way to assess the effectiveness of desmopressin is to analyse its ability to stop active bleeding. In this material there were 14 such episodes. **Nine** were bleedings connected with vaginal deliveries, out of which seven have already been mentioned above (Description of Adverse Events and Table 2). The remaining two had a blood loss of 400 and 550 ml. We have reduced the number of doses of desmopressin on this indication from initially 3-5 to 1-2. **Two** patients had vaginal bleeding, not connected with delivery, one of which was mentioned under Description of Adverse Events. Both got a single dose of desmopressin with prompt effect on the bleeding. **One** patient with vWD type IIA and active bleeding from the mouth had an immediate effect of one dose of desmopressin. The same patient received three doses of desmopressin in connection with a major gastrointestinal hemorrhage, at which the hemoglobin had dropped to 74 g/l, and recovered without the use of factor concentrates or other blood products.**One** patient with a platelet function defect caused by acetylsalicylic acid and maybe also by a myeloproliferative disease had been bleeding quite intensively for one day after a bone marrow biopsy, but this stopped after one dose of desmopressin.

Heparin-Induced Bleeding

We have recently demonstrated, that desmopressin induces a partial reversal of the effect of heparin on the bleeding time (Schulman and Johnsson 1991). We have had the opportunity to give desmopressin in seven cases with hemorrhage, caused by heparin alone or in combination with other factors. Three of those, including a patient mentioned in that paper, bled in connection with hemodialysis and prohylaxis with heparin or low molecular weigh heparin. Desmopressin stopped the hemorrhages without causing clot formations. Another patient had an aortic valve prosthesis and received heparin during surgery for a gynecological tumor. She bled profusely from the operation wound, and desmopressin had a prompt effect on this. Yet another patient, a Jehova's Witness, received heparin during pregnancy, due to pulmonary embolism during the first trimester. At the end of pregnancy she suddenly developed massive intra-abdominal hemorrhage. Emergency surgery was performed, but the baby could not be saved. The hemoglobin of the patient dropped to 30 g/l, but she refused blood products. She had already received protamin chloride. Desmopressin, given thereafter, seemed to stop the hemorrhage, and she recovered slowly with the additional help of injections of iron and erythropoetin.

CONCLUSION

It is obvious from the results presented here, that desmopressin will normalise or significantly reduce the bleeding time in the vast majority of patients with disorders of primary hemostasis. In the patients with vWD the response rate is 90%. Among those with vWD type I, which is by far the most common variant, it is as high as 97%. In the patients with a variety of platelet function disorders, including isolated prolonged bleeding time, 85% are responders.

We have not considered vWD type IIB an absolute contraindication for desmopressin, and we actually test the effect of desmopressin at an early stage of the investigation, before we have the results of the vWf multimers and thus knowledge of the subtype. Even in this group there are a few responders, who may benefit from desmopressin as an alternative to blood products in connection with surgery, as experienced by us (Schulman et al., 1991) or described by others (Kyrle et al., 1988 and Fowler et al., 1989).

The adverse events reported here had in several cases a natural explanation for the increased bleeding tendency, such as operation in tumor tissue or obstetric complications. Other events were of minor importance with more bleeding than normally observed during surgery but with excellent hemostasis postoperatively, and in none of those cases was transfusion with blood products necessary.

Since we were unable to perform a randomized, placebo-controlled study on the effect of desmopressin in these patients, we thought that a comparison of matched events, using the patients as their own controls would give us the best information in this respect. The outcome was better with than without desmopressin in every single one of the 18 cases. However, there are also other aspects than the blood loss itself. Massive bleeding during or after surgery can affect the result of the procedure. One example is the patient, who underwent breast surgery four times without desmopressin (Table 2), until she was referred to us. The reason for repeated surgery was that the cosmetic outcome each time was unacceptable, and this was clearly related to the bleeding complications. When she finally was correctly diagnosed and received prophylaxis with desmopressin, plastic surgery could be performed with a satisfactory result.

Still, the most important implication of the possibility to replace blood products with desmopressin is the elimination of risk of viral transmission. Although screening of blood donors with serology for HIV, hepatitis B and C is available and routinely carried out in many countries, there is a dark window from the time an individual is infected until antibodies are detectable. With the epidemic of especially HIV spreading from traditional risk groups to the general population, exclusion of the former will not provide complete additional protection to the serologic screening. The socioeconomic effects of chronic hepatitis developing into liver cirrhosis as a result of a transfusion related hepatitis C has only lately been realized. The use of desmopressin as prophylaxis against postoperative hemorrhage should result in a reduction of total costs for health care as well as elimination of individual suffering due to the above mentioned reasons. For patients with disorders of the primary hemostasis, travelling in countries of the third world, we have routinely prescribed a sufficient amount of desmopressin and taught them the injection technique, so that they could treat themselves immediately in case of hemorrhage.

A conclusion from these observations is, that it is crucial to identify and correctly diagnose the patients with disorders of primary hemostasis as early as possible, in order to avoid the condition's remaining undetected until after the patient has bled and has required transfusions after surgery. A history of hemorrhagic diathesis (in the patient or close relatives) or abnormal results in the preoperative hemostatic screening should lead to a consultation with a specialist in blood coagulation or a hematologist experienced in this field. With emergency surgery this consultation is still valuable, even if time will not permit a detailed investigation, since desmopressin can be given *ex juvantibus* and if the bleeding time is normalised, surgery can be performed with less delay than an hour after the test dose. The only contraindications we have considered against giving desmopressin are clinically important arteriosclerotic lesions and thrombotic disease, although we are aware of the fact that desmopressin has actually been used in many patients of this kind without convincing detrimental effects (Mannucci and Lusher, 1989).

ACKNOWLEDGEMENT

Financial support from the Karolinska Institute is greatfully acknowledged.

REFERENCES

Burroughs, A.K., Matthews, K., Qadiri, M. et al, 1985, Desmopressin and bleeding time in patients with cirrhosis, *Br Med J* 291:1377.

Fowler, W.E., Berkowitz, L.R. and Roberts, H.R., 1989, DDAVP for type IIB von Willebrand disease, *Blood* 74:1859.

Gader, A.M.A., da Costa, J. and Cash, J.D., 1973, A new vasopressin analogue and fibrinolysis, *Lancet* 2:1417.

Kobrinsky, N.L., Israels, E.D., Gerrard, J.M. et al, 1984, Shortening of the bleeding time by 1-deamino-8-D-arginine vasopressin in various bleeding disorders, *Lancet* 1:1145.

Kyrle, P.A., Niessner, H., Dent, J. et al, 1988, IIB von Willebrand's disease: pathogenetic and therapeutic studies, *Br J Haematol* 69:55.

Mannucci, P.M., Ruggeri, Z.M., Pareti, F.I. et al., 1977, 1-deamino-8-D-arginine vasopressin: a new pharmacological approach to the management of haemophilia and von Willebrand's disease, *Lancet* 1:869.

Mannucci, P.M., Remuzzi, G., Pusineri, F. et al., 1983, Deamino-8-D-arginine vasopressin shortens the bleeding time in uremia, *N Engl J Med* 308:8.

Mannucci, P.M. and Lusher, J.M., 1989, Desmopressin and thrombosis, *Lancet* 2:675.

Ruggeri, Z.M., Pareti, F.I., Bintadish, P. et al., 1974, Clotting factors in von Willebrand's disease, *Lancet* 2:105 (letter).

Schulman, S., Johnsson, H., Egberg, N. et al, 1987, DDAVP-induced correction of prolonged bleeding time in patients with congenital platelet function defects, *Thromb Res* 45:165.

Schulman, S., Johnsson, H. and Lindstedt, M., 1991, Desmopressin as a hemostatic agent in patients with disorders of primary hemostasis, *Eur J Surg* 157:647.

Schulman, S. and Johnsson, H., 1991, Heparin, DDAVP and the bleeding time, *Thromb Haemostas* 65:242.

DISCUSSION

Lusher: How frequently did you give the DDAVP to persons with platelet function disorders, and on what basis?

Schulman: We gave a few doses to start with: 4 - 5 doses in 8 - 12 hour intervals. Two patients had fluid problems and were given frusemide. Now we only give 1 or 2 doses at most in more major surgery: that seems enough.

Harris: How consistent is your protocol in using tranexamic acid? Do you always use it, or do you restrict its use? Can you recommend a regimen for it?

Schulman: We always use it in surgery of the mucous membranes, but not in microscopic surgery or where mucous membranes are not involved. We have used it in breast surgery on the basis that it has a high content of glandular tissue.

Kohler: Were the failures non-responders?

Schulman: No. We did not give DDAVP to non-responders. Failures were responders on first testing. In most of these cases local factors caused the bleed.

Kohler: You mentioned one dose. Was that true even for vW disease?

Schulman: No. We gave between one and three doses in vWf. Mild cases have one dose only: it works well.

Kohler: There are reports of late bleeds in mild vWf, and others recommend several DDAVP doses to prevent it. One perhaps should give it longer in vW disease.
Schulman: We continue with tranexamic acid for one week in mucous membrane surgery. That may prevent late bleeding.

Cattaneo: Were these complications related to long bleeding times in heparinized patients?
Schulman: They had prolonged APTT. It was difficult to arrange the measurement of bleeding times before we gave desmopressin. We know this is shortened by DDAVP infusion. In animal experiments there is no increase in thrombosis when DDAVP is added. We have not been worried by the thrombogenic risk.

CLINICAL EFFICACY OF DESMOPRESSIN AND CONSISTENCY OF RESPONSES TO SEPARATE INFUSION IN PATIENTS WITH PROLONGED BLEEDING TIME DUE TO CONGENITAL PLATELET DEFECT

Giancarlo Castman and Francesco Rodeghiero

Department of Hematology
Hemophilia and Thrombosis Centre
San Bortolo Hospital
I-36100 Vicenza

INTRODUCTION

Desmopressin (DDAVP) is able to shorten or normalize the prolonged bleeding time (BT) in the majority of patients with von Willebrand disease (vWD) by inducing an increase of factor VIII/von Willebrand factor measurements in plasma through mechanisms still unknown[1]. Recently, this agent proved also successful in correcting the BT and in the prevention of bleeding in several platelet function defects[2-5], with the exception of Glanzmann Thrombasthenia[2,6], and in patients with prolonged BT of undefined etiology[7]. The precise mechanism by which DDAVP acts in these disorders remains elusive. Despite several patients with congenital platelet disorders have been infused with DDAVP for experimental purpose, clinical experience is still limited. Moreover, it is not established if the response to the drug, in terms of BT correction, is consistent in time. If this holds true, a test-infusion with DDAVP could predict the usefulness of the drug in the individual patient.

In this study, we report the clinical experience with DDAVP in 11 patients with congenital platelet defect and prolonged BT. Moreover, the results of the consistency in time to separate DDAVP infusion is also reported.

PATIENTS AND METHODS

A) Patients

Twelve patients (10 female and 2 male) with inherited platelet disorders having been infused with DDAVP for experimental purposes, clinical experience is still limited. moderate lifelong bleeding history and prolonged BT, with other members symptomatic in their families. Case n° 11 (see Table 1) was a male with a platelet defect associated to mild hemophilia A (factor VIII:C 25-30 U/dL). In this case it was not possible to test any relative. Case n° 8 had a platelet defect associated to von Willebrand disease (Ristocetin cofactor activity 25 - 37 U/dL) and mild factor VII deficiency (F VII 40-55%). Specific defect was defined by the pattern of abnormalities on platelet aggregation studies. All the patients had normal aggregation response to arachidonate, thus excluding aspirin-like defects. Six of them had abnormal response to ADP, with second wave absent and disaggregation; abnormality to collagen-induced aggregation was also evident. Five out of them had normal aggregation to ADP, but low serotonine content and abnormal ATP/ADP ratio were suggestive for storage-pool defect in 3. Thus it was possible to consider storage pool disease for 9 patients and apparently isolated prolonged BT in 2. In addition, a young boy, aged 12, with Bernard-Soulier syndrome was also evaluated (case n° 12). This patient had severe bleeding diathesis, moderate to severe thrombocytopenia (platelet count 7 - 85 x $10^3/\mu L$), giant platelets on peripheral blood smear and complete absence of ristocetin-induced platelet agglutination. A cell sorter (FACS) analysis of the patient's platelets using a murine monoclonal anti-glycoprotein IB antibody (Beckton-Dickinson, USA) showed the complete absence of this platelet membrane protein.

Methods

Platelet aggregation was assayed in platelet-rich plasma (PRP), obtained by centrifuging citrated blood samples at 800 rpm for 15 minutes. ADP (2 μM), arachidonate (500 μg/mL), adrenalin (2.5 μM) and collagen (2 μg/mL) were the agonists used. Ristocetin-induced platelet aggregation (RIPA) was determined by measuring the concentration of ristocetin able to induce 30 % of aggregation 3 minutes later. BT was measured using a Simplate II device (General Diagnostic, Morris Plains, NJ, USA) by making two standardized vertical incision on the forearm.

DDAVP Infusion

After informed consent, DDAVP (Minirin, Valeas, Milano) was infused at 0.3 μg/kg b.w. diluted in 100 ml of isotonic saline over 30 minutes. Bleeding times and Factor VIII/von Willebrand Factor measurements were carried out before and at the end of infusion.

RESULTS

The results of the studies before and after DDAVP infusion are summarized in table 1.

As can be seen, all the patients had their BT shortened after DDAVP. In five of them, BT was normalized at the end of infusion and in 3 the normalization persisted up to 120 minutes. Two additional patients had their BT normalized at 120 minutes. In the patient with mild hemophilia A, VIII:C rose to 66 U/dl post-DDAVP, whereas in patients with von Willebrand disease, VIII/vWF measurements were normalized

Table 1. Bleeding times before and after DDAVP infusion

Patients	Bleeding time (minutes)		
	Before	End of infusion	120 minutes
1) P.O.	17.5	6	9.5
2) T.DB.	10	9	6
3) P.R.	12	7.2	6.5
4) M.F.	15	8.5	7.5
5) P.A.	14	12	8
6) G.E.	17	9	9.5
7) M.P.	25	7	6.5
8) Z.M.*	11.2	7.5	9.5
9) U.M.	18	9.7	10
10) U.A.	9	6.7	6
11) D.M.B.#	16	9.5	17
12) B.L.°	>30	>30	-
Normal range	3 - 7.5		

* von Willebrand disease
# mild hemophilia A
° Bernard-Soulier Syndrome

after infusion. The patient with Bernard-Soulier syndrome was completely unresponsive to DDAVP, with BT > 30 minutes after infusion.

Aggregation studies and measurements of serotonine content were repeated after DDAVP in 3 patients and no improvement was observed (data not shown).

DDAVP was repeated for clinical use in 8 patients (Table 2). The time from first infusion ranged from 1 to 30 months (median 9 months). As can be seen, a fairly consistent response was obtained, with a magnitude of departure from average BT less than 10 % in about 75 % of cases. DDAVP was used for prevention of bleeding during miomectomy, thyroidectomy, curettage, dental extraction, resection of stiloid process, saphenectomy and removal of a foreign body from leg. All these interventions proved successful with a single DDAVP infusion and no blood products were needed. in one of them it was administered on three separate occasions for clinical reasons. Case n° 2 underwent thyroidectomy, with three DDAVP infusions during a 36-hour period. Post-infusion BT was always normalized. Case n° 7 underwent stiloid process removal. She was infused also 12 hours later and on the 6th day from intervention for removal of sutures.

CONCLUSION

DDAVP is able to shorten or normalize BT of patients with congenital bleeding disorders, such as von Willebrand's

Table 2. Consistency of bleeding time to separate DDAVP infusions.

Patients	Bleeding time (minutes)	
	Before	After*
1) P.O.	17.5	6
	>20	11
2) T.DB.	10	6
	10	6.5
3) P.R.	12	6.5
	10	7
5) P.A.	14	8
	13	7
6) G.E.	17	9
	>20	10
7) M.P.	25	6.5
	>20	7
	>20	9
9) U.M.	18	9.7
	17	8
11) D.M.B.	16	9.5
	15.5	10

* nadir of bleeding time post-infusion.

disease (vWD)[1], platelet function defect[8] or apparently isolated prolonged BT[7]. The only notable exception is represented by Glanzmann Thrombasthenia[2,6], an autosomal recessive disorder characterized by the absence or the abnormality of GP IIb/IIIa complex on platelet membrane[9]. Our study confirms the effectiveness of DDAVP in shortening BT in patients with storage pool disease and patients with isolated prolonged BT.

The effect in storage pool disease is not related to improvement of platelet aggregation or increased serotonine content in platelets after DDAVP. In fact, in the three patients tested before and after DDAVP, no improvement of basal abnormality was observed. These latter findings have been previously observed in other studies, regardless the effect of DDAVP on BT[2,4]. In some cases, such as for example Bernard-Soulier syndrome not completely lacking Gp Ib, the raise of vWF elicited by DDAVP has been given a possible role in BT shortening by increasing the interaction with Gp Ib on platelet surface10 . However, in another report no BT shortening was observed in a patient with Bernard-Soulier syndrome[11]. In our patient BT remained markedly prolonged post-infusion. His platelets completely lacked Gp Ib. Thus in this disorder, traces of Gp Ib might be sufficient as to allow a partial shortening of BT after DDAVP infusion.

In a previous study in patients with von Willebrand disease and mild hemophilia A, we have demonstrated an excellent consistency of responses, in terms of VIII:C and BT, to separate DDAVP infusions[12]. No data are available for consistency of BT in congenital platelet function defects. Nieuwenhuis and Sixma[3] mentioned that the effect of DDAVP on the BT was reproducible in three patients who were tested in a second occasion. This is of more than academic interest. In fact, provided good consistency, a single test-infusion will predict the future usefulness of the drug in the individual patient. Eight of our patients were given a separate DDAVP infusion and the magnitude of departure from average BT nadir obtained with the separate infusions was below 10 % in almost all cases (table 2). Clinical experience with the use of DDAVP in these disorders is still limited. Some authors[2,3,5,13] reported an excellent clinical benefit for all treated patients. In our patients, similar results were obtained, with a major intervention (thyroidectomy for multinodular goitre) successfully carried out in a patient, by giving three DDAVP infusions, at 8 hour intervals.

In conclusion, we confirm the usefulness of DDAVP for the management of patients with prolonged BT due to congenital platelet defects. Moreover, since the consistency in time is very good in these patients, a test-infusion with DDAVP is advisable in these patients to predict its future usefulness.

REFERENCES

1. F.Rodeghiero, G.Castaman, P.M.Mannucci, Clinical indications for Desmopressin in congenital and acquired von Willebrand's disease, Blood Reviews 5: 155 (1991).
2. S.Schulman, H.Johnsson, N.Egberg, M.Blomback, DDAVP -induced correction of prolonged bleeding time in patients with congenital platelet function defects, Thromb. Res. 45: 165 (1987).
3. H.K.Nieuwenhuis, J.J.Sixma, 1-Desamino-8-D-arginine Vasopressin (Desmopressin) shortens the bleeding time in Storage Pool Deficiency, Ann. Int. Med. 108: 65 (1988).
4. D.M.Dimichele, W.M.Hathaway, Use of DDAVP in inherited and acquired platelet dysfunction, Am. J. Haematol. 33: 39 (1990).
5. N.L.Kobrinsky, E.D.Israels, J.M.Gerrard, M.S.Cheang, C.M.Watson, A.J.Bishop, M.L.Schroeder, Shortening of bleeding time by 1-deamino-8-D-arginine vasopressin in various bleeding disorders, Lancet 1: 1145 (1984).
6. P.M.Mannucci, V.Vicente, L.Vianello, M.Cattaneo,

I.Alberca, M.P.Coccato, M.P., E.Faioni, D.Mari, Controlled trial of Desmopressin in liver cirrhosis and other conditions associated with a prolonged bleeding time, Blood 67, 1148: (1986).
7. H.C.Kim, K.Salva, P.L.Fallot, G.I.Karp, J.Eisele, L.Matts, I.Heller, P.Saidi, Patients with prolonged bleeding time of undefined etiology, and their response to desmopresssin, Thromb. Haemostas. 59: 221: (1988).
8. P.M.Mannucci, Desmopressin: a nontranfusional form of treatment for congenital and acquired bleeding disorders, Blood 72: 1449 (1988).
9. I.N.George, J.P.CAEN, A.T.Nurden, Glanzmann's Thrombasthenia: the spectrum of clinical disease, Blood 75: 1383 (1990).
10. R.J.G.Cuthbert, H.H.K.Watson, S.I.Handa, I.Abbott, C.A.Ludlam, DDAVP shortens the bleeding time in Bernard -Soulier syndrome, Thromb. Res. 49: 649 (1988).
11. M.J.Mant, DDAVP in Bernard-Soulier syndrome, Thromb. Res. 52: 77 (1988).
12. F.Rodeghiero, G.Castaman, E.Di Bona, M.Ruggeri, Consistency of responses to repeated DDAVP infusions in patients with von Willebrand's disease and hemophilia A, Blood 74: 1997 (1989).
13. T.B.Kentro, R.Lottenberg, C.S.Kitchens, Clinical efficacy of desmopressin acetate for hemostatic control in patients with primary platelet disorders undergoing surgery, Am. J. Haematol. 24: 215 (1987).

DISCUSSION

Kobrinsky: What is the practical value of bleeding times?
Castaman: Some say that bleeding times are not useful predictors of bleeding. I rely more and more on the patient's history, as prolongation of bleeding times is not reliable in predicting severity of bleeding. It is useful for diagnosis only. When we have a convincing bleeding history, with a long bleeding time and aggregation difficulties, we feel we are justified in doing test infusions.

Kobrinsky: In someone going to surgery with a bleeding time of, say, 25, and the test is negative, what do you do?
Castaman: We assume that if the bleeding time is under 15, we give the drug and do not test. Over 15, we test and use the drug if it works. We would find it uncomfortable to rely on DDAVP if the test were negative. Then we would use DDAVP plus ethamsylate. In elective surgery we would give 0.6 mg/kg conjugated estrogen, starting 5 days before surgery. Ethamsylate induces shortening of bleeding time in most platelet disorders.

Kobrinsky: Dr Barth, what happens when oxytocin is ineffective in post-partum bleeding. Is desmopressin effective then? Would the presence of pharmacological doses of oxytocin prevent the effect?
Barth: I only have experience of rats, and it is difficult to extrapolate the data to women. In rat uterus DDAVP has 100 times less affinity to the receptor than oxytocin, so there should be no difficulty, and no induction of uterine atony. It may be better to use glypressin to constrict the vessels in the uterus.

Bichet: In women, n the non-pregnant uterus, there is no mRNA for the oxytocin receptor. This changes in pregnancy, so that there are formidable numbers of oxytocin receptors immediately before and for a few days after delivery. So I doubt that the contracting effect of oxytocin can be inhibited by DDAVP.
Kinter: DDAVP is an oxytocin agonist. It should not matter whether DDAVP or oxytocin is given first.
Bichet: I would certainly give oxytocin first.

DESMOPRESSIN, VON WILLEBRAND FACTOR AND SURGERY

Mark J. Weinstein

Department of Biochemistry
Boston University School of Medicine
Boston, MA 02118

INTRODUCTION

The synthetic vasopressin analogue desmopressin acetate (DDAVP) can induce a broad spectrum of physiological reactions that have hematological consequences. These include release of tissue plasminogen activator, depletion of plasminogen activator inhibitor, and activation of plasminogen[1-3]. Also, DDAVP can benefit hemostasis by stimulating the secretion of factor VIII coagulant protein (FVIII:C)/von Willebrand factor (vWF) from endogenous storage sites[1]. The latter hemostatic property forms the basis for the widespread therapeutic use of DDAVP to treat mild hemophilia and mild von Willebrand's disease[4,5]. DDAVP also benefits hemostasis by an unknown mechanism in many hematological and nonhematological diseases, including congenital and acquired platelet defects[6,7-8], and surgical bleeding[9,10], where FVIII:C/vWF concentrations are in the normal range.

The ill-defined bleeding diathesis associated with cardiopulmonary bypass (CPB) has some of the same characteristics as diseases that are amenable to treatment with DDAVP. During bypass, platelets exposed to the surface of the extracaporeal circuit become unresponsive to adenosine diphosphate and epinephrine, degranulate, lose fibrinogen receptors, and synthesize and release thromboxane A_2[11-13]. Thrombocytopenia and activation of plasminogen also occur during CPB.

To extend the therapeutic utility of DDAVP, and to further elucidate the mechanism of its salutary effect on hemostasis, Salzman et al[11] initiated a trial of DDAVP on patients undergoing complex cardiac surgery with cardiopulmonary bypass. We postulated that DDAVP would reduce blood loss in CPB, and that DDAVP would benefit hemostasis though its capacity to modulate vWF activity.

DDAVP might reduce perioperative blood loss by inducing the release of more hemostatically active forms of vWF than are usually present in the circulation. vWF normally appears in plasma as a series of oligomers ranging from $1 - 15 \times 10^6$ D. Larger sized multimers, contained within the Weibel-Paladie bodies of endothelial cells, are secreted after DDAVP infusion[14,15]. These unusually large multimers have 5-15 times the specific activity of normal size oligomers in mediating shear-induced platelet aggregation[16], and are presumably more active in promoting platelet attachment to damaged vessel surfaces. Infusion of DDAVP can raise vWF antigen concentration two or more fold above resting levels. The high concentration

Desmopressin in Bleeding Disorders, Edited by G. Mariani *et al.*
Plenum Press, New York, 1993

of more hemostatically active multimers might counterbalance the loss of platelet binding sites induced by CPB.

The outcome of the trial by Salzman et al[11] did in fact demonstrate that DDAVP could reduce bleeding in complex cardiac bypass operations, and that blood loss was greatest in patients who had relatively low concentrations of vWF[17]. In subsequent trials of DDAVP, I sought to verify the apparent relationships among vWF concentration, multimer distribution and bleeding in another cohort of adult cardiac bypass patients[18], and in patients undergoing hip replacement[19]. New insights were gained about properties of vWF that are characteristic of these patient groups, but DDAVP did not reduce bleeding, and blood loss did not correlate with vWF. In the following report I will compare these three investigations and emphasize features that distinguish the study showing a hemostatic effect of DDAVP from the others.

DDAVP AND COMPLEX CARDIAC BYPASS SURGERY: STUDY I

Salzman et al[11] examined the influence of DDAVP on blood loss in cardiopulmonary bypass by measuring the amount of intra and postoperative hemorrhage in 35 patients treated with DDAVP (0.3 ug/kg) and 34 who received a placebo. The patient population (Table 1) consisted primarily of individuals undergoing complex bypass procedures. Thirty one percent of these patients had repeat operations for recurrent valvular dysfunction or coronary occlusive disease, procedures known to have a high risk of excessive hemorrhage. Patients undergoing primary uncomplicated coronary-artery bypass grafting were excluded because of the potential that DDAVP might induce a prothrombotic state through the release of excessive amounts of high molecular weight vWF multimers. Also, the capacity of

Table 1. Patient characteristics in two trials of DDAVP in adult cardiac bypass operation[1]

	Salzman et al[11]		Ansell et al[18]	
	D	P	D	P
Patients	35	35	41	42
Valve Replacement	19	21	41	42
CABG	10	6	0	0
Valve + CABG	5	7	8	5
Other	1	1	8	8
Repeat Heart Surgery	22		10	9
Duration of Surgery (min)	373	392	261	242
Duration of Bypass (min)	144	159	119	112
Blood Loss Measured	Intra[2] + Post		Post	
Blood Loss: (ml)				
Intraoperative	592	993		
0 - 12 hr	510	803	792	608
12 - 24 hr	215	414	273	252
0 - 24 hr	1317	2210	1065	830

[1]From Ansell et al[18]
[2]"Intra" indicates blood loss measured from point of drug administration to the end of surgery.

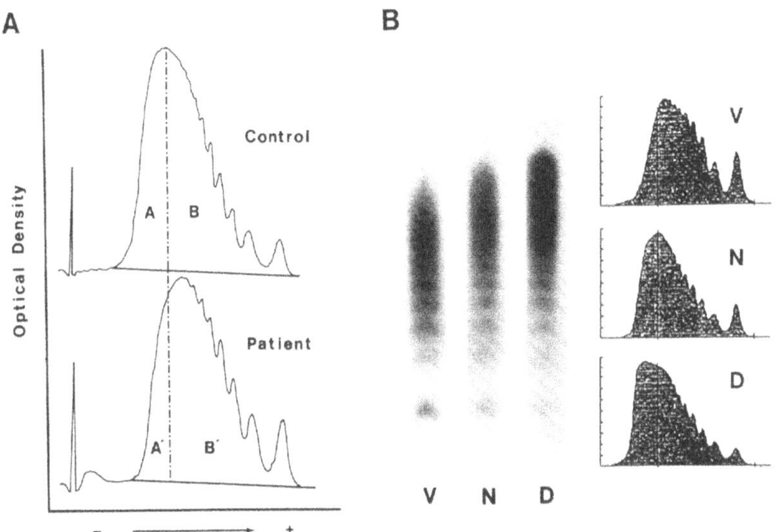

Figure 1. Measurement of normalized HMW multimer ratio from densitometry of vWF autoradiograms. (A) For a given sample, the integrated optical density area of HMW multimers (A'), (multimers with Mr greater than those at the maximum OD of control plasma), was divided by the total multimeric area (A'+B'). The normalized HMW multimer ratio was calculated by dividing this ratio by the ratio obtained from a normal pool control electrophoresed on the same gel. (B) Autoradiograph and densitometric scan of vWF from a patient with coronary valve disease (V); normal pool plasma (N); and 90 min after DDAVP (D). (from [17])

DDAVP to reduce blood loss would most likely be seen in patients who had substantial bleeding, especially if the effect was slight. The diagnoses of the two groups were similar except that the DDAVP group had fewer cases of combined aortic and mitral valvular disease.

The drug or placebo was administered following neutralization of heparin by protamine after disconnection from the extracorporeal circuit. Intraoperative blood loss, measured from the time of administration of the drug or placebo, and blood loss in the first 24 hours after operation were determined by weighing sponges and measuring the suction drainage. Samples of blood for assaying vWF were collected 1 or more days before operation, immediately after bypass, 90 minutes after drug treatment, and 24 hours post operation.

Results

Blood losses during the operation and 24 hours postoperatively were 40% less in the group receiving DDAVP (Table 1), and transfusion requirements were 34% less. A total of 14 patients had blood loss greater than 2 L; 11 of these were in the placebo group and 3 had received DDAVP. Of the 11 patients in the high blood loss placebo group, 4 underwent coronary artery bypass surgery, and 7 had valve replacement. The few thrombotic complications were evenly distributed among the drug and placebo recipients. In the placebo group, there was one intraoperative myocardial infarction and one postoperative stroke; in the DDAVP group one patient had a myocardial infarction and two had postoperative strokes.

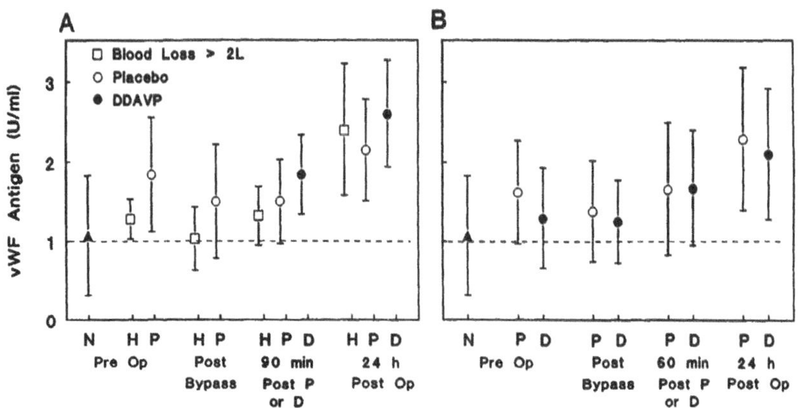

Figure 2. vWF antigen in Study I[11] (A) and Study II [18] (B) of DDAVP in CPB. N, healthy controls; H, blood loss > 2 L; P, placebo group; D, DDAVP group. In Study I, before bypass, patients who lost > 2 L of blood tended to have less vWF than other patients. After medication, the placebo group in Study I had significantly (p <.02) less vWF antigen than the DDAVP group. No such differences were noted in Study II.

vWF antigen was quantified by ELISA[18] or electroimmunoassay[17]. The relative proportion of high molecular weight vWF multimers were measured by separating vWF electrophoretically on SDS-agarose gels, labeling the protein with ^{125}I-anti vWF, and analyzing autoradiographs of the gel by densitometry. High molecular weight (HMW) multimers were defined as those with molecular weights greater than multimers at the maximum optical density of a normal pool plasma standard (Mr ~8 x10^6). The percentage of HMW multimers for a given patient was normalized to the percentage in the standard[17] (Figure 1).

vWF antigen. Prior to surgery, the mean concentration of vWF in the patient population, 1.8 ± 0.8 (SD) U/ml, was high compared to that of healthy controls (1.07 ± 0.76 U/ml, p <.05)(Figure 2A). The highest blood loss occurred in patients who had concentrations of vWF below the mean of the patient population before surgery and whose level remained low after bypass (Figure 2, 3). Of 22 patients in the placebo group who had vWF concentrations below the population mean, 11 had more than 2 L of intra and postoperative blood loss. Only 1 of 10 who had a concentration above the mean had this same amount of loss (Figure 4).

During bypass, hemodilution tended to decrease vWF antigen concentration. However, in 14 patients with initial vWF concentrations below the mean, vWF release during bypass was sufficient to overcome hemodilution, and their antigen concentration increased above initial levels. In the placebo group of patients, of 8 who had preoperative levels of vWF <1.8 U/ml, and who had an increase in vWF during bypass, only one bled >2 L. In contrast, of 12 placebo patients who had preoperative vWF levels <1.8 U/ml and whose vWF decreased during bypass, 8 bled >2 L. Similar results were obtained in patients who eventually received DDAVP[17]. Since these changes occurred before DDAVP or placebo were infused, they suggest that factors that influence vWF concentration during bypass, irrespective of drug treatment, are related to total blood loss.

After bypass, vWF concentration rose in most patients, regardless of DDAVP infusion (Figure 2A). Although the vWF concentration (1.8 ± 0.5 U/ml) of the DDAVP group was statistically different (p <0.02) from the placebo group (1.5 ± 0.65 U/ml, blood loss <2L; 1.3 ± 0.5 U/ml, blood loss >2 L) at 90 min post drug infusion, the increase was much less than the 2-4 fold rise observed in healthy control subjects or hemophiliacs treated with the drug. Twenty four hours after surgery, vWF concentration was high in all patients, regardless of whether they received DDAVP or placebo, or if blood loss was >2 L. These results indicate that surgery alone stimulates release of vWF and that the magnitude of the DDAVP effect is marginal. All patients, before, during and after bypass had concentrations of vWF far above those normally considered adequate for hemostasis.

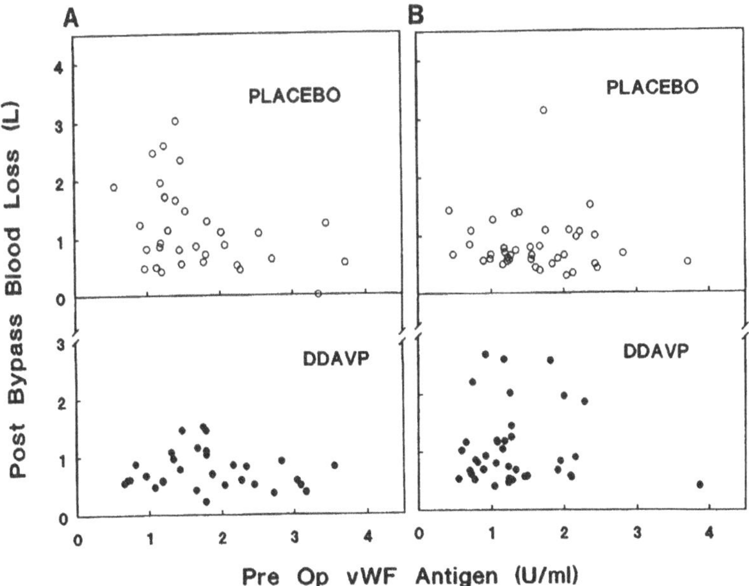

Figure 3. Post bypass blood loss in Study I (A) and Study II (B) plotted as a function of preoperative plasma levels of vWF for patients receiving a placebo or DDAVP.

vWF Multimers. Unexpectedly, the vWF multimeric distribution of coronary valve disease patients was found to be abnormal before surgery (Figs. 1, 5). The HMW multimer ratio of these patients,(0.67 ± 0.21), was significantly ($p < .001$) less than either healthy controls (0.93 ± 0.17) or coronary artery disease patients (0.91 ± 0.17)[17], but higher than that of patients with Type II von Willebrand's disease (0.2 ± 0.15). Coronary valve disease patients did not have abnormal bleeding times or ristocetin cofactor activities. The cause and hemostatic significance of this depletion is unknown but may be related to increased gastrointestinal bleeding reported in some patients with aortic valvular disease. The deficiency of large multimers did not correlate with subsequent blood loss, and the multimer distribution of valvular disease patients became like that of the other subjects during bypass (Figure 5A).

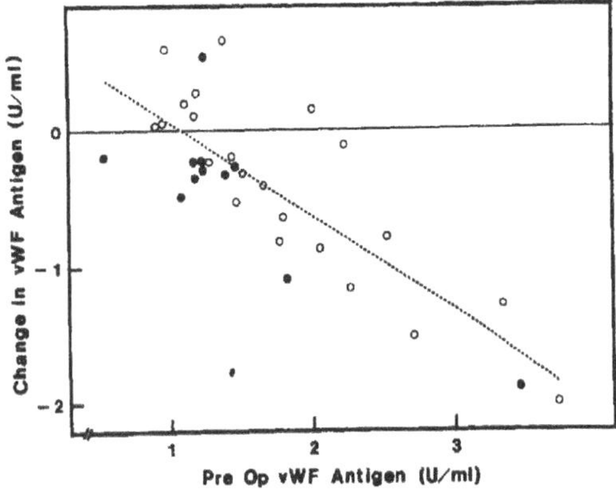

Figure 4. Initial vWF concentration plotted against difference in vWF concentration before and after bypass (change in vWF antigen) from Study I. Values above 0 indicate an increase in vWF above preoperative levels. Patients with intra plus postoperative blood loss > 2L (●) or < 2 L (○) (from [17]).

Infusion of DDAVP did not affect vWF multimer distribution beyond changes induced by surgery alone. Ninety minutes after medication, the multimer ratio was uniformly high for placebo and DDAVP recipients; 24 h after surgery the ratio had declined only slightly and was still above that of healthy controls (Figure 5A). Thus, the beneficial effect of DDAVP on hemostasis in bypass cannot be ascribed to the exclusive production of large vWF multimers not seen in the placebo group.

CARDIAC BYPASS SURGERY IN ADULTS: STUDY II

In 1987, Ansell et al[18] undertook another prospective, randomized, double blind, placebo-controlled trial of DDAVP to assess its potential of reducing postoperative hemorrhage in CPB patients undergoing valvular heart surgery. Five institutions participated in the protocol. The study population consisted of patients scheduled for cardiac valve surgery with or without concomitant coronary artery bypass. Exclusion criteria included recent myocardial infarction, unstable angina, deep vein thrombosis, pulmonary embolism, platelet defects or a history of hemorrhagic diathesis. Forty one patients received 0.3 ug/kg DDAVP and 42 a placebo (Table 1), after administration of protamine sulfate to neutralize heparin. The study included 19 patients (21%) undergoing repeat open heart surgery. Blood loss was measured by chest tube drainage in the first 6, 12 and 24 hours after surgery. In contrast to Salzman et al[11], blood shed between drug administration and chest closure was not considered. vWF multimers and concentration, and factor VIII activity were measured in samples taken before surgery, during and after bypass, 1, 6, 24, and 48 hours after drug treatment.

Results

No significant differences were found in the amount of bleeding or the transfusion requirements between the DDAVP and placebo groups (Table 1) in this trial. In fact, the mean of total blood loss was slightly higher in the DDAVP recipients. In the DDAVP group, 5 patients had blood loss greater than 2 L, compared to 1 in the placebo group (Figure 3). The same number of possible thrombotic complications were noted in the two groups, indicating that DDAVP did not increase the risk of thrombosis.

vWF antigen. Intra and post operative changes in vWF concentration were generally similar to those of the study by Salzman et al[17]. Before bypass, vWF concentration, 1.45 ± 0.67 U/ml, was higher than that of normal healthy controls. After bypass, hemodilution lowered the mean concentration to 1.1 ± 0.7 U/ml. Sixty

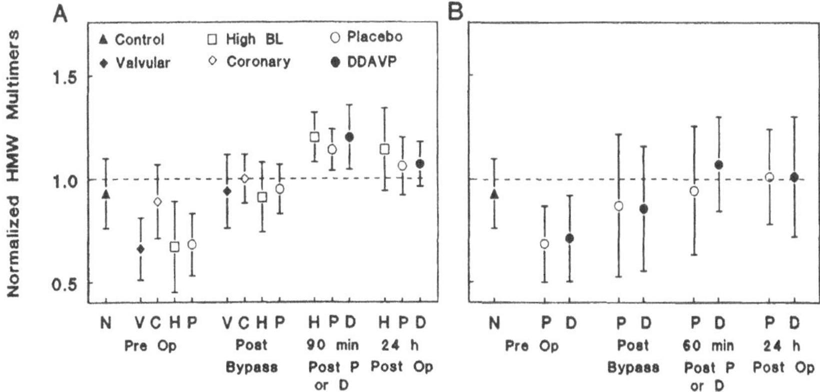

Figure 5. Normalized HMW multimer distribution in Studies I (A) and II (B) of DDAVP in CPB. In Study I, patients with valvular heart disease (V) had significantly less high molecular weight multimers before operation than those with coronary artery disease (C), or healthy controls (N). All patients in study II had valvular heart disease. H, blood loss >2L; P, placebo group; D, DDAVP group.

minutes after infusion of DDAVP or placebo, vWF concentration rose, but, in contrast to Study I, the DDAVP treated group had the same mean vWF concentration (1.67 U/ml) as the placebo group. Twenty four hours after the start of surgery, the DDAVP and placebo groups had high vWF concentrations, 2.09 and 2.29 U/ml respectively (Figure 2B). High blood loss was not associated with relatively low preoperative vWF concentrations or with the change in vWF concentration from pre to post bypass.

vWF Multimers. Changes in vWF multimer distribution were analogous to those found in Study I[17] but somewhat lower in magnitude (Figure 5). Preoperatively, the normalized multimer ratio was low, 0.68 ± 0.2, concomitant with the diagnosis of valvular heart disease for all patients. After bypass the ratio of large multimers increased to normal levels. An hour after drug infusion, the multimer ratio was slightly higher in the DDAVP group, 1.07 ± 0.2, compared to the placebo group, 0.94 ± 0.3. Twenty four hours after surgery both groups had the same normal multimer distribution. Multimeric composition did not correlate with blood loss.

Table 2. DDAVP in total hip replacement (from[19])

Treatment	n	Total* Blood Loss (ml)	% Reduction by DDAVP	+DVT	-DVT	%DVT	95% CI
Placebo	36	1427 ± 672	6.17% (NS)	12	24	35	15-45%
DDAVP	37	1340 ± 1103		13	24	35	20-50%

DDAVP Treatment Group	Placebo Treatment Group
1 unconfirmed DVT	4 unconfirmed DVT
6 confirmed by venogram	5 confirmed by venogram
4 confirmed by U/S	3 confirmed by U/S
2 by intention to treat	

*No statistically significant differences.

DDAVP IN HIP REPLACEMENT SURGERY

This frequently performed surgical procedure is associated with a high risk of blood loss requiring transfusion, and, following surgery, with venous thrombosis or thromboembolism. Deep vein thrombosis occurs in 40% of hip replacement patients who have received prophylactic antithrombotic treatment, while thromboembolism takes place in 20% who are given warfarin prophylactically[20]. To test the potential of DDAVP to reduce blood loss or possibly to induce thrombotic complications in these patients, we[19] undertook a prospective randomized double-blind trial of DDAVP in patients undergoing total hip replacement. We postulated that vWF concentration or multimer distribution might correlate with the occurrence of DVT.

Patients were administered the medication immediately after anesthesia. Blood loss was measured operatively and postoperatively. Warfarin was given to all patients postoperatively to achieve a prothrombin time of 15 to 17 seconds. The presence of deep vein thrombosis was determined by scanning of lower extremities for labelled fibrinogen and by impedance plethysmography. Positive diagnosis was confirmed by phlebography and ultrasound. vWF concentration and multimer distribution were measured in samples taken before surgery, 90 min, 5 h and 24 h after drug treatment.

Results

Although patients treated with DDAVP lost slightly less blood on average than the placebo group, this difference was not statistically significant (Table 2). The The occurrence of DVT was also similar in the two groups, demonstrating that DDAVP does not induce a prothrombotic state, supporting the survey by Mannucci and Lusher[21] that DDAVP is not associated with the risk of thrombosis.

DDAVP also had surprisingly little effect on either the concentration or multimer distribution of vWF (Figure 6). The concentration of vWF in these patients was in the normal range before surgery. Ninety minutes after drug treatment, the vWF antigen concentration of the DDAVP group (1.5 ± 0.45 U/ml) was not statistically different from the placebo recipients (1.2 ± 0.48 U/ml). Twenty four hours later the DDAVP and placebo groups had relatively high antigen levels of 1.6

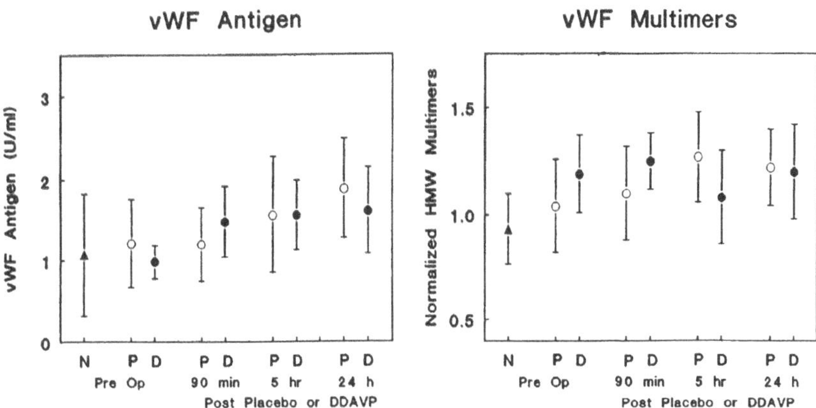

Figure 6. vWF antigen and normalized HMW multimer distribution in patients undergoing hip replacement surgery. N, healthy controls; P, placebo group; D, DDAVP group.

± 0.53 U/ml and 1.9 ± 0.6 U/ml respectively. The proportion of large multimers was high in these patients before and after surgery, averaging between 1.1 and 1.3; no significant differences were found between the DDAVP and placebo groups. Also, neither the concentration of vWF, nor multimer distribution correlated with subsequent development of thrombotic complications. The high antigen and multimer distribution may, however provide an environment that promotes thrombosis in conjunction with other stimulating factors.

CONCLUSION

Of the three trials testing the capacity of DDAVP to reduce intraoperative and postoperative bleeding reviewed here, a therapeutic effect was seen only in patients undergoing the most complex cardiac bypass operations. Other investigators also have had success using DDAVP to reduce postoperative[22,23] and intraoperative[24] hemorrhage in CPB, but most reports[25-29] have described results similar to those of Ansell et al[18] showing no effect, or a trend toward more blood loss with DDAVP[28,29]. The most obvious feature that distinguishes the investigation of Salzman et al[11] from the others was in the choice of patients. In most other trials, the the effect of DDAVP on hemostasis was tested in primary coronary artery bypass graft or simple valve replacement operations. In Salzman et al[11], many patients underwent complex repeat cardiac surgery, were on extracaporeal circulation for an extended period, and had high blood loss if not treated with DDAVP. The combined outcome of these three studies, and others, support the concept that the prophylactic use of DDAVP is not warranted in cases where blood loss is normal and hemostasis is adequate. DDAVP may be useful under conditions where bleeding is excessive or of obscure origin.

The study of Salzman et al[11] was the only one of the three to correlate a parameter related to vWF with blood loss. Patients with the highest blood loss tended to have less vWF than others before surgery, intraoperatively, and after placebo. The mechanism underlying this correlation is unclear, given that the concentration of vWF was far above that generally considered sufficient for hemostasis, and the differences between vWF in the placebo and DDAVP groups after medication, although statistically significant, were minor. Possibly, the association between vWF and bleeding was an epiphenomenon and not causally related. The intraoperative and postoperative concentration of vWF in the high blood loss group may have been low simply because vWF was not released from endogenous storage pools at a rate fast enough to sustain a high circulating concentration of the protein as blood was being lost through hemorrhage.

In the same vein, rather than there being a direct association between vWF concentration and blood loss, the relatively low preoperative and post bypass vWF concentration may be indicative of an overall inability of endothelial cells to express factors that could benefit hemostasis but were not measured in our studies. These include vWF directed towards the subendothelial matrix, and changes in the endothelial cell surface as vWF is released from the , and the Weibel-Paladie body membrane protein GMP-140 is transiently expressed on the cell surface[30].

Alternatively, under conditions of high blood loss, slight variations in the concentration of vWF may more profoundly influence hemostasis than at other times. Platelet surface proteins GPIb and GPIIb-IIIa are less accessible to their ligands after bypass[12]. If binding constants of these proteins become elevated after bypass, greater than normal levels of vWF may be required for hemostasis. DDAVP may provide a threshold amount of vWF needed for adequate platelet-vessel wall interaction.

In all three trials, DDAVP had much less of an effect on vWF concentration and multimer form than was expected from its ability to release vWF in mild hemophilia, von Willebrands disease or in healthy individuals. Other investigators have reported modest[24,25] or no increase[28] in vWF after DDAVP infusion in CPB. Presumably, the stress of surgery alone can substantially increase vWF concentration and HMW multimers by depleting the same storage pools that would otherwise respond to DDAVP. By analogy, DDAVP has little capacity to stimulate additional release of vWF after strenuous exercise[32] or after repeated usage of the drug over a short period of time[3].

While these studies did not demonstrate the anticipated relationship among DDAVP, vWF concentration, multimer distribution, and bleeding, several new observations were made about naturally occuring variations in vWF concentration and structure. vWF concentration was higher in patients with mitral stenosis than in others. Further analysis[32] showed that vWF concentration strongly correlates with hemodynamic factors including pulmonary vascular resistance and pulmonary arterial pressure and inversely with cardiac output. Whether high vWF concentrations are the product of shear-induced stimulation of vWF release from lung endothelial cells or the result of some hormonal agonist is under investigation.

Patients with coronary valve disease had reduced levels of large multimers. The etiology and pathophysiological significance of this abnormality is unknown, but the observed degree of multimer loss was not sufficient in itself to cause a bleeding diathesis. This information can be used in other studies to test the hypothesis that a given hemorrhagic disorder is caused by a deficiency of large multimers. If the normalized multimer ratio is in the range of the valvular disease population, it is unlikely to be solely responsible for bleeding.

These studies have also shown that the deficiency of large multimers is the result of extracellular modification of vWF. vWF released by DDAVP or surgical stress from patients with low multimer levels had the same distribution as that from patients with preoperative normal distribution. Possibly, the abnormal hemodynamics of coronary valve disease plays a role in this depletion because large multimers remain in the circulation for at least 48 hours after surgical correction of the valve defect.

In summary, these investigations have helped to better define the conditions under which DDAVP can be used to reduce perioperativer bleeding and the need for transfusion. They have also provided new information about the structure, function and concentration of vWF as it exists in vivo. More work is needed, however, to elucidate the mechanisms underlying the hemostatic effect of DDAVP, and to optimize its therapeutic efficacy.

ACKNOWLEDGEMENTS

I am most grateful to Drs. Edwin Salzman, J. Anthony Ware and Jack Ansell for giving me the opportunity to participate in these studies, and I thank them for their helpful comments in preparing this manuscript.

REFERENCES

1. P.M. Mannucci, M. Aberg, I.M. Nilsson, and B. Robertson, Mechanism of plasminogen activator and factor VIII increase after vasoactive drugs, *Br. J. Haematol.*, 30:81 (1975).
2. I.R. MacGregor, E. Roberts, C.V. Prowse, N.A. Booth, A. Broomhead, and P. Litka, Changes in plasma t-PA, PAI and factor VIII following I.V. and S.C. injection of DDAVP in healthy volunteers, *Thromb. Haemost.*, 58:366 (Abst) (1987).
3. M. Levi, J.P. de Boer, D. Roem, J.W. ten Cate, and C.E. Hack, Plasminogen activation in vivo upon intravenous infusion of DDAVP. Quantitative assessment of plasmin- 2-antiplasmin complex with a novel monoclonal antibody based radioimmunoassay, *Thromb. Haemostas.*, 67:111 (1992).
4. B. de la Fuente, C.K. Kasper, F.R. Rickles, and L.W. Hoyer, Response of patients with mild and moderate hemophilia A and von Willebrand's disease to treatment with desmopressin, *Ann. Internal. Med.*, 103:6 (1985).
5. P.M. Mannucci, M.T. Canciani, L. Rota, and B.S. Donovan, Response of factor VIII/vWF to DDAVP in healthy subjects and patients with haemophilia A and von Willebrand disease. *Br. J. Haem.*, 47:283 (1981).
6. D.M. DiMichele, and W.E. Hathaway, Use of DDAVP in inherited and acquired platelet dysfunction, *Am. J. Hematol.*, 33:39 (1990).
7. N.L. Kobrinsky, E.D. Israels, J.M. Gerrard, M.S. Cheang, C.M. Watson, A.J. Bishop, and M.L. Schroeder, Shortening of bleeding time by 1-deamino-8-D-arginine vasopressin in various bleeding disorders, *Lancet*, 1:1145 (1984).
8. P. Mannucci, Desmopressin: A novel nontransfusion form of treatment for congenital and acquired bleeding disorders, *Blood*, 72:1449 (1988).
9. N.L. Kobrinsky, M. Letts, L.R. Patel, E.D. Israels, R.C. Monson, N. Schwetz, and M.S. Cheang, 1-Desamino-8-d-arginine vasopressin (Desmopressin) decreases operative blood loss in patients having Harrington rod spinal fusion surgery, *Ann. Int. Med.*, 107:446 (1987).
10. R.G. Johnson, and J.M. Murphy, The role of desmopressin in reducing blood loss during lumbar fusions, *Surgery*, 171:223 (1990).
11. E.W. Salzman, M.J. Weinstein, R.M. Weintraub, J.A. Ware, R.L. Thurer, L. Robertson, A. Donovan, T. Gaffney, V. Bertele, J. Troll, M.S. Smith, and L.E. Chute, Treatment with desmopressin acetate to reduce blood loss after cardiac surgery, *N. Eng. J. Med.*, 314:1402 (1986).
12. R.W. Colman, Platelet and neutrophil activation in cardiopulmonary bypass, *Ann. Thorac. Surg.* 49:32 (1990).
13. R.K. Wenger, H. Lukasiewicz, B.S. Mikuta, S. Niewiarowski, and L.H. Edmunds, Loss of platelet fibrinogen receptors during clinical cardiopulmonary bypass, *J. Thorac. Cardiovasc. Surg.*, 97:235 (1989).
14 M. Takeuchi, H. Nagura, and T. Kaneda, DDAVP and epinephrine-induced changes in the localization of von Willebrand factor antigen in endothelial cells of human oral mucosa, *Blood*. 72:85 (1988).
15. Z.M. Ruggeri, P. Mannucci, R. Lombardi, A.B. Federici, and T.S. Zimmerman, Multimeric composition of factor VIII/von Willebrand factor following administration of DDAVP: implications for pathophysiology and therapy of von Willebrand disease subtypes, *Blood*, 59: 1272 (1982).

16. J.L. Moake,N.A. Turner, N.A. Stathopoulos, L.H. Nolasco, J.D. Hellums, Involvement of large plasma von Willebrand Factor (vWF) multimers and unusually large vWF forms derived from endothelial cells in shear stress-induced platelet aggregation, *J. Clin. Invest.*, 78:1456, (1986).
17. M. Weinstein, J.A. Ware, J. Troll, and E. Salzman, Changes in von Willebrand factor during cardiac surgery: Effect of desmopressin acetate, *Blood*, 71:1648 (1988).
18. J. Ansell, V. Klassen, S.B. Lew, M.J. Weinstein, T. VanderSlam, I. Gratz, J. Leslie, A. Roberts, and N. Fleming, Does desmopressin acetate prophylaxis reduce blood loss after valvular heart surgery? A randomized, double blind study, *J. Thorac. Cardiovas. Surg.*, In press.
19. E. Salzman, M. Weinstein, J.A. Ware, Adventures in hemostasis: DDAVP in cardiac surgery, *Archives of Surg.*, In press.
20. E.W. Salzman, and W.H. Harris, Prevention of venous thromboembolism in orthopaedic patients, *J. Bone and Joint Surg.*, 58:903 (1976).
21. P.M. Mannucci, and J.M. Lusher, Desmopressin and thrombosis. *Lancet*, ii:675 (1989).
22. L.S. Czer, T.M. Bateman, R.J. Gray, M. Raymond, M.E. Stewart, S. Lee, D. Goldfinger, A. Chaux and J.M. Matloff, Treatment of severe platelet dysfunction and hemorrhage after cardiopulmonary bypass: reduction in blood product usage with desmopressin, *J. Am. Coll. Cardiol.*, 9:1139 (1987).
23. R.B. Chard, C.A. Kam, G.R. Nunn, D.C. Johnson, and W. Meldrum-Hanna, Use of desmopressin in the management of aspirin-related and intractable haemorrhage after cardiopulmonary bypass, *Aust. N. Z. J. Surg.*, 60:125 (1990).
24. E. Rocha, R. Llorens, J.A. Paramo, R. Arcas, B. Cuesta, and A.M. Trenor, Does desmopressin acetate reduce blood loss after surgery in patients on cardiopulmonary bypass?, *Circulation*, 77:1319 (1988).
25. T.L.G. Andersson, J.O. Solem, L. Tengborn, and E. Vinge Effects of desmopressin acetate on platelet aggregation, von Willebrand factor, and blood loss after cardiac surgery with extracorporeal circulation. *Circulation*, 81:872 (1990).
26. W.D. Lazenby, I. Russo, B.J. Zadeh, J.A. Zelano, W. Ko, C.C. Lynch, O.W. Isom, and K.H. Krieger, Treatment with desmopressin acetate in routine coronary artery bypass surgery to improve postoperative hemostasis, *Circulation*, 82:IV-413 (1990).
27. T.J. Spyt, M.A. Weerasena, W.H. Bain, G.D.O. Lowe, and A. Rumley, The effects of desmopressin acetate (DDAVP) on haemostasis and blood loss in routine coronary bypass surgery: a randomized, double-blind trial, *Perfusion*, 5(supl):57 (1990).
28. T. Hackmann, R.D. Gascoyne, S.C. Naiman, G.H. Growe, L.D. Burchill, W.R.E. Jamieson, S.B. Sheps, M.T. Schechter, and G.E. Townsend, A trial of desmopressin (1-desamino-8-D-arginine vasopressin) to reduce blood loss in uncomplicated cardiac surgery, *N. Eng. J. Med.*, 321:1437 (1989).
29. M.D. Seear, L.D. Wadsworth, P.C. Rogers, S. Sheps, and P.G. Ashmore, The effect of desmopressin acetate (DDAVP) on postoperative blood loss after cardiac operations in children, *J. Thorac. Cardiovasc. Surg.*, 98:217 (1989).
30. R. Hattori, K.K. Hamilton, R. Fugates, R.P. McEver, and P. Sims, Stimulated secretion of endothelial von Willebrand factor is accompanied by rapid redistribution to the cell surface of the intracellular granule membrane protein GMP-140, *J. Biol. Chem.*, 264:7768 (1989).
31. V. Vicente, I. Alberca, and P.M. Mannucci, Reduced effect of exercise and DDAVP on factor VIII-von Willebrand factor and plasminogen activator after sequential application of both the stimuli. *Thromb. Haemostas.*, 51:129 (1984).
32. W. Penny, M.J. Weinstein, J.A. Ware,and E. Salzman, Correlation of circulating von Willebrand factor levels with cardiovascular hemodynamics, *Circulation*, 83:1630 (1991).

DISCUSSION

Cattaneo: Were the methods of blood loss in the two trials comparable?
Weinstein: Yes: we used sponges and intrathoracic drainage.

Rao: Why was the blood loss so different in the two studies?
Weinstein: Intraoperative blood loss was included in the Salzman study but not in the Ansell

study. Even correcting for this, blood loss in the placebo group of the Salzman study was greater, presumably because there were more "redo" coronary artery bypass grafts, which produce higher losses.

Sassetti: I am always suspicious abut blood loss assessment. Was it corrected for infusions of therapeutic fluids, hematocrit, and so on?
Weinstein: We corrected for the dilution effect of hematocrit and resuscitative fluids, and the blood losses were still different.

Schulman (Sweden): How much of the loss occurred before DDAVP was given?
Weinstein: We do not have the numbers.

Berrettini (Italy): How did you assess deep vein thrombosis?
Weinstein: Screening for DVT was by labelled fibrinogen scanning of the calves and impedance phethysmography. There was the same incidence in the placebo and desmopressin groups.

DESMOPRESSIN IN CARDIAC SURGERY WITH EXTRA-CORPOREAL CIRCULATION

E. Rocha[1], J.A. Páramo[1], R. Llorens[2] and F. Hidalgo[3]

[1]Haematology, [2]Cardiovascular Surgery and [3]Anaesthesia Services
University Clinic, Faculty of Medicine, University of Navarra
Pamplona (Spain)

INTRODUCTION

Patients who undergo cardiopulmonary bypass (CPB) for open heart surgery have an increased susceptibility to postoperative bleeding[1]. They often require blood component therapy, reoperation for bleeding control is sometimes necessary and occasionally life-threatening hemorrhage occurs during the postoperative period. The majority of patients primarily bleed from the operative site and the excessive bleeding is related to the surgical damage to blood vessels.

However, in some patients, diffuse systemic bleeding[2,3] suggests an acute acquired hemostatic defect. The basic pathophysiology of altered hemostasis associated with CPB remains confusing because of the complexity of the hemostatic process and the many uncontrolled variables associated with CPB, such as the surgical procedure, type of anaesthesia, drug administration, transfused blood products, hypothermia, hemodilution and the type of oxigenator. The abnormalities most frequently found include heparin and protamin excess, heparin rebound, low platelet count, low fibrinogen and other coagulation factors, primary fibrinolysis, and disseminated intravascular coagulation[4-16]. However, the major contributor to abnormal haemostasis is the alteration of platelet function[2,3,17-28].

Platelet dysfunction is consequent to transient platelet activation and appears to be dependent on contact of blood with the nonphysiological surfaces. Platelet abnormalities include secondary release and partial depletion of platelet α-granules, but not dense granules, as well as an increase of the plasma levels of platelet factor 4 and β-thromboglobulin.

Desmopressin in Bleeding Disorders, Edited by G. Mariani *et al.*
Plenum Press, New York, 1993

Although the exact mechanism responsible for this platelet dysfunction remains unknown, several lines of evidence suggest a reversible membrane abnormality. In vitro studies have demonstrated that platelets exposed to the oxygenator apparatus show a reduced binding to fibrinogen and α-adrenergic agonists[19,20,25]. Indeed, a defect in ristocetin-induced platelet aggregation has been described in these patients[3], suggesting a role for von Willebrand factor in the hemostatic defect[27]. Moreover, George et al[24] have reported significant decreases in the amount of membrane antigen for glycoproteins Ib, IIb and IIIa on circulating platelets following CPB. These functional abnormalities progressively increase with the duration of cardio-pulmonary bypass, the level of hypothermia and the use of various drugs. The platelet dysfunction is usually reversible within one hour following cardiopulmonary bypass, but in some patients a persistent functional platelet defect may occur.

Since a significant platelet function defect may be the primary cause of hemorrhage, sometimes bleeding can be controlled and the bleeding time shortened by platelet transfusions. However, very often no clinically significant benefit can be demonstrated. Although prostacyclin protects platelets from activation during cardiopulmonary bypass in primates[29], such an effect has not been proven in human patients[30].

Another alternative for the treatment of this hemostatic defect could be to increase the plasma concentration of von Willebrand factor (vWF), since the increase of high molecular weight multimers of von Willebrand factor has been shown to shorten the prolonged bleeding time under diverse conditions, including uremia, chronic liver disease and aspirin ingestion[31-35]. Such an effect can be achieved by cryoprecipitate administration or by the infusion of desmopressin acetate (DDAVP) which is known to shorten the bleeding time and increase the level of factor VIII, von Willebrand factor and their high molecular weight multimers.

CLINICAL STUDIES

The hemostatic properties of DDAVP in patients undergoing open heart surgery with CPB were first studied by Czer et al[36,37] in a prospective nonrandomized clinical study. Patients who had excessive bleeding more than two hours after CPB as well as a prolongation of the bleeding time were treated with blood products, either alone or in combination with 0.3 μg/kg of desmopressin. Patients treated with DDAVP needed significantly less transfusion of blood products, specially red blood cells and platelets (table I), without detectable adverse effects. Moreover, desmopressin infusion shortened the bleeding time from 17 to 12.5 minutes ($p < 0.05$), and significantly increased F VIII:C and vWF levels ($p < 0.05$) which could contribute to the clinical benefit, despite the fact that the recovery of platelet function is not complete, as indicated by the prolongation of the bleeding time.

Salzman et al[38] performed a double-blind, prospective, randomized trial to study the effect of intraoperative DDAVP in 70 patients undergoing cardiac operations requiring CPB. Those with primary uncomplicated coronary-artery bypass grafting were not included because of the risk of early graft occlusion subsequent to the effects of DDAVP on von Willebrand factor in plasma. Patients were randomized to DDAVP (0.3 µg/kg) or placebo. Treatment was given intravenously in a 50-ml saline solution over 15 minutes when CPB had been concluded and inmediately after administration of protamine. The duration of extracorporeal circulation was similarly prolonged in both groups (144 ± 38 and 159 ± 66 minutes, respectively). The desmopressin-treated patients showed a significant reduction in intraoperative, 24 hours postoperative, and total blood loss and lower red-cell transfusion requirements (table II), without detectable adverse effects. All three patients that required reoperation for control of bleeding and 11 of the 14 patients that lost more than 2000 ml of blood during and in the first 24 hours after operation were in the placebo group. Patients receiving DDAVP showed significantly higher vWF:Ag levels 90 minutes after infusion than those who received the placebo. An interesting finding was the possible relation between the preoperative plasma vWF:Ag level and the total blood loss.

Table I. Blood requirements and reoperation for hemorrhage in Czer's study[37]

	Desmopressin (n = 23)	Control (n = 16)	p value
Blood products used			
Red blood cells	4.8 ± 3.0	7.9 ± 4.7	0.015
Platelets	4.0 ± 6.7	11.8 ± 9.1	0.004
Plasma	2.7 ± 2.8	4.2 ± 2.6	NS
Total	15.3 ± 13.4	29.2 ± 19.3	0.02
Reoperation	2 (9 %)	12 (75 %)	0.001

In the light of these results it seemed that the beneficial effect of the DDAVP in cardiopulmonary bypass was probably related to an elevation of von Willebrand factor in plasma, perhaps mediated by a change in the distribution of multimers of von Willebrand factor, with an increase of high molecular weight multimers. However, the effectiveness of DDAVP in reducing blood loss could not be related to the increase of large vWF multimers in another study[39], and these authors think that the effectiveness of DDAVP might be due to a rise in F VIII:C, or the exposure of new binding sites on endothelial cells. Although the beneficial effects of desmopressin remain unclear, Harker[27] states that if the results of these trials are confirmed and can be applied to other types of cardiac operations, mainly primary coronary-artery bypass grafting, treatment with DDAVP could produce substantial savings in blood supplies, reduce the risk of transfusion-transmitted diseases and diminish the rate of reoperation for hemorrhage.

Table II. Results of Salzman's trial[38]

	Desmopressin (n = 35)	Placebo (n = 35)	p value
Red cells used (unit)	2.6 ± 2.1	3.7 ± 3.3	0.079
Blood loss (ml)			
Intraoperative	592 ± 358	993 ± 858	0.015
From 0-12 hr	510 ± 289	803 ± 471	0.003
From 12-24 hr	215 ± 113	414 ± 429	0.013
Total	1,317 ± 487	2,210 ± 1415	0.001
vWF:Ag (U/ml)			
Before operation	1.85 ± 0.76	1.79 ± 0,78	NS
After treatment	1.80 ± 0.53	1.46 ± 0.55	0.02

A year later our group[40] carried out a double-blind, randomized, prospective trial involving 100 patients undergoing CPB for valvular heart disease or atrial septal defects, who were randomly assigned to receive DDAVP (0.3 μg/kg) or a placebo. Patients on coronary-artery bypass grafting were excluded. Treatment was administered intravenously in a 50 ml saline solution for 15 minutes on completion of CPB and immediately after administration of protamine. Both groups were similar with regard to the baseline clinical characteristics, the main diagnoses and the types of surgery as well as in the duration of extracorporeal circulation (93 ± 43 vs. 94 ± 40 minutes). As shown in table III, no significant differences in either the postoperative or the total blood loss were observed between groups. Only intraoperative blood loss was significantly lower ($p < 0.02$) in the DDAVP group (131 ± 106 ml/m^2) than in the placebo group (193 ± 137 ml/m^2). The volume of red cell transfused in the first 3 days was similar in both groups and only one patient in the placebo group required surgical reoperation to control bleeding. There was a significant increase of F VIII:C and vWF:Ag and a shortening of the bleeding time

90 minutes after therapy in the desmopressin group as compared to the placebo group ($p < 0.001$). Whereas no correlation between bleeding time, F VIII:C and vWF:Ag with the total blood loss was observed in the samples obtained preoperatively and 90 minutes after treatment, a significant negative correlation ($r = -0.36$, $p < 0.001$) between the concentration of F VIII:C in the sample obtained 90 minutes after administration of treatment and intraoperative blood loss was able to be demonstrated.

Table III. Blood loss, transfusion requirements and laboratory results in the sample obtained 90 minutes after treatment in patients studied by Rocha et al.[40]

	Desmopressin (n = 50)	Placebo (n = 50)	p value
Blood loss (ml/m^2)			
Intraoperative	131 ± 106	193 ± 137	0.02
0-24 hr	249 ± 144	253 ± 224	NS
24-72 hr	78 ± 58	89 ± 89	NS
Total	458 ± 206	536 ± 304	NS
Red cells used (ml)	1,642 ± 705	1,574 ± 645	NS
Laboratory tests			
Bleeding time (min)	9.4 ± 0.7	13.8 ± 1.1	0.001
F VIII:C (U/ml)	1.6 ± 0.1	1.0 ± 0.1	0.001
vWF:Ag (U/ml)	1.7 ± 0.1	1.0 ± 0.1	0.001

Therefore, we cannot confirm that DDAVP reduces total blood loss and transfusion requirements, although it was observed to significantly reduce intraoperative blood loss. The characteristics of patients included in our study and in Salzman's study[38] were similar with respect to age, sex, diagnosis and operative procedure, except that in the latter study a small patient group with coronary artery disease, known to have high perioperative bleeding complications, was included. Thus, it seems unlikely that differences in characteristics of the patients in these studies are responsible for the disparate findings. A significant difference was that the blood loss observed in Salzman's study[38] was higher than in our study, which could be related to the longer duration of extracorporeal circulation. The difference in the total blood loss between both studies can be important. It has been argued that the good results found by Salzman et al.[38] may be related to the high postoperative blood loss reported in their patients[41,42].

We found a significant negative correlation between intraoperative blood loss and the plasma concentration of F VIII:C 90 minutes after treatment, suggesting that the reduction might be related to an increase in factor VIII:C induced by DDAVP, as was previously indicated by Weinstein et al[39].

Since the administration of DDAVP in patients placed on CPB surgery for valvular heart disease or atrial septal defects is effective in reducing intraoperative bleeding, with no side effects, we conclude that this drug may be useful only intraoperatively in patients with excessive intraoperative hemorrhage, which might be related to the short duration of the effect of desmopressin.

Hackmann et al.[43] performed a double-blind, randomized trial to determine if DDAVP is useful in all elective cardiac surgical procedures involving CPB. They studied 150 consecutive patients undergoing uncomplicated elective cardiac surgery, including primary coronary-artery bypass grafting, who were randomly assigned to receive either 0.3 μg/kg of desmopressin or placebo. The study drug was infused in 25 ml of saline solution, over 15 minutes, after CPB was terminated and protamine administered. The two treatment groups were homogeneous in their baseline characteristics, the types of surgery performed, the concomitant medication and the duration of the operation. The duration of bypass (168 ± 58 vs. 161 ± 52 minutes) was similar to that reported in Salzman's trial[38] but longer than in our study[40]. As shown in table IV no significant differences in either intraoperative or postoperative and total blood loss were observed between the desmopressin and placebo groups. The proportion of patients who received blood products intra and postoperatively was similar in both groups except for the administration of plasma postoperatively which was higher in the DDAVP group than in the placebo group (58 % vs. 41 %, p = 0.05). Among those patients who received blood products, the distribution of amounts received during and after operation was similar in the two groups. Five patients in the DDAVP group and two in the placebo group needed reoperation for hemorrhage. Mortality rate was similar in both groups. The level of ristocetin cofactor and the concentration of vWF multimers 90 minutes and 24 hours after treatment were similarly increased in both groups with respect to basal value, and there was no selective increase of large multimers of von Willebrand factor . A negative correlation between total blood loss and the ristocetin-cofactor level at 90 minutes was found.

There was a discrepancy between the results of this study and those previously published. Hackman et al.[43] conclude that the use of desmopressin in an unselected group of patients who underwent cardiac surgery, including primary coronary-artery bypass grafting, did not appear to confer any benefit in terms of a reduction of blood loss or the need for blood replacement. The different method of selection of patients may provide at least a partial explanation. Salzman et al.[38] included in their study patients undergoing valve replacement or complex cardiac procedures, perhaps subject to higher blood loss, and we[40] studied patients undergoing valve repair or replacement or repair of an atrial septal defect, whereas in these two studies patients with primary coronary-artery bypass grafting were excluded. In contrast, in Hackman's study[43], 69 % of the patients underwent this last procedure. The mean blood loss in the placebo group of Salzman's study was significantly higher than in the other two studies. Moreover, Hackman et al.[43] found a similar increase of ristocetin cofactor in patients treated with DDAVP or placebo. They suggest that the severe stress associated with cardiac surgery alone served to increase von Willebrand factor values even when desmopressin had not been given. However, we and others[38,39,44] did find a significant increase in vWF:Ag 90 minutes after DDAVP treatment with respect to placebo group.

Table IV. Results of Hackman's study[43]

	Desmopressin (n = 74)	Placebo (n = 76)	p value
Blood loss (ml)			
Intraoperative	200	200	NS
Postoperative	865	738	NS
Total	1,138	1,010	NS
Patients transfused (%)			
Intraoperative: red cells	46	41	NS
plasma	22	22	NS
Postoperative: red cells	50	54	NS
plasma	58	41	0.05
all products	77	75	NS
Ristocetin cofactor (%)			
Basal	136.4 ± 68.4	136,1 ± 59,5	NS
90 minutes	241.3 ± 97.9	218,1 ± 85,4	NS
Multimers increased (%)			
Basal	11	24	0.04
90 minutes	75	63	NS

As shown in table V four recent studies have confirmed the results of Hackman et al[43]. One was performed in cardiac operations in children[45] and three in coronary-artery bypass surgery[44,46,47]. Another study has even shown that the total postoperative blood loss ($p < 0.0001$) and the red cell transfusion rates ($p < 0.005$) were significantly higher in the DDAVP group than in the control group[48], which could be related to the fibrinolytic state produced as a result of DDAVP-induced increase in tissue plasminogen activator. These authors suggest that DDAVP may be of no benefit in patients undergoing cardiopulmonary bypass surgery.

Table V. Analysis of five trials using desmopressin

	Desmopressin	Placebo or control	p value
Sear MD et al.[45]			
No. patients	30	30	
Total blood loss (ml/kg)	40.0 ± 33,1	30.5 ± 37.9	NS
Anderson TLG et al.[44]			
No. patients	10	9	
Total blood loss (ml)	852 ± 223	1,020 ± 422	NS
Lazenby WD et al.[46]			
No. patients	30	30	
Total blood loss (ml): 0-12 h	465 ± 207	511 ± 221	NS
12-24 h	236 ± 127	260 ± 112	NS
Red cells used (unit)	2.8 ± 2.1	2.2 ± 1.8	NS
Hedderich GS et al.[47]			
No. patients	31	31	
Total blood loss (ml)	1,716 ± 688	1,826 ± 849	NS
Red cells used (unit)	3.6 ± 0.8	3.4 ± 1.3	NS
LoCicero J et al.[48]			
No. patients	74	91	
Total blood loss (ml)	1,306 ± 688	896 ± 33	0.001
Red cells used (unit)	1.23 ± 0.8	0.35 ± 0.8	0.005

A further prospective, randomized trial, was recently carried out by our group to establish whether a second dose of DDAVP could improve the results of our first study. Ninety patients undergoing various cardiac surgical procedures, including primary coronary-artery bypass grafting, were randomly assigned to one of the following groups: (1) 30 patients received 0.3 μg/kg of DDAVP intravenously in a 50 ml saline solution for 15 minutes on completion of CPB and immediately after administration of protamine; (2) 30 patients received two doses of DDAVP, the first as in the previous group and the second 6 hours later; (3) 30 patients received no treatment. The baseline characteristics, the main diagnoses, the types of surgery and the duration of surgery and extracorporeal circulation were similar in the three groups. Results of blood loss and transfusion requirements are shown in table V. There were no significant differences in any of these parameters, and no side effects were observed. We conclude that a second dose of DDAVP given 6 hours after surgery does not reduce the postoperative bleeding.

No side effects as a result of DDAVP administration have been reported in the different studies performed so far, except for a serious reaction to desmopressin in a child with cyanotic heart disease[49].

Table VI. Blood loss and transfusion requirements in relation to various therapeutic methods.

	Group 1	Group 2	Group 3	p value
Blood loss (ml/m^2)	515 ± 310	465 ± 228	432 ± 236	NS
Red cells used (ml)	1,258 ± 894	1,206 ± 1,074	1,216 ± 1,088	NS

CONCLUSIONS

There is evidence that the administration of DDAVP may be effective in reducing hemorrhage in patients at high risk such as those undergoing valve replacement combined with coronary-artery bypass grafting or reoperations[50,51] or in those with aspirin-related bleeding after bypass[52] or in patients with severe platelet dysfunction and excessive mediastinal bleeding more than 2 hours after termination of cardiopulmonary bypass[53]. However, the majority of patients who undergo cardiac surgery without complications will have only moderate blood loss, and in these cases desmopressin does not appear to offer any advantages beyond those of conventional techniques for reducing the use of blood products. Thus, desmopressin could be administered to patients who are at particular high risk of bleeding but not routinely to all patients undergoing cardiopulmonary bypass surgery.

It has recently been reported that the intraoperative administration of aprotinin significantly reduces postoperative blood loss in patients undergoing cardiac operations. The protease inhibitor aprotinin seems to constitute a better alternative than DDAVP in the reduction of bleeding associated with CPB when given prophylactically.

REFERENCES

1. F. Bachmann, R. McKenna, E.R. Cole and H. Najafi. The hemostatic mechanism after open-heart surgery. I. Studies on plasma coagulation factors and fibrinolysis in 512 patients after extracorporeal circulation. J. Thorac. Cardiovasc. Surg. 70:76 (1975).
2. R.L. Bick. Hemostasis defects associated with cardiac surgery, prosthetic devices, and other extracorporeal circuits. Semin. Thromb. Hemost. 11:249 (1985).
3. E.F. Mammen, M.H. Koets, B.C. Washington et al. Hemostasis changes during cardiopulmonary by-pass surgery. Semin. Thromb. Hemost. 11:281 (1985).
4. N. Ellison, C.P.Beaty, D.R. Blake, H.A. Wurzel and H. Mac Vaugh III. Heparin rebound: studies in patients and volunteers. J. Thorac. Cardiovasc. Surg. 67:723 (1974).
5. M.N. Andersen, M. Mendelow and G.A. Alfano. Experimental studies of heparin-protamine activity with special reference to protamine inhibition of clotting. Surgery 46:1060 (1959).
6. S.V. Kevy, R.M. Glickman, W.F. Bernhard, L.K. Diamond and R.E. Gross. The pathogenesis and control of the hemorrhagic defect in open heart surgery. Surg. Gynecol. Obstet. 123:313 (1959).
7. R. McKenna, F. Bachmann, B. Whitaker, J.R. Gilson and M.J. Weinberg. The hemostatic mechanism

after open-heart surgery. II. Frequency of abnormal platelet functions during and after extracorporeal circulation. J. Thorac. Cardiovasc. Surg. 70:298 (1975).

8. J.D. Milam, S.F. Austin, R.F. Martin, A.B. Keats and D.A. Cooley. Alteration of coagulation and selected clinical chemistry parameters in patients undergoing open heart surgery without transfusions. Am. J. Clin. Pathol. 76:155 (1981).

9. J. Umlas. Fibrinolysis and disseminated intravascular coagulation in open heart surgery. Transfusion 16:460 (1976).

10. O. Kucuk, H.C. Kwaan, J. Frederickson, L. Wade and D. Green. Increased fibrinolytic activity in patients undergoing cardiopulmonary bypass operation. Am. J. Hematol. 23:223 (1986).

11. R.L. Bick, N.R. Arbegast, L. Crawford, L. Holterman, T. Adams and W.R. Schmalhorst. Hemostatic defects induced by cardiopulmonary bypass. Vasc. Surg. 9:28 (1975).

12. R.L. Bick, W.R. Schmalhorst and N.R. Arbegast. Alterations of hemostasis associated with cardiopulmonary bypass. Am. J. Clin. Pathol. 63:588 (1975).

13. R.G. Kladetsky, S. Popov-Cenic, W. Buttner, N. Muller and H. Egli. Studies of fibrinolytic and coagulation factors during open-heart surgery with ECC. Thromb. Res. 7:579 (1975).

14. J.A. Páramo, J. Rifón, R. Llorens, J. Casares, M.J. Paloma and E. Rocha. Intra- and postoperative fibrinolysis in patients undergoing cardiopulmonary bypass surgery. Haemostasis 21:58 (1991).

15. J. Stibbe, C. Kluft and E.J. Brommer. Enhanced fibrinolytic activity during cardiopulmonary bypass in open heart surgery in man is caused by extrinsic (tissue type) plasminogen activator. Eur. J. Clin. Invest. 14:373 (1984).

16. J. Rifón, J. Fernandez, J.A. Páramo, B. Cuesta and E. Rocha. Fibrinogen and fibrin degradation products in patients undergoing open-heart surgery. Blood Coag. Fibrinol. 1:509 (1990).

17. L.A. Harker, T.W. Malpass, H.E. Branson, E.A. Hessel and S.J. Slichter. Mechanism of abnormal bleeding in patients undergoing cardiopulmonary bypass: acquired transient platelet dysfunction associated with selective-granule release. Blood 56:824 (1980).

18. C. Beurling-Harbury and C.A. Galvan. Acquired decrease in platelet secretory ADP associated with increased postoperative bleeding in post-cardiopulmonary bypass patients and in patients with severe valvular heart disease. Blood 52:13 (1978).

19. J. Musial, S. Niewiarowski, D. Hershock, T.A. Morinelli, R.W. Colman and L.H. Edmunds Jr. Loss of fibrinogen receptors from the platelet surface during simulated extracorporeal circulation. J. Lab. Clin. Med. 105:514 (1985).

20. Y.T. Wachtfogel, J. Musial, B. Jenkin, S. Niewiarowski, L.H. Edmunds Jr. and R.W. Colman. Loss of platelet$_2$-adrenergic receptors during simulated extracorporeal circulation prevention with prostaglandin E_1. J. Lab. Clin. Med. 105:601 (1985).

21. V.P. Adonizio Jr., J.F. Strauss III, R.W. Colman and L.H. Edmunds Jr. Effects of prostaglandin E_1 on platelet loss during in vivo and in vitro extracorporeal circulation with a bubble oxygenator. J. Throac. Cardiovasc. Surg. 77:119 (1979).

22. V.P. Addonizio, J.B. Smith, J.F. Straus, R.W. Colman and L.H. Edmunds Jr. Thromboxane synthesis and platelet secretion during cardiopulmonary bypass with bubble oxygenator. J. Thorac. Cardiovasc. Surg. 79:91 (1980).

23. L.H. Edmunds, N. Ellison, R.W. Colman et al. Platelet function during cardiac operation. Comparison of membrane and bubble oxygenators. J. Thorac. Cardiovasc. Surg. 83:805 (1982).

24. J.N. George, E.B. Pickett, S. Saucerman et al. Platelet surface glycoproteins. Studies on resting and activated platelets and platelet membrane microparticles in normal subjetcs and observations in patients during adult respiratory distress syndrome and cardiac surgery. J. Clin. Invest. 78:340 (1986).

25. R.K. Wenger, H. Lukasicwicz, B.S. Mikuta, S. Niewiarowski and L.H. Edmunds Jr. Loss of platelet fibrinogen receptors during clinical cardiopulmonary bypass. J. Thorac. Cardiovasc. Surg. 97:235 (1989).

26. W.R. Friedenberg, W.O. Myers and E.D. Plotka. Platelet dysfunction associated with cardiopulmonary bypass. Ann. Thorac. Surg. 25:298 (1978).
27. L.A. Harker. Bleeding after cardiopulmonary bypass. N. Engl. J. Med. 314:1446 (1986).
28. V.L. Hennessey, R.E. Hicks, S. Niewiarowski et al. Function of human platelets during extracorporeal circulation. Am. J. Physiol. 232:622 (1977).
29. T.W. Malpass, S.R. Hanson, B. Savage, E.A. Hessel and L.A. Harker. Prevention of acquired transient defect in platelet plug formation by infused prostacyclin. Blood 57:736 (1981).
30. T.W. Malpass, D.W. Amory, L.A. Harker, T.D. Ivey and D.B. Williams. The effect of prostacyclin infusion on platelet hemostatic function in patients undergoing cardiopulmonary bypass. J. Thorac. Cardiovasc. Surg. 87:550 (1984).
31. P.M. Mannucci, M.T. Canciani, L. Rota and B.S. Donovan. Response of factor VIII/von Willebrand factor to DDAVP in healthy subjects and patients with haemophilia A and von Willebrand's disease. Br. J. Haematol. 47:283 (1981).
32. V. Vicente, I. Alberca, J.F. Macias and A. Lopez-Borrasca. DDAVP in uremia. Nephron. 36:145 (1984).
33. G.L. Vigano, P.M. Mannucci, A. Lattuada, A. Harris and G. Remuzzi. Subcutaneous desmopressin (DDAVP) shortens the bleeding time in uremia. Am. J. Haemat. 31:32 (1989).
34. N.L. Kobrinsky, E.D. Israels, J.M. Gerrard et al. Shortening of bleeding time by 1-deamino-8-D-arginine vasopressin in various bleeding disorders. Lancet 1:1145 (1984).
35. G. Agnelli, M. Berettini, M. De Cunto and G.M. Nenci. Desmopressin-induced improvement of abnormal coagulation in chronic liver disease. Lancet 1:645 (1983).
36. L. Czer, T. Bateman, R.J. Gray et al. Prospective trial of DDAVP in treatment of severe platelet dysfunction and hemorrhage after cardiopulmonary bypass. Circulation 72 (suppl. III): III-130 (1985).
37. L.S.C. Czer, T.M. Bateman, R.J. Gray et al. Treatment of severe platelet dysfunction and hemorrhage after cardiopulmonary bypass: reduction in blood product usage with desmopressin. J. Am. Coll. Cardiol. 9:1139 (1987).
38. E.W. Salzman, M.J. Weinstein, R.M. Weintraub et al. Treatment with desmopressin acetate to reduce blood loss after cardiac surgery: a double-blind randomized trial. N. Engl. J. Med. 314:1402 (1986).
39. M. Weinstein, J.A. Ware, J. Troll and E. Salzman. Changes in von Willebrand factor during cardiac surgery: effect of desmopressin acetate. Blood 71:1648 (1988).
40. E. Rocha, R. LLorens, J.A. Páramo, R. Arcas, B. Cuesta and A. Martín Trenor. Does desmopressin acetate reduce blood loss after surgery in patients on cardiopulmonary bypass?. Circulation 77:1319 (1988).
41. F. Millard. Desmopressin acetate to reduce blood loss after cardiac surgery (Letter). N Engl. J. Med. 315:834 (1986).
42. G. Allen. Desmopressin acetate to reduce blood loss after cardiac surgery (Letter). N. Engl. J. Med. 315:835 (1986).
43. T. Hackmann, R.D. Gascoyne, S.C. Naiman et al. A trial of desmopressin (1-deamino-8-D-arginine vasopressin) to reduce blood loss in uncomplicated cardiac surgery. N. Engl. J. Med. 321:1437 (1989).
44. T.L.G. Anderson, J.O. Solem, L. Tengborn and E. Vinge. Effects of desmopressin acetate on platelet aggregation, von Willebrand factor, and blood loss after cardiac surgery with extracorporeal circulation. Circulation 81:872 (1990).
45. M.D. Seear, L.D. Wadsworth, P.C. Rogers, S. Sheps and P.G. Ashmore. The effect of desmopressin acetate (DDAVP) on postoperative blood loss after cardiac operations in children. J. Thorac. Cardiovasc. Surg. 98:217 (1989).
46. W.D. Lazenby, I. Russo, B.J. Zadeh et al. Treatment with desmopressin acetate in routine coronary

artery bypass surgery to improve postoperative hemostasis. Circulation 82 (suppl. IV):413 (1990).

47. G.S. Hedderich, D.J. Petsikas, B.A. Cooper et al. Desmopressin acetate in uncomplicated coronary artery bypass surgery: a prospective randomized clinical trial. Can. J. Surg. 33:33 (1990).

48. J. LoCicero, M. Massad and J. Matano. Effect of desmopressin acetate on hemorrhage without identifiable cause in coronary bypass patients. Am. Surg. 57:165 (1991).

49. S.J. Israels and N.L. Kobrisky. Serious reaction to desmopressin in a child with cyanotic heart disease (letter). N. Engl. J. Med. 32:1563 (1989).

50. E.W. Salzman. Desmopressin and surgical hemostasis (letter). N Engl J. Med. 322:1085 (1990).

51. E. Rocha, R. Llorens, J.A. Páramo. Desmopressin and surgical hemostasis (letter). N. Engl. J. Med. 322:1085 (1990).

52. L.S.C. Czer and S.M. Capon. Clinical experience in disorders of haemostasis. Drug Invest. 2 (suppl. 5):32 (1990).

53. R.B. Chard, C.A. Kam, G.R. Nunn, D.C. Jhonson and W. Meldrum-Hanna. Use of desmopressin in the management of aspirin-related and intractable haemorrhage after cardiopulmonary bypass. Aust. N. Z. J. Surg. 60:125 (1990).

DISCUSSION

Kobrinski: In one study, five patients on desmopressin and two on placebo had to return to surgery. This suggests a possible surgically correctable cause for the bleeding. If you removed these patients from the group, would that make a difference to the analysis?
Rocha: No.

Harris (Sweden): In view of the heterogeneous trial results, would it be worth forming a committee to pool the results of all the controlled trials? The studies in Scotland, England, Sweden and Belgium would give a considerable data base to identify the associated factors - not just to make a meta-analysis.
Rocha: The studies are not easily comparable.
Harris: That is so, but we can learn so much by setting up a larger data base.

Schulman: What is your opinion of the use of aprotinin? Dr Rocha: The possible decrease of fibrinolytic activity after aprotinin is not confirmed.

DESMOPRESSIN CORRECTS THE HEMOSTATIC DISORDER INDUCED BY DEXTRAN AND REGIONAL ANESTHESIA IN TOTAL HIP REPLACEMENT

Per Anders Flordal

Department of Surgery
Danderyd Hospital
S-182 88 Danderyd, Sweden

INTRODUCTION

Blood loss is an important problem in total hip replacement and most patients receive blood transfusions (Flordal and Neander, 1991). The topics of this paper are: (1) is there a hemostatic disorder, possibly contributing to the extensive blood loss (Flordal et al., 1991b). and (2) may desmopressin correct such a disorder (Flordal et al., 1991b) and / or reduce blood loss (Flordal et al., 1991a)?

Regional anaesthesia is often used in relation with total hip replacement because it has been shown to reduce blood loss (Modig and Karlström, 1987) and prevent postoperative deep vein thrombosis (Modig et al., 1986) in this procedure. Dextran also prevents postoperative thromboembolic complications (Bergqvist, 1983; National Institutes of Health, 1986) and may reduce transfusion requirements serving as a plasma expander (Thorén and Wiklund, 1983; Messmer, 1988).

BIOCHEMICAL TEST AND DRUG ADMINISTRATION

Eight women, with mean age 63 (range 43–72) years, and four men, with mean age 67 (range 55–73) years, scheduled for total hip replacement, were studied with respect to coagulation parameters. Patients above the age of 80 years or with severe vascular, hepatic or renal disease were not included. The indication for surgery was primary arthrosis in eight, sequelae to hip fractures in two patients, repeated hip prosthesis dislocations in one and prosthesis loosening in one patient. Methyl-metacrylate cement was used in all patients. In a double-blind fashion each patient received an infusion of placebo or desmopressin (Ferring AB, Sweden) 0.3 µg/kg body weight diluted in 50 ml saline at the start of surgery. The same infusion was repeated 6 hours later, on both occasions at an infusion rate of 20–30 minutes.

Venous samples were taken at 8.00 (before the induction of anesthesia), at about 12.00 (1 hour after the end of the operation), at 15.00 and on the following day at 8.00. Analyses were made for platelet count and hemoglobin concentration (Hb), activated partial thromboplastin time (APTT, Cephotest, Nycomed, Sweden), factor VIII procoagulant activity (FVIII:C, Coatest S-2222, Kabi Vitrum Diagnostica, Sweden) and von Willebrand factor antigen (vWF:Ag, electroimmunoassay (Laurell, 1972) with rabbit antibody, Dakopatts, Denmark).

Desmopressin in Bleeding Disorders, Edited by G. Mariani *et al.*
Plenum Press, New York, 1993

Table 1. Descriptive data on 50 total hip replacement patients studied with respect to blood loss.

	Control	Desmopressin	Difference
Men	12	12	n.s.
Women	13	13	n.s.
Age [years]	68±9	64±9	n.s.
Body weight [kg]	71±15	75±12	n.s.
Body height [cm]	171±11	172±9	n.s.
Body mass index [kg/m^2]	24±3	25±3	n.s.
Primary arthrosis	21	23	n.s.
Secondary arthrosis	2	0	n.s.
Revision arthroplasty	2	2	n.s.
Cemented prosthesis	17	21	n.s.
- BiMetric	9	11	n.s.
- Charnley	3	7	n.s.
- Stanmore	5	3	n.s.
Uncemented prosthesis (BiMetric)	8	4	n.s.
Operation time [min]	104±20	106±23	n.s.
Preoperative			
- Hb [g/l]	134±12	135±11	n.s.
- platelet count [10^9/l]	258±53	257±50	n.s.
- prothrombin complex [%]	97±17	103±19	n.s.
- APTT [s]	24±2	25±2	n.s.
- Ivy bleeding time [min]	3.7±1.3	3.7±1.1	n.s.

Numbers, or means ±SD.

The bleeding time was determined preoperatively and 1 hour after surgery, according to a modification of Ivy's method with the Simplate II device (General Diagnostics) and 40 mmHg stasis.

Another fifty patients (Table 1) were studied with respect to blood loss. On the afternoon before surgery venous blood was taken for Hb, platelet count, prothrombin complex assay (Diagnostica Stago, France), APTT and Ivy bleeding time. Hb and platelet count were again determined on the third postoperative day.

These patients too were randomly allocated to receive desmopressin 0.3 µg/kg body weight or placebo (saline) at the start of surgery and again 6 hours later.

ANESTHETIC AND SURGICAL TECHNIQUE

All patients were assessed in hospital two weeks preoperatively by an anesthetist and an orthopedic surgeon. The aim was to identify patients requiring further preparation or treatment before surgery and to ascertain that no prostaglandin synthesis inhibitors were in use.

Operations started at 9.15–9.30. Ringer acetate 500 ml was infused before induction of spinal anesthesia with plain bupivacaine 0.5% (Astra AB, Sweden). All but one patient in the coagulation study and all but seven patients in the blood loss study also had an epidural catheter for postoperative pain relief with bupivacaine and morphine. Ephedrine was administered pre- or intraoperatively to prevent the systolic blood pressure from falling below 100 mmHg.

Total hip replacements were performed with the patients in the lateral position. Both cemented and uncemented prostheses were used (Table 1).

During surgery all patients received an intravenous infusion of 6% dextran 70 (Pharmacia AB, Sweden) 500–1000 ml for thrombosis prophylaxis and plasma expansion, the volume infused depending on the amount of blood loss. Hapten dextran 1 (Pharmacia AB, Sweden) 3 g was infused before dextran 70 to prevent allergic reactions. A balanced isotonic crystalloid solution was infused intra- and postoperatively for the first 24 hours. A further 500 ml dextran was infused on the first postoperative day.

Table 2. Infusions, injections, blood pressures and urine production during the perioperative 24 hour period in the patients studied with respect to blood loss.

	Control (n=25)	Desmopressin (n=25)	Difference
Ephedrine [mg]	22 ±22	35 ±27	n.s.
Dextran 70 [ml, 60 mg/ml]	760 ±255	760 ±255	n.s.
Crystalloids [ml]	3640 ±940	3820 ±620	n.s.
Mean systolic blood pressure [mmHg]			
– before anaesthesia	146 ±16	148 ±22	n.s.
– during surgery	117 ±13	111 ±14	n.s.
– postoperatively	113 ±12	114 ±16	n.s.
Urine production [ml]	2040 ±600	2070 ±590	n.s.
Furosemide [mg]	8 ±9	12 ±10	$p<0.05$

Means ±SD.

The mean operation time in the 12 patients in the coagulation study was 101 (range 75–135) minutes, intraoperative blood loss 640 (range 225–1750) ml and postoperative drainage loss up to the following morning 560 (range 150–1400) ml. Erythrocyte concentrate corresponding to a mean of 560 (range 0–1800) ml donor blood and balanced crystalloid solutions at a mean of 4070 (range 3200–5300) ml were infused during surgery and postoperatively. One patient received 300 ml plasma and 200 ml 20% albumin.

In the patients whose blood loss was studied the amounts injected and infused were as shown in Table 2. Seven patients also received 100–600 ml 20% albumin, without any significant difference between groups. Plasma was not used.

ASSESSMENT OF BLOOD LOSS

All swabs used during surgery were weighed on a ±0.1 g scale as soon as they were taken from the wound. At the end of surgery the contents of the suction bottle were also weighed and a reduction was made from the irrigation fluid used. Paper drapings were used, absorbing negligible amounts of fluid, and any fluid accumulated in folds was collected in the suction bottle. The compilation of these data defined intraoperative blood loss.

A drain was placed in the wound before closure and connected to a vacuum drainage device. The drainage loss was defined as the blood loss into the drainage bag up to the morning of the first postoperative day.

If there has been no blood transfusions, the total blood loss, L (including hematomas, intravascular thrombus formation and hemolysis), may be calculated (Bourke and Smith, 1974) as $L=BV*{}^{e}\log(Hb_{pre}/Hb_{post})$, where Hb_{pre} is preoperative and Hb_{post} postoperative hemoglobin concentrations and BV the blood volume (estimated according to Nadler et al. (1962)). However, if blood has been transfused, some of the hemoglobin included in Hb_{post} would be derived from transfused blood. Hemoglobin that has been transfused, Hb_{transf}, is to some extent lost intraoperatively, in the drainage, and in hematoma formation. Hb_{post} should therefore be reduced by $Hb_{transf}*(1-e^{-L/BV})/L$. Consequently the total blood loss (L) of each patient is obtained from the non-linear equation

$$L=BV*{}^{e}\log\frac{Hb_{pre}}{Hb_{post}-Hb_{transf}*(1-e^{-L/BV})/L}$$

This equation assumes isovolaemia and that blood transfusions, if any, were given at approximately the same rate as blood was lost.

Blood transfusions were given as microaggregate-poor erythrocyte concentrate, in units made from 450 ml donor blood, suspended in SAGM solution (Högman et al., 1983) to 300 ml, with a mean Hb of 200 g/l. The units had been stored at +4°C for a mean of two weeks. According to the regular quality control of the blood bank, 90–95% of such erythrocytes are alive 24 hours after transfusion. Thus, Hb_{transf} for use in the formula above was 60 g/unit, necessitating assessment of the influence of 5–10% hemolysis.

STATISTICS

Analysis of variance with a repeated measurement design (Winer,1971; Brain Power, 1986) was used to compare differences between groups when repeated measurements had been done over time or with different methods. Other differences were tested using the Mann-Whitney *U* test with correction for ties (Siegel and Castellan, 1989). A *p* value less than 0.05 was taken as the criterion of statistical significance.

COAGULATION PARAMETERS

The FVIII/vWF complex normally rises after trauma and surgery (Rem et al., 1981; Paramo and Rocha, 1985). Dextran has been known to depress FVIII/vWF (Batlle et al., 1985). Epidural block postpones the FVIII/vWF increase otherwise induced by trauma (Rem et al., 1981; Bredbacka et al., 1986; Modig, 1988), as it blocks the nociceptive afferents responsible for this reflex. Furthermore, blood loss includes a proportional loss of FVIII/vWF.

Accordingly, FVIII:C (Fig. 1) and vWF:Ag (Fig. 2) were found to be low in total hip replacement patients treated according to our routine. Half of them had values in the subnormal range, as in mild hemophilia, possibly promoting blood loss. The mean postoperative bleeding time was also at the limit of pathological levels (Table 3).

FVIII:C and vWF:Ag increased in all six desmopressin treated patients during surgery and were within or above the normal range during the whole postoperative period (FVIII:C 92–290%, vWF:Ag 93–231%, Figs. 1 and 2). The postoperative bleeding time in the desmopressin treated patients was significantly shorter than it was in the control group (p=0.01, Table 3). The difference before surgery was not significant. The changes in vWF:Ag and bleeding time were correlated (r=–0.72, p=0.01) and the rise in vWF is the probable reason for the shorter postoperative bleeding time in desmopressin treated patients than in controls.

All APTTs were within the normal range (20–30 s, Table 3). FVIII:C and APTT changes were correlated (r=–0.64, p=0.03). The platelet counts did not differ significantly between groups (Table 3). Two values just below the normal range (150–400 x 10^9/l) were registered in each group.

Table 3. Ivy bleeding time, APTT and platelet count in total hip replacement patients (n=6 in each group) and statistical significance of change during treatment (over time) and of difference between treatments.

	Time of day				Within	Between
	08.00	12.00	15.00	08.00	treatment	treatments
Bleeding time [min]						
placebo	5.0 ±0.6	8.5 ±1.0			p<0.05	p=0.01
desmopressin	3.7 ±0.5	5.1 ±0.6			p<0.05	
APTT [s]						
placebo	24 ±1	26 ±1	25 ±1	26 ±1	n.s.	n.s.
desmopressin	26 ±1	23 ±1	23 ±1	24 ±1	n.s.	
Platelet count [x 10^9/l]						
placebo	240 ±16	192 ±21	199 ±17	202 ±19	p<0.01	n.s.
desmopressin	264 ±9	224 ±12	191 ±17	196 ±15	p<0.001	

Means ±SEM.

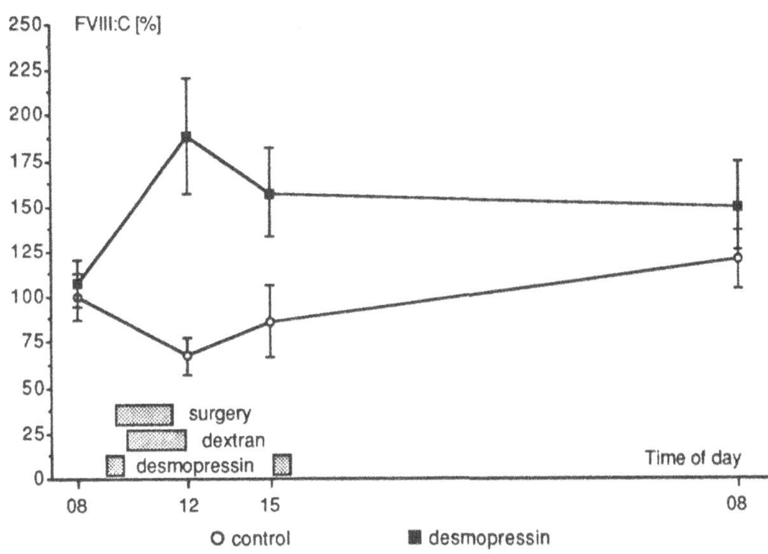

Fig. 1. Factor VIII:C as percentages of the mean of a healthy reference population. Means and SEM, six total hip replacement patients in each group. Changes were significant in both groups ($p<0.05$ and $p<0.01$, respectively). The difference between groups was significant ($p<0.001$).

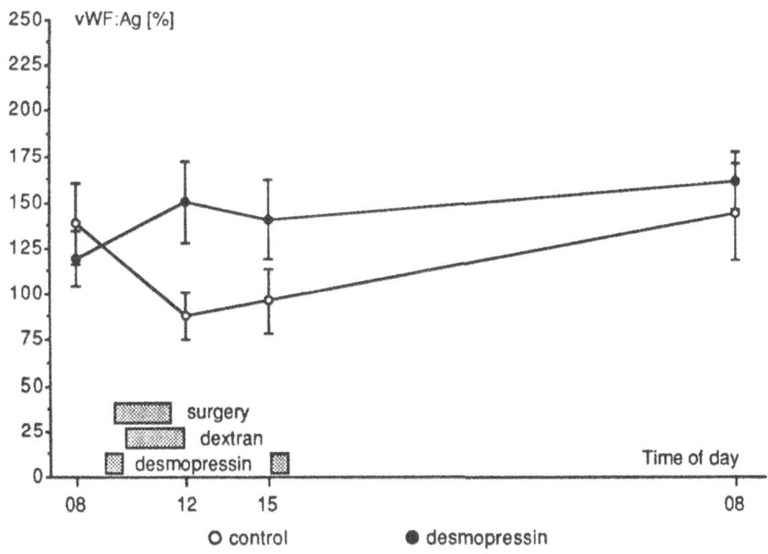

Fig. 2. VWF:Ag as percentages of the mean of a healthy reference population. Means and SEM, six total hip replacement patients in each group. Changes were significant in both groups ($p=0.01$ and $p=0.001$, respectively). The difference between groups was significant ($p<0.01$).

BLOOD LOSS

The total blood loss was reduced by 310 ml (17%) in patients who received desmopressin ($p<0.05$, Table 4). The total blood loss relative to estimated blood volume was reduced from 42% to 33% ($p=0.02$). Transfusion requirements were not significantly reduced (0.3 units, n.s.).

Intraoperative blood loss and postoperative drainage loss did not differ between groups. If intraoperative blood loss plus drainage loss is treated as one blood loss measurement and the calculated total blood loss as another independent measurement, statistical evaluation of both measurements in one single test confirms that the reduction of blood loss by desmopressin was statistically significant, also when taking all data into consideration.

The total blood loss was greater in patients who received uncemented prostheses (mean 2350 ml vs. cemented 1500 ml, $p<0.001$). There were eight uncemented procedures in the control group (mean blood loss 2180 ml) and four in the desmopressin group (2700 ml, n.s.). If these were excluded from analysis, desmopressin was still seen to reduce the mean total blood loss by 380 ml ($p<0.05$).

Table 4. Blood loss and transfusion requirements.

	Control (n=25)	Desmopressin (n=25)	Difference
Intraoperative blood loss [ml]	900 ±300	880 ±430	n.s.
Drainage loss [ml]	730 ±340	640 ±300	n.s.
Total blood loss [ml]	1860 ±710	1550 ±900	$p<0.05$
Total relative blood loss [%]	42 ±17	33 ±18	$p=0.02$
Blood transfusions [units]	1.5 ±1.2	1.2 ±1.0	n.s.
Hb decrease [g/l]	27 ±14	22 ±15	n.s.
Platelet count decrease [10^9/l]	56 ±34	26 ±45	$p<0.01$

Means ±SD.

The total blood loss takes into account all forms of blood loss that the patient is subjected to – including hematoma and thrombus formations and hemolysis. The formula that was defined and used here has the limitation that it assumes a constant blood volume. From data provided by Schött et al. (1985), who studied patients in similar circumstances, mean perioperative blood volume can be calculated to be 98 % of preoperative. Recalculating the total blood losses with perioperative blood volumes randomly assumed to be 90–100% of estimated preoperative blood volumes did not disturb the statistical significance of the difference.

The formula for total blood loss accounts for hemolysis of the patient's own erythrocytes, but not of transfused erythrocytes. According to our quality control, such hemolysis is 5–10% after 24 hours and then about the same on the third postoperative day (Mollison et al., 1987). The introduction of as much as 20% hemolysis of transfused erythrocytes in the blood loss calculations did not disturb the significance of the difference between groups.

Thus, the conclusion of significantly reduced blood loss does stand up to abundant violations of the primary assumption as to isovolemia and hemolysis of transfused erythrocytes.

The total blood loss differed significantly between the groups, but the intraoperative blood loss did not. The reduction of postoperative blood loss was not seen as a significantly reduced drainage loss; postoperative bleeding seems to have been more efficiently drained in the desmopressin group, possibly explained by the fact that desmopressin is a potent fibrinolysis activator (Mannucci et al., 1975).

Transfusion requirements may be the most significant parameter, especially in the era of hepatitis, HIV and other contagious agents that are still unknown to us. The effect of desmopressin on blood transfusions was not significant. However, if blood had been transfused to make both groups end up on the same mean Hb drop (Table 4) the difference would have been 0.7 instead of 0.3 units and possibly significant.

The blood loss reduction by desmopressin is compatible with its normalizing the otherwise prolonged bleeding time and increasing the otherwise low factor VIII and von Willebrand factor levels, as was shown in identically treated patients.

The platelet count decreased significantly less in the desmopressin group (Table 3), which was also the case in the study of Salzman et al. (1986). A possible explanation could be that the rise in von Willebrand factor levels induced by desmopressin improved platelet function (Mannucci, 1988), so that haemostasis was achieved with less platelet consumption.

SUMMARY AND CONCLUSIONS

In total hip replacement using regional anesthesia, dextran infusion and ephedrine injections, the present study has shown a platelet function defect, reflected in a prolonged bleeding time. This may be what makes desmopressin effective in this context (Salzman, 1990). The defect may be caused by the low vWF levels seen instead of the increased levels which are the normal response to trauma, and possibly also by platelet function inhibitory effects of dextran (Bergqvist 1983). Moreover, both ephedrine (Flordal and Svensson, 1991) and local anesthetics used for regional anesthesia (Borg and Modig, 1985; Henny et al., 1986; Bovill and Odoom, 1987) inhibit platelet function.

Desmopressin reduced blood loss with 310 ml. The effect may be more pronounced in procedures where more blood loss is to be expected (for instance, revision arthroplasties), or, especially, when anti-inflammatory drugs are not as strictly excluded as they were in this study.

In this study desmopressin was administered twice, in most other studies only once. In volunteers, the half-life of the FVIII increase after a single dose is 3–6 hours and that of the vWF increase 5–9 hours (Schulman, 1991). The half-life in surgical patients is not known, but it seems to be about the same (Lethagen et al., 1991; Figs. 1 and 2). It may be shortened by dextran (Flordal et al., 1991c). The duration of a single dose may not be enough to achieve significant improvement of hemostasis.

REFERENCES

Batlle, J., del Río, F., López Fernández, M.F., Martín, R., and López Borrasca, A., 1985, Effect of dextran on factor VIII/von Willebrand factor structure and function, *Thromb Haemost*. 54:697–9.

Bergqvist, D., 1983, "Postoperative Thromboembolism", Springer-Verlag, Berlin.

Borg, T., and Modig, J., 1985, Potential anti-thrombotic effects of local anaesthetics due to their inhibition of platelet aggregation, *Acta Anaesthesiol Scand*. 29:739–42.

Bourke, D.L., and Smith, T.C., 1974, Estimating allowable hemodilution, *Anesthesiology* 41:609–12.

Bovill, J.G., and Odoom, J.A., 1987, The influence of epidural anesthesia with bupivacaine on platelet function and correlation with plasma bupivacaine concentration, *Anesthesiology* 67(suppl 3A):A273.

Brain Power, Inc., 1986, "StatView 512+", Abacus Concepts Inc., Calabasas.

Bredbacka, S., Blombäck, M., Hägnevik, K., Irestedt, L., and Raabe, N., 1986, Per- and postoperative changes in coagulation and fibrinolytic variables during abdominal hysterectomy under epidural or general anaesthesia, *Acta Anaesthesiol Scand*. 30:204–10.

Flordal, P.A., and Neander, G., 1991, Blood loss in total hip replacement. A retrospective study, *Arch Orthop Trauma Surg*. 111:34–8.

Flordal, P.A., and Svensson, J., 1991, Haemostatic effects of ephedrine, submitted for publication.

Flordal, P.A., Ljungström, K.-G., Fehrm, A., Ekman, B., and Neander, G., 1991a, Desmopressin in total hip replacement – effects on blood loss and thromboembolism, submitted for publication.

Flordal, P.A., Ljungström, K.-G., Svensson, J., Ekman, B., and Neander, G., 1991b, Effects on coagulation and fibrinolysis of desmopressin in patients undergoing total hip replacement, *Thromb Haemost*. 66:562–6.

Flordal, P.A., Svensson, J., and Ljungström, K.-G., 1991c, Effects of desmopressin and dextran on coagulation and fibrinolysis in healthy volunteers, *Thromb Res*. 62:355–64.

Högman, C.F., Rosén, I., Andreen, M., Åkerblom, O., and Hellsing, K., 1983, Haemotherapy with red-cell concentrates and a new red-cell storage medium, *Lancet* i:269–72.

Henny, C.P., Odoom, J.A., ten Cate, H., ten Cate, J.W., Oosterhoff, R.J.F., Dabhoiwala, N.F., and Sih, I.L., 1986, Effects of extradural bupivacaine on the haemostatic system, *Br J Anaesth*. 58:301–5.

Laurell, C.-B., 1972, Electroimmuno assay, *Scand J Clin Lab Invest*. 29 (suppl 124):21–37.

Lethagen, S., Rugarn, P., and Bergqvist, D., 1991, Blood loss and safety with desmopressin or placebo during aorto-iliac graft surgery, *Eur J Vasc Surg.* 5:173–8.
Mannucci, P.M., 1988, Desmopressin: a nontransfusional form of treatment for congenital and acquired bleeding disorders, *Blood* 72:1449–55.
Mannucci, P.M., Åberg, M., Nilsson, I.M., and Robertson, B., 1975, Mechanism of plasminogen activator and factor VIII increase after vasoactive drugs, *Br J Haematol.* 30:81–93.
Messmer, K.F.W., 1988, Hemodilution – possibilities and safety aspects, *Acta Anaesthesiol Scand.* 32(suppl 89):49–53.
Modig, J., 1988, Influence of regional anesthesia, local anesthetics and sympathicomimetics on the pathophysiology of deep vein thrombosis, *Acta Chir Scand.* suppl 550:119–27.
Modig, J., and Karlström, G., 1987, Intra- and post-operative blood loss and haemodynamics in total hip replacement when performed under lumbar epidural versus general anaesthesia, *Eur J Anaesthesiol.* 4:345–55.
Modig, J., Maripuu, E., and Sahlstedt, B., 1986, Thromboembolism following total hip replacement. A prospective investigation of 94 patients with emphasis on the efficacy of lumbar epidural anesthesia in prophylaxis, *Regional Anesth.* 11:72–9.
Mollison, P.L., Engelfreit, C.P., and Contreras, M., 1987, "Blood transfusion in clinical medicine", 8th ed., Blackwell Scientific Publications, Oxford.
Nadler, S.B., Hidalgo, J.U., and Bloch, T., 1962, Prediction of blood volume in normal human adults, *Surgery* 51:224–32.
National Institutes of Health, Consensus conference, 1986, Prevention of venous thrombosis and pulmonary embolism, *JAMA.* 256:744–9.
Paramo, J.A., and Rocha, E., 1985, Changes in coagulation and fibrinolysis after total hip replacement and their relations with deep vein thrombosis, *Haemostasis* 15:345–52.
Rem, J., Feddersen, C., Brandt, M.R., and Kehlet, H., 1981, Postoperative changes in coagulation and fibrinolysis independent of neurogenic stimuli and adrenal hormones, *Br J Surg.* 68:229–33.
Salzman, E.W., 1990, Desmopressin and surgical hemostasis, *N Engl J Med.* 322:1085.
Salzman, E.W., Weinstein, M.J., Weintraub, R.M., Ware, J.A., Thurer, R.L., Robertson, L., Donovan, A., Gaffney, T., Bertele, V., Troll, J., Smith, M., and Chute, L.E., 1986, Treatment with desmopressin acetate to reduce blood loss after cardiac surgery. A double-blind randomized trial, *N Engl J Med.* 314:1402–6.
Schött, U., Thorén, T., Sjöstrand, U., Berséus, O., and Söderholm, B., 1985, Three per cent dextran-60 as a plasma substitute in blood component therapy. II. Comparative studies on pre- and postoperative blood volume, *Acta Anaesthesiol Scand.* 29:775–81.
Schulman, S., 1991, DDAVP – the multipotent drug in patients with coagulopathies, *Transfusion Medicine Reviews* V:132–44.
Siegel, S., and Castellan, N.J.J., 1989, "Nonparametric Statistics for the Behavioral Sciences", 2nd ed., McGraw-Hill, Singapore.
Thorén, L., and Wiklund, L., 1983, Intraoperative fluid therapy, *World J Surg.* 7:581–9.
Winer, B.J., 1971, "Statistical Principles in Experimental Design", Mc Graw-Hill, New York, pp 514–603.

DISCUSSION

Kobrinsky: Would you comment on the improved drainage function on desmopressin, in view of the results in the cardiac studies?
Flordal: I estimate that it is the same as with total hip replacement. The drains do not release all the blood loss, and desmopressin may help the drainage, leading to the false impression that more blood is lost.

Kohler (Germany): As for cost analysis, the risks of blood transfusion have decreased dramatically. Also, you use both dextran to decrease hemostasis, and desmopressin to increase it. Should you not use no drug at all?
Flordal: If we abandoned this we would have a very high incidence of deep vein thrombosis (around 50%), and that would not be acceptable. As for hepatitis, it may be a low risk now, but there is still hepatitis non-A, non-B infection, and there may be new future risks.

Cattaneo: What about the thromboses we see on dextran?
Flordal: Thromboses are seen, but they are often of no clinical significance.
Rocha: Low molecular weight heparin is preferable to dextran.
Flordal: The blood loss from dextran and low molecular weight heparin regimens is very similar. It is safe to combine them.

EFFECTS OF DESMOPRESSIN ON NORMAL DONORS IN PLASMA EXCHANGE DONATIONS

Richard J. Sassetti, Medical Director
Bruce C. McLeod, Associate Medical Director
Blood Center
Rush-Presbyterian-St. Luke's Medical Center, Chicago, IL 60612

INTRODUCTION

The use of desmopressin (DDAVP) to stimulate increased factor VIII in plasmapheresis donors was an evolutionary step in our efforts to use cryoprecipitate produced by repetitive large volume (2-3 L) plasma exchange of dedicated donors for treatment of hemophilia A.[1,2,3] The donation procedure evolved from our experience in the treatment of cryoglobulinemia by plasmapheresis.[4] To reduce replacement fluid cost and minimize the risk of disease transmission for patients undergoing repeated plasmapheresis we had explored the feasibility of using the cryoglobulin-depleted plasma from a previous donation as the replacement fluid in a therapeutic plasma exchange. Being persuaded of the efficacy and safety of the procedure, we were led to consider an analogous procedure, performed on dedicated blood donors, as a source of large quantities of cryoprecipitate. The principle advantage perceived for such a program was a reduction in the risk of disease transmission by minimizing the number of donors to which a hemophilic patient is exposed. Awareness that desmopressin should raise donor factor VIII to levels 3 to 4 times baseline suggested that it might enhance the performance of the donation, resulting in higher yields and lower per-unit cost.

In this presentation we will review the status of this program, emphasizing our observations of the effects of repeated desmopressin stimulation on individual donors. Plasma exchange donations were first reported in 1980 and the first desmopressin stimulated donations took place in July, 1984. The data presented herein are derived from 615 plasma exchange donations by 50 individuals between January, 1982 and May, 1990.

METHODS

A. Donor Recruitment and Selection

Donors participating in the study came from two groups: 1) Medical Center employees and students who volunteered as research subjects and 2) relatives or friends who have served as dedicated donors for patients with Hemophilia A. All donors passed

Desmopressin in Bleeding Disorders, Edited by G. Mariani *et al.*
Plenum Press, New York, 1993

the standard blood donor pre-screening and had a spontaneous factor VIII level greater than .8 IU/ml.

B. Plasma Exchange Donation

The method for plasma exchange donation is described in detail elsewhere[2] and outlined schematically in Figure 1. Briefly, the process begins with three plasma donations of 0.5 L each, to provide an inventory of autologous plasma. A 2 liter exchange donation is then possible (2 L of plasma are removed, 1.5 L stored autologous plasma plus 0.5 L saline are returned using an automated apheresis device). Cryoprecipitate is produced from the fresh plasma and the cryo-supernatant is available as replacement fluid for the next plasma exchange donation, and so on. At any subsequent donation the exchange volume can be increased by 0.5 L (up to 3 L) by including an extra 0.5 L saline in the replacement fluid formula. In a "stimulated donation" desmopressin is infused intravenously in a dose of 0.3ug/kg (up to a maximum of 20 ug) over a period of 15 to 30 minutes just prior to the donation. Further cost efficiency was subsequently achieved by simultaneous production of a single donor platelet transfusion; this is given to another patient and partially subsidizes the factor VIII harvest.

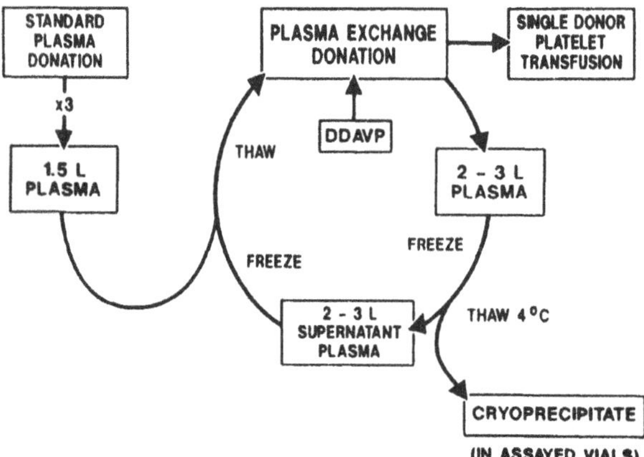

Figure 1. Schematic diagram of plasma exchange donation.

Plasma was collected in 0.5 L increments in sterile plastic bags and immediately frozen in an ethanol-solid carbon dioxide bath. Most cryoprecipitate was prepared by the thaw-siphon technique.[5,6] In the earliest phase of the study each bag was analyzed separately for factor VIII:C content and dispensed individually. In later phases all cryoprecipitate from a single donation was pooled. The pool volume was measured and aliquots were removed after thorough mixing for analysis of factor VIII:C activity in a single stage assay (dilutions made with hemophilic plasma or 5% albumin). The pool was then dispensed aseptically in 10 to 20 equal portions into sterile 30 ml plastic vials, which were sealed with rubber diaphragm caps, labeled and frozen. When the factor VIII analysis was complete the factor VIII content per vial was calculated and added to the label.[3] The resulting product has proven comparable, in terms of convenience of administration, to commercially available concentrates and, when maintained in a suitable home freezer, is perfectly compatible with home therapy. Availability in small and variable dose increments allows administration of the desired dose with minimum wastage. Families who have had prior experience with lyophilized commercial concentrates in home therapy find that our preparation compares favorably in terms of both logistics and hemostatic effectiveness.

C. Donor Data Collected

Prior to each donation donors were interviewed to assess side effects of the previous donation, paying special attention to bleeding tendency and fluid retention. During most of the study period it was possible to follow a number of screening laboratory tests during periods of donation activity. Every second donation was preceded by the following studies: hemoglobin, hematocrit, platelet count, white blood cell count and differential, urinalysis, serum protein electrophoresis, activated partial thromboplastin time, prothrombin time, thrombin time, fibrinogen, fibrin split products and serum multichannel analysis which included sodium, potassium, chloride, carbon dioxide, blood urea nitrogen, creatinine, total protein, albumin, calcium, phosphate, cholesterol, glucose, uric acid, bilirubin, alkaline phosphatase, lactic acid dehydrogenase (LDH), serum glutamic oxaloacetic transaminase (SGOT), and serum glutamic pyruvate transaminase (SGPT). Factor VIII antigen (factor VIII:Ag) and von Willebrand factor (vWF) were measured at every fourth donation. Blood was drawn for factor VIII:C analysis, and pulse rate and blood pressure were measured just before and just after each desmopressin infusion and at the end of desmopressin stimulated donations.

D. Statistical Analysis

Statistical analyses were performed on a personal computer with commercial software (ABSTAT, Anderson-Bell, Parker, CO) using the student's t test, correlation and regression analysis where appropriate.

RESULTS

A. Donors

Ten female and 40 male donors participated. All gave informed consent as approved by the institutional review board. Females ranged in age from 18 to 49 years with a mean of 28 and a median of 24; males ranged from 23 to 60 with a mean of 33 and a median of 31. Eighteen individuals donated without desmopressin stimulation on 173 occasions and with it on 200 other occasions for a total of 373 donations; 32 individuals received desmopressin on all occasions for 242 donations.

For a variety of reasons twenty donors left the program after 5 or fewer donations. Early in the study research subjects were recruited for a limited number of donations. Later several parental donors made long trips to our facility to begin a dedicated donor program, anticipating transfer to a similar program being organized nearer their homes.

B. Donation Intervals and Exchange Volumes

While the planned minimum interval between donations was 7 days (unstimulated) or 14 days (stimulated), there is a wide range of donation frequencies. Donation intervals range from 3 to 869 days, with a mean of 50, a median of 21 and a mode of 14 days. Exclusion of the donor with an 869 day interval alters the maximum to 435 days; the mean drops to 49 days, but the median and mode remain at 21 and 14 days, respectively. There are peaks in the donation interval plot between 5 and 9, and between 13 and 15 days, but these account for only 42% of donations. On 87 occasions the interval between donations exceeded 100 days. The wide range of variation can be attributed to several factors. At the low end, donors recruited as research subjects were required to adhere to the prescribed interval. The long tail of the frequency distribution up to 869 days reflects the activity of dedicated (usually parental) donors serving children with lower factor requirements.

Table I depicts the change in the volume of plasma exchanged that occurs with an increasing number of donations. In the early phase of the study, all exchanges were 2 liters. Later we explored escalating exchange volume by 0.5 liters after 4-6 successful donations at 2.0 or 2.5 liters. Currently, new donors are escalated from 2 liters to 3 liters as quickly as possible, usually over the first 3 exchange donations. Smaller exchange volumes in the early phase of a given donor's participation affect the total yield of factor VIII, while the smaller total number of donors at higher donation numbers is due to variation in factor requirements among dedicated donors and dropout for the reasons mentioned above.

Table 1. Liters of Plasma Per Donation

	Number of Donations at Stated Exchange Volume							
Liters of Plasma	1 %(N)	2 %(N)	3 %(N)	4 %(N)	5 %(N)	10 %(N)	15 %(N)	20 %(N)
2	100(50)	66(29)	55(22)	53(18)	45(14)	30(6)	31(4)	33(2)
2.5	0(0)	34(15)	15(6)	18(6)	26(8)	40(8)	15(2)	17(1)
3	0(0)	0(0)	30(12)	29(10)	29(9)	30(6)	54(7)	50(3)
(Total N)	50	44	40	34	31	20	13	6

Some differences in donation frequency between male and female donors are notable. The ratio of male to female donors was 4 to 1. Of the 613 donations studied only 92 were made by females, for a male to female donation ratio of 6.8 to 1. The overall mean donation number for the 50 participants was 24.5 with a maximum of 146 and a median of 10. For the males the total was 523 with a mean of 27, a maximum of 146 and a median of 11. For the 92 donations by females, the mean was 10, the maximum 35 and the median 7. If the male with 146 and the female with 35 donations are eliminated, the values for the mean number of donations converge but remain different. For the males the mean becomes 10 ± 8.5, the maximum 44, and the median 7. For females the mean becomes 6 ± 4.2, the maximum 16 and the median 4. These trends are probably related, in a roundabout fashion, to the genetics of hemophilia. For dedicated donor support of a hemophilic child we have emphasized fathers who, presumably, are unaffected. By contrast all but 2 of the female donors were "research subjects" and donated only a limited number of times. This also means that female donors are represented by smaller exchanges with lower factor VIII yields.

C. Total Program Factor VIII Production

Overall we harvested 2,544,044 IU of factor VIII by plasma exchange donation from the 613 donations. Of that amount 2,338,054 IU came from a total of 1230 liters of plasma obtained in 477 stimulated donations or an average of 1901 IU per liter of plasma or 4878 IU per donation as compared to 205,990 IU from 304 liters of plasma in 136 unstimulated donations for an average of only 390 IU per liter or 871 IU per donation. The use of desmopressin clearly enhanced the provision of factor VIII in this way.

D. Analysis of Factor VIII Yield Data

Six hundred thirteen of the 615 plasma exchange donations had at least partial valid data that could be analyzed for variables related to factor VIII yield. Regression analysis was used to investigate trends over time, while the two-tailed Student's t test was used to analyze differences between outcomes of stimulated and unstimulated donations.

Table II presents descriptive statistics for seven data elements considered most likely to contribute to donation performance. As expected, there was no difference between the pre-donation factor VIII levels for stimulated (122±43%) and unstimulated (117±37%) donors. Mean factor VIII immediately after the 30 minute desmopressin infusion was 265±133%, a highly significant 225% increase. This rapid rise is consistent with the 3-400% maximal increase over baseline observed by others in a 2-3 hour interval.[7,8]

Mean factor VIII yield (4961 IU) in the stimulated donations was 325% that of the unstimulated donations (1525 IU), a highly significant difference ($p < .0001$ by unpaired t test). The coefficients of variation for these two means are 50 and 45%, respectively. This wide variability could be due, in part, to variation in exchange volume (Table I). However analysis of subsets with the same exchange volumes, shown in Table III, while it illustrates the expected influence on yield, does not significantly alter the variability.

The yield per liter for the 3 liter exchanges in unstimulated donors is relatively low. The number of donations is small so this may simply be a statistical aberration; however, it may also reflect the fact that, as exchange volume increases beyond 2 liters, the reinfused

Table 2. Descriptive statistics for key donation variables

Variable	DDAVP[1]	N	Mean	SD[2]	CV[3]
Liters of plasma	N	136	2.2	0.35	16
	Y	477	2.6	0.43	17
Factor VIII pre donation (%)	N	21	117	37	32
	Y	385	122	43	35
Factor VIII post DDAVP (%)	N	ND[4]	ND	ND	ND
	Y	401	265	133	50
Factor VIII Rise[5]	N	ND	ND	ND	ND
	Y	360	225	116	92
Factor VIII in cryo (IU/ml)	N	78	8.9	3.9	44
	Y	469	33	15	45
Factor VIII Yield (IU)	N	78	1525	692	45
	Y	469	4961	2478	50

[1]Y = desmopressin stimulation, N = no desmopressin stimulation; [2]Standard Deviation; [3]Coefficient of variation; [4]Not Done; [5]The ratio of post to pre desmopressin expressed as a percent

Table 3. Factor VIII Yield Corrected For Volume of Donation

Volume (L)	DDAVP[1]	N	Mean Yield (IU)	SD[2]	CV[3]
2.0	N	33	687	281	40
	Y	124	1641	816	50
2.5	N	28	813	218	27
	Y	138	1870	722	39
3.0	N	13	411	146	35
	Y	203	2076	871	42

[1]Y = desmopressin stimulation, N = no desmopressin stimulation
[2]Standard Deviation; [3]Coefficient of Variation

factor VIII poor plasma becomes an increasingly significant component of the harvested plasma (greater than 50% for a 70 kg donor), leading to a real decrease in yield per liter. In stimulated donations, this tendency would be offset by the continued mobilization of factor VIII during donation.

Initial analysis of the raw data suggested significant differences between sexes in factor VIII yield at p less than .01 (unstimulated male 1605±643 IU, unstimulated female 1325±694; stimulated male 5154±2554, stimulated female 3882±1643). However these differences can be at least partially explained by the smaller exchange volumes for women mentioned above. When the factor VIII yield is normalized for differences in the volume of plasma processed and expressed as factor VIII per liter of plasma exchanged, differences in factor VIII yield cease to be statistically significant (unstimulated male 665±267, unstimulated female 663±242; stimulated male 1940±847, stimulated female 1687±1492). Thus males and females seem to perform equally well in plasma exchange donation and to have equivalent responses to desmopressin.

In a further effort to understand variability in yield, all of the donor variables mentioned in the Methods section were analyzed as independent variables in a regression analysis of factor VIII yield (partially normalized to yield per liter exchanged) as the dependent variable using Pearson's multiple correlation matrix. Unstimulated and stimulated donations were analyzed separately. The data displayed in Table IV are the correlation coefficients (the limits of which are -1 and +1) and their signs for variables found to have statistically significant ($p < .01$) regression coefficients.

Table 4. Correlation Coefficient Of Factors Potentially Affecting Factor VIII Yield

	Yield Per Liter			
	Unstimulated		Stimulated	
	CC[1]	Sign	CC	Sign
Volume of Donation	ins[2]		.43	+
Number of Donations	.38[3]	+	.32	+
Spontaneous factor VIII Level	ins		.32	+
Post-Desmopressin factor VIII Level	ND[4]		.28	+

[1]Correlation Coefficient; [2]Absolute Value of CC < .0001
[3]Exclusion of a Single Donor Reduces CC to < .001; [4]Not Done

Two aspects of this data are noteworthy. First, the correlation coefficients are relatively low. In unstimulated donations, factor VIII yield has virtually no correlation with either volume of donation or pre-donation factor VIII level. This unlikely prediction may reflect the contribution of other uncontrolled variables, such as donor size or efficiency of cryoprecipitate processing, to total yield. The coefficient of .38 for the number of unstimulated donations is reduced to insignificance by the exclusion of a donor with a high spontaneous factor VIII level who made the largest number of unstimulated donations. Second, there seems to be a positive correlation between the number of donations and the yield in both unstimulated and stimulated donors. However when the t test is used to compare yields from donations early in the series to those of later donations there is no significant difference, suggesting that the correlation is spurious.

Further analysis of the relationship between factor VIII yield and factor VIII levels was carried out by dividing the stimulated donations into two groups based on a pre-donation factor VIII parameter. The donations were divided into two groups - those with values above and those with values below the median for the parameter. The relationship to donation yield was assessed with the t test. This kind of analysis was done for pre-donation factor VIII, post-desmopressin factor VIII and the percent rise in factor VIII. The mean yields for donors with spontaneous factor VIII levels above and below the median value of 118% were 1859±830 and 1967±843 IU, respectively. This difference was not statistically significant. The differences between yields around the post-desmopressin levels (median = 240, low mean = 1736±766, high mean = 2133±877) was significant ($p < .0001$), as was the difference around the percentage rise in factor VIII (median = 101, low mean = 1809±766, high mean = 2025±927, $p < .01$).

E. Donor Well-being and Adverse Effects

In our experience desmopressin administration has generally been well tolerated. While virtually all donors develop facial flushing, most are not aware of it. There have been no associated hypertensive episodes. No donors complained of palpitations, nor were any episodes of tachycardia noted during or after donation. No donor complained of fluid retention in the day after a dose.

Our study of donors' well-being included longitudinal repetition of a number of coagulation tests as well as hematologic and biochemical screening tests, as described in the methods section. Sequential values were available for 445 donations by 37 donors (mean = 12 donations). These were normalized by expressing each value as a percentage of the baseline value for the donor and analyzed in a correlation matrix versus the number of donations. Trends might represent long term effects of either the donation procedure or desmopressin stimulation. Since the most active donor had undergone 72 donations before we began to monitor these parameters, he was excluded from this analysis. His values were, however, analyzed separately and are discussed below.

While the regression analysis produced some p values less than .01, all regression coefficients are small relative to the magnitude of the constant term of the regression line. Further analysis was therefore carried out to interpret the significance of these small regression coefficients. If the p value for the regression coefficient was less than .01, the ratio of the regression coefficient (the slope of the regression line) to the constant term (the intercept of the regression line, which is the value of the variable at zero donations) was calculated to determine the fractional increment per donation for the variable in question. Table V displays the data for hematologic and coagulation parameters, none of which showed a significant trend.

Table 5. Regression Analysis of Hematologic and Coagulation Variable in Donor Undergoing Repeated Donation/Desmopressin Stimulation

	CC[1]	RC[2]	p Value
Hematocrit	.04	.02	.45
White Cell Count	.05	.13	.33
Absolute Lymphocyte Count	.01	.03	.86
Prothrombin Time	.04	.09	.53
Partial Thromboplastin Time	.04	.03	.59
Thrombin Time	.09	.15	.17
Fibrinogen	.06	.14	.33
Factor VIII:Ag	.26	-.38	.29
vWF	.14	-.002	.62

[1]Correlation Coefficient; [2]Regression Coefficient

Table VI displays similar data for various biochemical indicators of renal and hepatic physiology. All 15 analytes have small correlation coefficients. Only two, the calcium and cholesterol, had significant p values in the regression analysis; for both of these the table lists a ratio of the regression coefficient to the constant term. In both cases the ratio is .003 or less indicating that if donation or desmopressin has an effect, the value of the parameter would decrease in these cases by less than 3.6% over the average course of 12 donations. This suggests that the correlation is spurious and like the remainder of the variables there is no clinically important change detected.

Table 6. Correlation of Biochemical Variables With Donation Number

	CC[1]	RC[2]	p Value	Ratio[3]
Blood Urea Nitrogen	.08	.25	.22	
Creatinine	.16	.21	.02	
Uric Acid	.12	-.18	.07	
Calcium	.39	-.23	.001	-.002
Phosphate	.03	-.05	.65	
Cholesterol	.22	-.41	.002	-.003
Glucose	.17	.64	.02	
Total Protein	.16	-.09	.15	
Albumin	.14	-.09	.84	
Gamma Globulin	.12	-.29	.11	
Bilirubin	.05	-.26	.44	
Alkaline Phosphatase	.12	.57	.09	
LDH	.10	-.18	.16	
SGOT	.0001	.024	.99	
SGPT	.01	.069	.85	

[1]CC = correlation coefficient; [2]RC = regression coefficient
[3]ratio of regression coefficient to constant term of regression equation

The most active donor in our program provided all the factor VIII needed by his adolescent son with severe hemophilia for over 6.5 years. He donated 675,750 IU of factor VIII in 386 liters of plasma in 146 donations (90 with desmopressin). The son, whose age ranged from 10 to 16 years over this time, required over 100,000 IU per year. The average interval between the father's donations was 17 days with a median of 14 days; however, with stimulated 3 liter donations he could keep pace with his son's needs by donating only once every 3 to 4 weeks. This interval conforms to U.S. Food and Drug Administration guidelines for platelet donors. His experience emphasizes the ability of plasma exchange donation to cope with heavy factor VIII use.

Likewise the data from his donations may provide information about the long term effects of plasma exchange donation. Figure 2 illustrates the dependence of factor VIII yield on both volume of donation and desmopressin stimulation for this donor's 146 donations. His mean factor VIII yield without stimulation was 2042 IU per donation. With stimulation the mean factor VIII yield was 6982 IU per donation. The mean yield per liter of plasma donated was 841 IU unstimulated and 2401 IU stimulated. His mean pre- and post-stimulated donation factor VIII levels were 157 and 342 IU. Laboratory data from his 73rd though 146th donations were normalized and subjected to a regression analysis as described above. None of the monitored parameters showed a significant trend. In particular, the regression line for his pre-donation factor VIII level was flat, suggesting that there was neither enhancement nor exhaustion of factor VIII production by repeated donation or desmopressin stimulation. There was a slight negative trend in both factor VIII antigen and vWF levels with repeated donation but the correlation was not statistically significant.

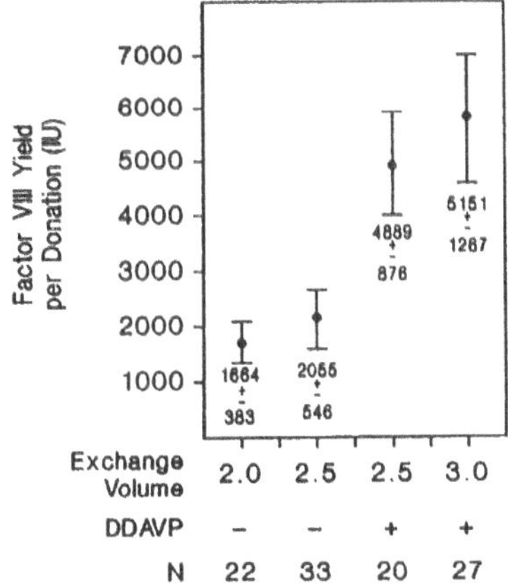

Figure 2. The effect of donation technique on yield in the most active donor.

The only individual to report any symptoms suggestive of thrombotic events during the period of donation was this highly prolific donor. He sustained a small myocardial infarction during his 146th donation, the 90th in which he received the standard dose of desmopressin.[9] The role of desmopressin in this event is problematic. The temporal sequence was striking but the subject had numerous independent risk factors for vascular disease (hypertension, a 50+ pack year smoking history, high cholesterol, high triglycerides, and a family history of premature vascular disease) and had tolerated desmopressin without difficulty on 89 prior occasions. In addition the day in question was particularly stressful for him because of events related to progression of his son's HIV infection (acquired from commercial concentrates prior to his participation in the single donor cryo program).

F. Clinical Experience

Cryoprecipitate from plasma exchange donation has been used extensively in a collaborative program with Children's Memorial Hospital of Chicago.[2,3] Recipients in that program have shown the expected post-infusion factor VIII increment of about 2% per IU per kg, and several half-life determinations were between 10 and 14 hours. The material has been given to over 40 hemophilic children in the Chicago metropolitan area, including over 20 who have been supported by a single donor for periods of 1 to 6 years. This experience encompasses well over a thousand infusions for the full gamut of bleeding manifestations both for inpatients and outpatients. Hemostatic effectiveness has always been comparable to that of commercially available products. To date we have achieved our goal of limiting donor exposure for the recipients, even those who require annual doses in excess of 100,000 IU, and continue to support several severely affected young people. Routine follow up of our recipients has revealed no evidence that hepatitis, HIV or other blood borne infections have been acquired during periods of single donor support.

Two preliminary observations of recipients concern different aspects of the immune response. In comparison to a control cohort of patients receiving dry heat treated factor VIII concentrates, recipients of dedicated donor cryoprecipitate our product seem to have maintained higher T4:T8 ratios and higher absolute CD4 + cell counts[10], suggesting that the nonspecific immunosuppression seen with commercial concentrates may not occur with plasma exchange donation produced cryoprecipitate. We have also looked at the question of inhibitor formation, combining data from our program and similar programs in Iowa City, Iowa, and Minneapolis-St. Paul, Minnesota. In these three programs, which encompass over 40 patients receiving only cryoprecipitate from a single parental donor, there have been no instances of inhibitor formation after a median duration of treatment that exceeds 2 years.[11]

CONCLUSION

Our effort to develop plasma exchange donation as a source of factor VIII was motivated by concern for recipient safety at a time when commercial factor VIII products carried a high risk of transmitting viral diseases. While the risks associated with commercial products have decreased in the intervening years, limitation of donor exposure remains a valid approach to reduction of recipient risk, and plasma exchange donation can provide this advantage, not only for hemophiliacs but also for patients with hypofibrinogenemia and von Willebrand's disease.[12]

Even in hemophilia A, where virus-inactivated lyophilized concentrates are widely available, there continues to be interest in this approach to replacement therapy because of cost considerations. The long term cost of factor VIII replacement with monoclonally purified or recombinant concentrates is now expected to exceed many patients' insurance limits. With the combination of desmopressin stimulation and a "subsidy" from the simultaneous platelet donation we have been able to provide single donor factor VIII for only $.20 per IU. For some families this makes plasma exchange donation a desirable option. In addition, no inhibitor to factor VIII has been detected to date and studies of cellular immune markers suggest a lesser immunosuppressive effect in patients using this product.

Our extensive past experience with use of desmopressin in this context has provided a substantial data base with which to evaluate the effects of repeated donation and desmopressin infusion on normal persons. We also have a continuing concern about the safety of desmopressin because we continue to use it in our program. We have therefore carried out a detailed analysis of data accumulated in several protocols that span six years, 50 donors and nearly 500 doses of desmopressin. The analysis confirms several conclusions drawn previously from individual protocols. The aggregate data document that exchange volume is an important determinant of factor VIII yield and confirm the supposition that desmopressin is highly effective in augmenting yield at any studied exchange volume. Further analysis focused on the variability in factor VIII yield and on potential effects of donation and/or desmopressin on donor health and well-being.

Variability of factor VIII yield per liter plasma donated both from time to time for a given donor and from donor to donor is very wide. Two factors potentially confounding the comparison of factor VIII levels, desmopressin response and factor VIII yield are the donors' levels of anxiety and the degree to which exercise influences their spontaneous factor VIII levels or their responses to desmopressin.[13,14] These variables were neither controlled for nor assessed. In addition, variability in the precision and accuracy of coagulant activity measurements make the interpretation of this wide variability in factor VIII yield difficult.

Our clinical observations of normal individuals who receive repeated doses of desmopressin prior to plasma exchange donation have generally coincided with the conclusions of other investigators that it is an innocuous drug. The one notable exception was the donor who suffered a myocardial infarction. While we remain uncertain of the significance of this event, we are cognizant of scattered reports of thrombotic incidents in patients who have received desmopressin, and of the ongoing debate regarding whether these rare events are simply coincidental or may in fact be caused by desmopressin. We look forward to definitive resolution of this question, perhaps by other participants in this symposium. In our own program we responded to the myocardial infarction incident by restricting the use of desmopressin to nonsmoking younger donors (males under 40, females under 45) who lack identifiable risk factors for vascular disease, including diabetes, hypertension, personal or family history of premature vascular disease, and cholesterol >250 mg/dl.

The laboratory data accumulated on donors in our program are reassuring. No donor developed markedly or persistently abnormal values for any of the parameters followed. Furthermore, the detailed statistical analysis presented in this paper revealed no clinically important trend toward a long term change in any of them. This was true for coagulation factors, including those most likely to be directly effected by desmopressin or the plasma exchange donation, such as factor VIII and fibrinogen. It also held for standard screening tests of renal and hepatic function, and for all the formed elements of the blood. The absence of any stimulatory or tachyphylactic effect would suggest that there is no permanent effect of donation or desmopressin stimulation and that an interval of approximately 14 days between donations is sufficient to allow recovery from any temporary effect. Removal of lymphocytes is an expected concomitant of platelet harvesting and the potential for inducing a cellular immune deficiency by net depletion of circulating T cells as a long term effect of harvesting circulating T-cells along with plasma and/or platelets is a concern.[15] We found no tendency for absolute lymphocyte count to decrease in our donors.

To summarize, desmopressin has been used in our program for 6.5 years and we have observed 50 normal donors who received desmopressin, including 30 who received 5 to 10 doses and 13 who received 20 to 90 doses. With only one significant and no minor untoward events in a total that now exceeds 500 stimulated donations we feel that desmopressin stimulated plasma exchange donation is a reasonably safe procedure, suitable for individuals in the role of a blood donor.

REFERENCES

1. McLeod BC, Sassetti RJ, Cole ER, Pierce MI. Factor VIII collection by pheresis. Lancet 1980; 2:671-673.
2. McLeod BC, Scott JP. Transfusion studies of "single donor" factor VIII from plasma exchange donation. JAMA 1984; 252:2726-2729.
3. McLeod BC, Sassetti RJ, Cole EP, Scott JP. A high-potency, single donor cryoprecipitate of known factor VIII content dispensed in vials. Ann Intern Med 1987; 106:35-40.
4. McLeod BC, Sassetti RJ. Plasmapheresis with return of cryoglobulin depleted autologous plasma (cryoglobulinpheresis) in cryoglobulinemia. Blood 1980; 55:866-870.
5. Mason EC. Thaw-siphon technique for production of cryopre-cipitate concentrate of factor VIII. Lancet 1987; 2:15-17.

6. Kang EP. An improved thaw-siphon method for cryoprecipitate preparation. Vox Sang 1980; 38:172-177.
7. Mannucci PM, Ruggeri ZM, Pareti FI, Capitanio A. 1-Deamino-8-D-arginine vasopressin: a new pharmacological approach to the management of hemophilia and von Willebrand's disease. Lancet 1977; 1:869-872.
8. Nilsson IM, Walter H, Mikaelsson M, Vilhardt H. Factor VIII concentrate prepared from DDAVP stimulated blood donor plasma. Scand J Haematol 1979; 22:42-46.
9. McLeod B. Myocardial infarction in a blood donor after administration of desmopressin. Lancet 1990; 336:1137-1138.
10. Scott JP, McGann K, Gill JS, McLeod BC, Gamerman S. Is immune function altered by the infusion of high protein load material in the treatment of hemophilia A? Ped Res 1988; 23:347A.
11. McLeod B, Kisker T, Hasegawa A, Edson R, Gamerman SA, Scott P. Incidence of inhibitors in hemophiliacs treated with single donor cryoprecipitate from plasma exchange donation. Blood 1989; 74(Suppl 1):37A.
12. McLeod BC, McKenna R, Sassetti RJ. Treatment of von Willebrand's disease and hypofibrinogenemia with single donor cryoprecipitate from plasma exchange donation. Am J Hematol 1989; 32:112-116.
13. Ingram GIC. Increase in antihemophilic globulin activity following infusion of adrenaline. J Physiol 1961; 156:217-224.
14. Egeberg O. Changes in the activity of antihemophilic A factor (f,VIII) and in the bleeding time associated with muscular exercise and adrenaline infusion. Scand J Clin Lab Invest 1963; 15:539-549.
15. Matsui Y, Martin-Alocio S, Doenges E, Christenson L, Shapiro HM, Yunis EJ, Page PL. Effects of frequent and sustained plateletpheresis on peripheral blood mononuclear cell populations and lymphocyte functions of normal plasma volunteer donors. Transfusion 1986; 26:446-452.

DISCUSSION

Lusher: I would like to congratulate you on your programme, especially at a time when transfusion transmitted viral diseases were of paramount concern. Despite your concluding remarks, now that plasma-derived clotting factor concentrates are less likely to infect and recombinant FVIII will soon be available, is it worthwhile to continue it? It seems to be costly to set up. Have you long range plans for the program?
Sassetti: I agree that its benefits have been attenuated, but it is still an alternative for families, and has less economic impact on their life than using commercial materials. I am also singularly impressed by the enthusiasm of the families to help their children. Although we no longer seek new patients, they continue to arrive.

Mannucci: You showed that the group treated with cryoprecipitate had CD4 cell counts of 1500, and the commercial group, 900. Were they a mixture of HIV+ and HIV- patients?
Sassetti: Yes.
Mannucci: These were values taken while they were in the programme? Could their baseline values of CD4 levels have differed before the study?
Sassetti: We do not have the baseline levels.

Mariani: Are there legal complications for this form of DDAVP usage?
Sassetti: The only constraint is of frequency of donation, which is a FDA mandate. The patient who donated most often was within the rules, in that the interval between donations was never less than three weeks.

Sultan: Are there ethical problems in giving a drug to donors?
Kohler: Two systems have been presented. Volunteers were given the drug intranasally, and families of patients were given high parenteral doses. Both only work if high doses are given, and there was a blood pressure fall in our donors at doses comparable to those given in the United States. They had a 1% incidence of vaso-vagal reactions, but a regular fall in blood pressure of 20% was needed to give a sufficient Factor VIII yield. We would expect more side effects than when it is given to patients with hemophilia or vW disease.
Sassetti: Since the donors were supine for 3 hours after the infusion, there were few vaso-vagal reactions in our group. It is different if they are up and about after 30-45 minutes.

Kohler: If DDAVP 0.3 mcg/kg is given, there are larger effects on blood pressure than with a blood donation of 500ml.
Kessler: In the United States it would not be practical to implement the system for parents of hemophiliacs, not only because of the thrombogenic possibilities, but because of seizures and hyponatremia in a small number of patients. Also, as a child grows older, the parent cannot keep up with his needs. Reimbursement may not be possible for families in a voluntary programme. The FDA has prevented such programmes except in cases like that of Dr Sassetti, which have evolved under FDA auspices.

Sassetti: It is certainly onerous to operate. Its preclusion by the FDA limits its usefulness, but the programme was never envisaged as a substitute to all the alternatives. We started it because of the high publicity about disease transmission: the people who approached us may have a distorted view of the risk, and we are trying to correct it, but there still remains a niche for it.

Bichet: The hyponatremia only appears in children, never in adults. In animals it is almost impossible for DDAVP alone to cause it; fluid intake has also to be forced. In a literature review there were no symptomatic hyponatremia cases except in neonates.
Mannucci: I agree with Dr Bichet: hyponatremia does not occur under these conditions. The system is only applicable to particular circumstances. Parents tend to compensate for their "guilt" by donating their blood, and are not entirely convinced that blood products are safe. In vW disease cryoprecipitate produced in this way may be more effective than commercial products. With DDAVP more complete multimers are formed. From the theoretical viewpoint it would be interesting to expand this programme.
Sassetti: The problem with cryoprecipitate from community blood centres is that the blood can remain in the whole state for 7 hours 59 minutes before it is processed, so that the yield can be very low. Our product is out of the body for less than 3 hours before processing. We have not looked at multimers.

THE USE OF DDAVP IN BLOOD DONORS TO INCREASE THE YIELD OF FACTOR VIII IN THE PREPARATION OF FACTOR VIII CONCENTRATES

Inga Marie Nilsson

Department for Coagulation Disorders
University of Lund
Malmö General Hospital
S-214 01 Malmö, Sweden

INTRODUCTION

The aim of national self-sufficiency with respect to factor VIII concentrates has been difficult to achieve, owing to the limited supply of source plasma and the poor yield of factor VIII in the production process. For low purity concentrates such as cryoprecipitate, the yield is rarely more than 30-40%; and for high purity concentrates, the final recovery rate is even lower. If domestic supplies of plasma were to be able to cope with the requirements of factor VIII concentrate, clearly methods had to be found to improve the yield. The effect of DDAVP on factor VIII prompted us to study its use in blood donors prior to blood collection, to increase the yield of factor VIII in the production of factor VIII concentrates. These studies were started in 1978.

In two preliminary studies (Nilsson et al., 1979 a,b), DDAVP was administered intravenously to blood donors who gave their informed consent - 40 donors in one study, and 80 in the other. The dosage given was 0.2 µg/kg body weight. Prior to the DDAVP injection, an inhibitor of fibrinolysis, tranexamic acid (Cyklokapron, 0.01 g/kg, Kabi, Sweden) was given to prevent any activation of the fibrinolytic system due to the release of plasminogen activator. Blood was collected 15 minutes after the injections. Fraction I-0 (AHF-Kabi) was prepared from the DDAVP plasma pool. A control fraction I-0 was prepared from the same group of blood donors under identical conditions except for the drug treatment (Figure 1). The DDAVP-fraction I-0 concentrates contained 2-3 times as much factor VIII clotting activity (VIII:C) as the control fractions. The von Willebrand

Desmopressin in Bleeding Disorders, Edited by G. Mariani *et al.*
Plenum Press, New York, 1993

Table 1. Factor VIII activity in concentrates prepared from blood donors given DDAVP intranasally and in control concentrates from the same group of blood donors

	Units VIII:C per mL	
	Control concentrate	DDAVP concentrate
AHF-Kabi (fraction I-0)	2.8	4.5
Cryoprecipitate	3.6	15.4
Octonativ, Kabi (high-purity F VIII conc)	42	112

factor (vWF) content of the DDAVP-fractions was about twice that of the control fractions. No difference in stability of VIII:C was seen. *In vivo* studies showed that infusion of the DDAVP fractions to patients with severe hemophilia A caused a 2-3 times higher increase in VIII:C than after infusion of the same volume of the control fractions. No difference in disappearance rate of VIII:C was seen. The DDAVP fraction was also found to correct the hemostatic defect in a patient with type III von Willebrand's disease.

In subsequent studies (Mikaelsson et al., 1982; 1984), intranasal instillation of DDAVP was chosen, since this route of administration was considered safe and feasible for routine use at blood centers. Up to 420 donors participated, receiving a dose of 325 µg DDAVP 60 minutes prior to blood donation. The DDAVP solution (0.25 ml, 1300 µg/ml) was applied in the nasal cavity by means of a calibrated catheter (Rhinyl, Ferring AB, Malmö, Sweden). Immediately after separation from the blood cells, 50 mg tranexamic acid was added to each plasma bag. Blood was collected twice from all donors with an interval of 6-8 weeks. On the first occasion DDAVP was given to half of the donors while the other half were not treated. On the second occasion the procedure was reversed, DDAVP being given only to previously untreated groups instead. The DDAVP and control plasma pools were used to prepare a low-purity factor VIII concentrate (fraction I-0, AHF-Kabi), cryoprecipitate, and a high-purity factor VIII concentrate (Octonativ, Kabi). The DDAVP factor VIII concentrates contained 2-4 times as much VIII:C as did the corresponding control concentrates (Table 1). The concentration of vWF:Ag was also increased. The *in vitro* properties of the DDAVP concentrates were otherwise identical to those of conventionally prepared concentrates. No DDAVP or tranexamic acid could be demonstrated in the concentrates (Table 2). It was not possible to demonstrate any fibrinolytic activity either in the DDAVP plasma or in the DDAVP concentrates. It was clear that the requirement of source plasma could be reduced by half, if DDAVP plasma was used.

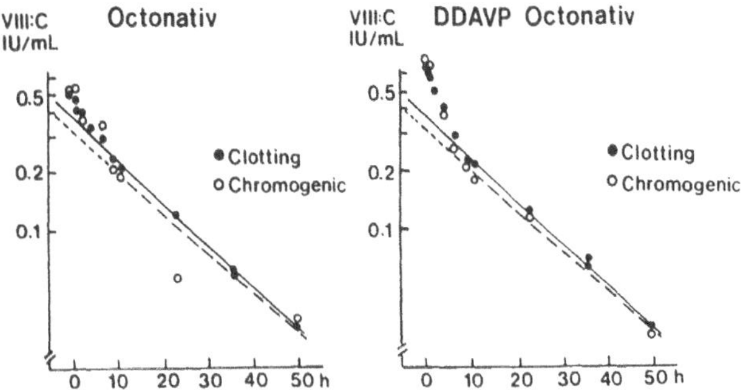

Figure 1. In vivo disappearance curves obtained in two patients with severe hemophilia A after injection of the Octonativ batches. A1 (control) and A2 (DDAVP). Dose 25 IU/kg body weight. Ordinate: log plasma level of VIII:C (n=2). Abscissa: time after injection. VIII:C was assessed both by one-stage assay and by a chromogenic subtrate method.

Controlled *in vivo* studies of DDAVP concentrates and control concentrates were then performed. Matched batches of DDAVP and control concentrates were always tested in the same patients. Figure 1 shows plasma concentrations of VIII:C in 2 hemophilia A patients after injection of DDAVP-Octonativ and control Octonativ at the same dosage of 25 IU/kg body weight. The pharmacokinetic data for the matched pairs of DDAVP and control batches are shown in Table 3. The *in vivo* recovery was in the range of 97-110% for all the batches, which is a normal finding. The half-life was 11-14 h, which is also within the normal range. There were no statistically significant differences between the DDAVP batches and their corresponding controls in any of the pairs of batches tested. The pharmacokinetic results were also analysed using non-compartmental methods (Matucci et al., 1985). Distribution volume, clearance and mean residence time showed no difference between the batches. Thus, our results showed both low- and high-purity factor VIII concentrates derived from DDAVP plasma to have the same pharmacokinetic properties as ordinary factor VIII concentrates.

In further studies (Jonsson et al., 1986), long-term safety and efficacy was investigated. Immediate side-effects were monitored in 319 blood and plasma donors after instillation of 300 µg DDAVP intranasally on at least two occasions. The predominant side-effect was a transient facial flush, which was reported in 4.8% of the administrations. Otherwise no adverse effects were noted. In an extended study, 42 plasma donors instilled 300 µg DDAVP intranasally twice monthly for nine months. Body weight, blood status, liver enzymes and plasma proteins were checked on each occasion, and hormonal response once at the end of the nine-month period. All the test results were normal. No circulating antibodies to DDAVP could be demonstrated. On the basis of these results, the application of DDAVP prior to plasma collection was licensed by the Swedish authorities in 1986.

Table 2. Analytical profile of factor VIII concentrates from blood donors given DDAVP intranasally and corresponding control concentrates

		Fraction I-0 (AHF-Kabi)		Octonativ[1] batch			
		Control	DDAVP	A1 Control	A2 DDAVP	B1 Control	B2 DDAVP
VIII:C	IU/mL	2.8	4.5	42	112	52	78
VIII:Ag	IU/mL	7.2	11.3	63	255	87	195
vWF:Ag	U/mL	10	15	101	175	146	232
Protein	g/L	17	15	21	40	25	28
Fibrinogen	g/L	15	13	11	10	10	11
Fibrinolytic activity	CU/mL	0.1	<0.1	<0.1	<0.1	<0.1	<0.1
Tranexamic acid	µg/mL	-	<0.5	-	<0.5	-	<0.5
DDAVP	ng/mL	-	<0.001	-	<0.001	-	<0.001

[1] High-purity F VIII conc.

Table 3. Pharmacokinetic data for the factor VIII concentrates (mean ± SD, n = 5)

	Octonativ batch no.			
	A1 control	A2 DDAVP	B1 control	B2 DDAVP
In vivo recovery, %	97±13	103±8	98±20	108±14
	p>0.05		p>0.05	
Half-life, h	13±4	13±3	11±4	11±2
	p>0.05		p>0.05	
Cl[1], mL/kg/h	3.6±1.1	3.5±1.1	3.1±0.5	4.1±1.0
MRT[2], h	16±5	17±4	16±6	14±3
Vss[3], mL/kg	59±3	52±7	47±10	54±5

[1] Cl = clearance
[2] MRT = mean residence time
[3] Vss = distribution volume

In further trials, however, the yield of VIII:C was sometimes lower than expected, and it was shown that several donors did not respond to intranasal DDAVP in the drop form on all occasions - probably due to inadequate application of DDAVP in the drop mode. This observation together with clinical reports on unpredictable response when DDAVP was administered by blowing into the nasal cavity drops of DDAVP by means of a catheter or single-dose pipette led to the development of a new delivery system for DDAVP in the form of a precompression, metered-dose spray.

The use of DDAVP in blood donors to increase the yield of factor VIII in the preparation above all of cryoprecipitate is particularly worth considering in developing countries such as India, which I recently visited. There almost the only treatment available treatment for hemophilia A patients is cryoprecipitate prepared from single donors - usually family members - at the blood banks of some of the largest hospitals. With the use of the new spray reproducibly increased yields could be obtained, and doubling the yield of VIII:C would mean a lot in such countries.

ACKNOWLEDGEMENT

This investigation was supported by grants from the Swedish Medical Research Council (00087).

REFERENCES

Jonsson, S., Harris, A., and Nilsson, I.M., 1986, A national self-sufficiency in FVIII supply. A long term study on the safety and efficAcy of administration of DDAVP in repeated plasma donation. *XIX Congr. Int. Soc. Blood Transf.* (Abstract).

Matucci, M., Messori, A., Donati-Cori, G., Longo, G., Vannini, S., Morfini, M., Tendi, E., and Rossi-Ferrini, P.L., 1985, Kinetic evaluation of four factor VIII concentrates by model-independent methods. *Scand. J. Haematol* 34:22.

Mikaelsson, M., Nilsson, I.M., Cedergren, B., Jonsson, S., Rydberg, L., and Wiechel., B., 1984a, The use of desmopressin (DDAVP) in the preparation of improved factor VIII concentrate. *Scand. J. Haematol.* Suppl. 40, 33:93.

Mikaelsson, M., Nilsson, I.M., Vilhardt, H., and Wiechel, B., 1982b, Factor VIII concentrate prepared from blood donors stimulated by intranasal administration of a vasopressin analogue. *Transfusion* 22:229.

Nilsson, I.M., Mikaelsson, M.,Vilhardt, H., and Walter, H., 1979, DDAVP factor VIII concentrate and its properties in vivo and in vitro. *Thromb. Res.* 15:263.

Nilsson, I.M., Walter, H., Mikaelsson, M., and Vilhardt, H., 1979, Factor VIII concentrate prepared from DDAVP stimulated blood donor plasma. *Scand. J. Haematol.* 22:42.

DISCUSSION

Kohler: Have you prior experience of using DDAVP without tranexamic acid.
Nilsson: Yes we got a very low yield of FVIII. It depends on the production of plasminogen activator and natural inhibitors of fibrinolysis being during the preparation procedure. We also tried to increase the yield by giving 0.4 mcg/kg body weight DDAVP and then we had a very poor yield of FVIII, because the given amount of tranexamic acid was not sufficient.

Mannucci: Did you have a chance to study the multimers?
Nilsson: Yes, the multimer pattern was identical to those in the controls. We had the same effect in the patients with vW disease.

Weinstein: What about the cost-effectiveness in obtaining higher yields?
Nilsson; We were upset with Ferring because of the high price. We hope that with competition they will decrease the price!

Sassetti: What is your level of donor acceptance?
Nilsson: We had no problems with the donors, but we did not ask new donors. Almost all accepted the regime.

EPIDEMIOLOGY OF MILD AND MODERATE HEMOPHILIA A AND VON WILLEBRAND'S DISEASE

Guglielmo Mariani[1] , Alessandro Ghirardini[2] and Nicola Schinaia[2]

[1]Hematology
Department of Human Biopathology
University of Rome
Rome
Italy

[2]AIDS National Operational Center
Istituto Superiore di Sanità
Rome
Italy

INTRODUCTION

Epidemiological studies of hemophilia have recently received an impulse following the appearance of the severest and most life-threatening complication of this disease, HIV infection. Studies of prevalence and incidence, cohort studies, studies aimed at evaluating the impact of treatments have been conducted. Since these studies required firmly established denominators the need for carefully analyzed prevalence and incidence figures for hemophilia has become of paramount importance.

The most suitable tools for obtaining such figures are National Registries or National and International Surveys of hemophilia cases. The features of these tools are quite different, but if surveys are carried out on a regular basis the final results may not differ. These tools have been in use for over a decade in countries where the management of hemophilia has been standardized and covers the whole national territory, as in Scandinavia, Holland, the United Kingdom, and the U.S.A. . More recently in Canada an accurate National Survey of the Canadian hemophilia population has been carried out [1] and in Italy a formal Registry has been created [2].

EPIDEMIOLOGY OF HEMOPHILIAS

The importance of the data deriving from these tools of epidemiological evaluation is

Desmopressin in Bleeding Disorders, Edited by G. Mariani *et al.*
Plenum Press, New York, 1993

such that in each country programmes aimed at studying the hemophilia population should be implemented.

Treatment is one of the aspects which would benefit most from accurate knowledge of the hemophilia population. In fact, hemophilia is not, phenotypically speaking, a homogeneous disease and the treatment may differ substantially in the context of the so-called "clinical variants". As a consequence, there is general agreement on the fact that blood derivatives should be used only in severe cases and, when indicated, in moderate forms of hemophila A. For most of the latter and for the mild cases a alternative treatment to blood products is available: Desmopressin. In hemophilia B, there is, however, no alternative to factor IX concentrates, whatever the severity of the clinical picture.

Two questions now emerge: how prevalent are the mild and moderate variants of hemophilia A and in what proportion within the population? These questions are of relevant importance since a wider use of Desmopressin may avoid the occurrence of side effects related to the use of factor concentrates, thus preventing morbidity and mortality.

Epidemiological studies have provided an answer. The prevalence of hemophilia has been calculated as being between 3.3 and 10 per 100,000 inhabitants, that is 6.6 to 20 per 100,000 males[3]. The most recent epidemiological studies, the Canadian[1] and the Italian[2], have provided figures which support the previously reported data: 13.6 and 9,7 / 100,000 males respectively. The proportion of hemophilia A/B cases is consistent within the various epidemiological studies, ranging from 78/22 (3.6/1) to 87/13 (6.7/1)1,2,4.

What is the proportion of the clinical variants within the general hemophilia population? This figure appears to vary to a certain extent with reference to the historical periods. In the early studies (before 1980) the proportion of severe hemophilia cases varied between 49 and 77 percent[5,6,7,8]; in the most recent studies[4,9,10,11], the reported prevalence of severe hemophilia is substantially lower, ranging from 29 to 43 percent and, conversely, moderate and mild cases of hemophilia are consistently reported as being in the vast majority . These findings were indirectly confirmed by Larsson[4] who found an increase of 2.5 fold in the prevalence of the mild cases versus only 0.5 fold in that of the severe; in this study the proportion of mild cases was reported as increasing from 35 percent in the sixties to 54 percent at the beginning of the eighties. This was confirmed by Ghirardini et al.[2] who described temporal trends in hemophilia incidence (from 1952 to 1987) suggesting that the diagnosis of mild and moderate hemophilia has improved. Less detailed data concerning the prevalence and the proportion of non-severe cases, that is to say moderate and mild forms of hemophilia, are available. Here again Larsson in his survey on Swedish hemophiliacs[12] provided precise data showing a prevalence of 30/16/54 percent for the severe/moderate/mild clinical variants respectively. These proportions were confirmed by Walker in his Canadian Survey[1] where severe cases were 38%, moderate 19% and mild 43%. These proportions deal with all cases of hemophilia (A + B), but no differences are apparent between hemophilia A and B in the occurrence of the clinical variants.

EPIDEMIOLOGY OF VON WILLEBRAND'S DISEASE

The evaluation of the prevalence of von Willebrand's disease in a given population is difficult to assess for a number of reasons, the most important of which are:

1.the ample phenotypic polymorphism;
2.the presence of asymptomatic subjects;
3.the diagnostic criteria ;
4.the lack of standardization of the diagnostic tools;
5.the influence of inherited characteristics on the levels of vWF;
6.the influence of acquired situations on the levels of vWD.

We will briefly analyze the above mentioned situations which can indeed influence any prevalence assessment of the disease. The disease is highly polymorphic in terms of both its clinical and its laboratory features. Several "types" and "subtypes" have been described reflecting the presence of numerous underlying gene alterations. A number of subjects, however, display only subtle laboratory changes and have never experienced bleeding episodes, even at advanced age. In this respect, Miller et al.[13], analyzing two large families with vWD, found that 11 out of 26 carriers seemed to be phenotypically normal. Diagnostic criteria for vWD are far from being uniformly accepted and the methods are not even standardized. In addition, the most accepted diagnostic tools (vWFactor antigen, Ristocetin cofactor) are influenced by congenital (blood group, race) or acquired situations (pregnancy, acute phase reaction, stress etc.).

The prevalence assessment of von Willebrand's Disease has been carried out following two methodologies, of which one is based on localized and formal epidemiological surveys and the other on the observation of subjects with clinically meaningful disease.

The first approach, which relies on the accurate screening of relatively small, geographically localized samples was pioneered by Rodeghiero et al.[14], who, by means of a careful , standardized prospective study carried out on 1,281 students resident in two different areas of the province of Vicenza, Italy, demonstrated an overall prevalence of 0.82% (90% confidence limits: 0.67 to 1.15). Werner et al.[15] also carried out a study on a composite population of school students, finding a 1.3% prevalence. Miller et al.[16], evaluating a cohort of 500 blood donors, found a prevalence of 1.6% . In a study conducted by Meriane et al.[17] in Algeria in which adults were also screened, a prevalence of 1.23% was found. A very recent Japanese study [18] has indicated a prevalence of 1.3% in apparently healthy individuals. Details of the above mentioned studies are set out in Tab.1.

The differences among these five studies, although small on epidemiological grounds, may be due to the criteria chosen to diagnose vWD. However, considering that they were carried out in different countries, on different ethnic groups and that they have found prevalences ranging from 0.8 to 1.6, a prevalence of the magnitude of 1 percent should be considered realistic and credible. All the subjects diagnosed in the above mentioned formal epidemiological surveys belonged to type I vWD. This comes as no surprise if one takes into account that the screened populations were unselected and considers the rarity of the other types. In fact vWD type I accounts for 70-80% of the whole vWD population 19,20.

The second approach used to determine the prevalence of vWD is based on clinical practice, that is to say by using questionnaires to collect cases diagnosed at the Centers. An example of this approach is the study by Bloom and Giddings[21] who carried out an international Survey on the prevalence of AIDS in vWD and, as a by-product, tried to obtain indications regarding the prevalence of vWD. The prevalences reported varied greatly among the various

Table 1. Formal epidemiological studies on vWD.

Author	year	Country	Studied subjects	Prevalence (%) adjusted	Blood Group vWF
Rodeghiero[14]	1987	Italy	1,218	0.82	yes
Werner[15]	1991	USA	600	1.30	yes
Miller[16]	1987	USA	500	1.60	yes
Meriane[17]	1991	Algeria	487	1.80	yes
Shinmyozu[18]	1991	Japan	1,512	1-2	?

geographical areas and their magnitude (varying from 3.7 to 239 subjects/ million) is quite different from that found in the formal epidemiological surveys. This was also true for areas with an efficient network of hemophilia care, such as in Scandinavia: here a prevalence of 0.0221% was reported, which appears to be underscored at least 50 times in comparison with that reported in the formal epidemiological surveys. This is not surprising considering that the main purpose of the survey was to analyze HIV infection in patients with vWD -that is to say treated patients- and that the target of the survey was the "clinical vWD".

CONCLUDING REMARKS

In conclusion, the prevalence of mild factor VIII deficiencies, which comprise mild & moderate hemophilia A and Type I vWD is higher than currently believed. Mild and moderate hemophilia A accounts for more than 50% of the total hemophilia A population, that is, in absolute terms, approximately 1/20,000 males. von Willebrand's disease has a prevalence of circa 1/100 individuals, according to the estimations derived from formally conducted epidemiological surveys.

These, therefore are the patients who are eligible for treatment with Desmopressin. Eligible subjects must of course be screened and the efficacy of the vasopressin analogue evaluated beforehand, even though limitations to the use of the drug are few. This synthetic analogue, therefore, represents a real opportunity for the treatment of a large number of potential bleeders. The most important advantage to be gained from the use of Desmopressin is, of course, the elimination of all risks connected with the use of blood derivatives.

REFERENCES

1. I. Walker. Survey of the Canadian hemophilia population, Can. J. Publ. Health 82:127 (1991).

2. A. Ghirardini, N. Schinaia, F. Chiarotti, N. Binkin and the GICC. Epidemiology of hemophilia and HIV infection in Italy. Submitted for publication.
3. S.A. Larsson.Hemophilia in Sweden. Studies on demography of hemophilia and surgery in hemophilia and von Willebrand's Disease in "Thesis" Medical Writing, Malmo (1984).
4. S.A. Larsson, I.M. Nilsson, M. Blomback. Current status of Swedish hemophiliacs I.A demographic survey, Acta Med. Scand.212:195 (1982).
5. J.J. Veltkamp, G. Schrijver, W. Willeumier, B.van de Putte, H. van Dijck. Hemophilia in the Netherlands. Results of a survey on the medical, genetic and social situation of the Dutch hemophiliacs, Acta Med. Scand. Suppl. 572:64 (1974).
6. J.P. Allain. Management of hemophilia in France, Thromb. Haemost. 35:553 (1976).
7. T. Mandalaki. Management of hemophilia in Greece, Thromb. Haemost. 35:522 (1976).
8. N.J. Brandt. Haemofili. Organisation af forebyggelse og behandling, Ugeskr Laeger. 141:1300 (1979).
9. H. Heger, P.F. Hjort, S.A.Evensen. Helseokonomisk analyse av blodersykdommen i Norge, Tidsskr Nor Laegeforen 100:948 (1980).
10. M.E. Eyster, J.H. Lewis, S.S. Shapiro, F. Gill, M. Kajani, D. Prager, I. Djerassi, S. Rice, C. Lusch, A. Keller, The Pennsylvania hemophilia program 1973-1978, Am. J. Hematol. 9:277 (1980).
11. C.R. Rizza and R.J.D. Spooner. Treatment of hemophilia and related disorders in Britain and Northern Ireland during 1976-80: Report on behalf of the directors of hemophilia centers in the United Kingdom, Br. Med. J. 286:929 (1983).
12. S.A. Larsson. Hemophilia in Sweden. Studies on demography of hemophilia and surgery in hemophilia and von Willebrand's disease, Acta Med.Scand. Suppl.684:1 (1984).
13. C.H. Miller, J.B. Graham, L.R. Goldin, R.C. Elston. Genetics of classic von Willebrand's disease 1: Phenotypic variation within families, Blood. 54:117 (1979).
14. F. Rodeghiero, G. Castaman, E. Dini. Epidemiological investigation of the prevalence of von Willebrand's disease. Blood. 89:454 (1987).
15. E.J. Warner, E.M. Broxson, E.L. Tucker, L.F. Amnsiac, D.S. Giroux, T.C. Abshire : Prevalence of von Willebrand disease in children: a multiethnic study, Blood. Suppl. (1987), abstract 262.
16. C.H. miller, R. Lenzi, C. Breen.Prevalence of von Willebrand's disease among U.S. adults, Blood. Suppl. (1987), abstract 1365.
17. F. Meriane, Y. Sultan, H. Arabi, O. Chafa, T. Chellali. Incidence of a low von Willebrand factor activity in a population of algerian students,Blood. Suppl. (1987), abstract 1928.
18. K. Shinmyozu, T. Okadome, Y. Maruyama, M. Osame, M. Tara. A study on the frequency of von Willebrand's deficiency state, Rinsho Ketsueki 32:67 (1991).
19. S.A. Berliner, U. Seligsohn, A. Zivelin, E. Zwang, G. Sofferman. A relatively high frequency of severe (type III) von Willebrand's disease in Israel, Br. J. Haematol. 62:535 (1986).
20. H. Link, I.M. Nilsson, L. Holmberg, G. Weissbach. Frequency of different types of von Willebrand's disease in the GDR, Acta Med Scand. 224:275 (1988).

21. A.L. Bloom and J.C. Giddings. HIV infection and AIDS in von Willebrand's disease. An international survey including data on the prevalence of clinical von Willebrand's disease. in: "Hemophilia and von Willebrand's disease in 1990s" J.M. Lusher and C.M. Kessler eds.,Elsevier Science Publishers B.V. (1991).

DISCUSSION

Kobrinsky: Distribution of the ABO blood groups differs in different centres. Does this have an impact on vWf incidence in different countries?
Mariani: They may pose problems for assessing normal ranges, but they have no influence on the prevalence of vW disease.

Kessler: There is interest in correlating vW disease with atherosclerosis and atherogenesis. Do mild-moderate vW disease patients have a lower incidence of them in communities where they are common?
Mariani : It is very difficult to assess prevalence of vW disease in general populations, and the relationship between it and atherosclerosis is not firmly established. There is only an indication that severe vW disease protects against severe atherosclerosis, and diet plays a role possibly more important than lack of vWf.

AN OVERVIEW OF GENE ALTERATIONS IN MILD HEMOPHILIA AND VON WILLEBRAND DISEASE

Francesco Bernardi, Patrizia Patracchini
Mirco Pinotti, Giovanna Marchetti

Centro Studi Biochimici delle Patologie del Genoma Umano
Istituto di Chimica Biologica
Università di Ferrara, Ferrara, Italy

INTRODUCTION

Several factors can account for the severity and heterogeneity of clinical phenotypes.

SEVERITY OF PHENOTYPES

- COPY NUMBER AND LOCALIZATION OF GENE(S)
- INTERACTIONS BETWEEN NORMAL AND MUTATED GENE PRODUCTS
- EPISTATIC EFFECTS OF OTHER LOCI
- REDUCED OR ALTERED GENE EXPRESSION

The number of copies per haploid genome does not account for differences in expression of altered coagulation factor genes, which are single copy genes or have inactive pseudogenes. Differently, the X chromosome localization plays a major role in factor VIII (FVIII) and factor IX (FIX) deficiency (hemophilia A and B).
An additional factor is represented by the interaction of mutant and normal gene products in quaternary structures (e.g. dimer or multimer formation). These interactions give rise to dominant phenotypes as observed in von Willebrand disease (VWD). Moreover, other genes seem to modify the expression of abnormal clotting factors through poorly understood epistatic effects.

This paper is focused on molecular lesions compatible with partial expression of coagulation factor genes.

The mutations could affect the nucleic acid (mRNA) transcription or processing,

Desmopressin in Bleeding Disorders, Edited by G. Mariani *et al.*
Plenum Press, New York, 1993

the translation efficiency or, most important, the processing, stability, secretion or activity of abnormal proteins. The protein activity includes the proteolytic cleavages as well as non-covalent interactions between factors and cofactors.

<u>GENE EXPRESSION</u>

-	NUCLEIC ACIDS	TRANSCRIPTION RNA PROCESSING
-	TRANSLATION EFFICIENCY	
-	PROTEIN	STABILITY SECRETION ACTIVITY

Transcription

The most important aspect is represented by the initiation complex formation, which is dependent on the promoter sequence, a large DNA region involved in polymerase and transcription factor interactions. A promoter mutation can alter the transcription rate and thus the amount of mRNA available for translation.

Splicing

The mRNA splicing is driven by consensus splicing sequences located between introns and exons. Mutations in these DNA regions can reduce the splicing rate or efficiency. In addition a new splicing site can be activated by mutations in cryptic sites.

Processing and secretion

Protein synthesis, maturation and secretion, which involve a huge number of steps, represent a major target in altered gene expression, and several examples are present in mutated clotting factors.

MILD HEMOPHILIA B

The FIX gene has been extensively studied and a large number of mutations hasve been described (Giannelli et al., 1990).

Different mutations have been found in the promoter region (-20, -6, 13) and some of them give rise to the Leiden phenotype, characterized by increasing of FIX expression after puberty (Reitsma et al., 1988; Crossley and Brownlee, 1990). Among the several splicing mutations described, only two seem to give rise to a mild phenotype.

Missense mutations are certainly the most frequent cause of mild hemophilia B and, apart from signal peptide, they are present in different protein domains. It is interesting to observe that they affect processing, carboxylation, activation and catalytic efficiency. The chemical properties of residues are conserved in the catalytic domain, while large changes are tolerated in other domains.

Table 1. Mutations in mild hemophilia B

PATIENT	CLOTTING	MUTATION	COMMENTS
Leyden	1-60	G->A	Promoter
Leyden		T->A	Promoter
HB13	32	A->G	Promoter
HB6	20	Del 4 bases	Splicing
Toronto13,15	10	A->G	Splicing
London, Ont1	6	Asn2->Asp	Processing?
Oxford b2	6	Glu7->Ala	Gla
HB2, Toronto17	30	Arg29->Gln	
Hoogeveen	14	Lys43->Glu	
Alabama	10	Asp47->Gly	
Hollywood, UK7	11	Pro55->Ala	
Durham	14	* Gly60->Ser	
UK6	8	Asp64->Gly	ß-OHAsp
Leamington	13	Gly114->Ala	
Chapel Hil	8	* Arg145->His	Activation
Cardiff2	15	Val182->Leu	
Wultschkau	7	Val211->Phe	
HB11	12	* Ala233->Thr	Catalytic
HB8	24	Asn260->Ser	Domain
Zoeterwoude	13	Leu279->Ile	
UK13	4-16	Ala291->Thr	
Liebenzel	6	* Thr296->Met	
Unnamed	5	Val307->Ala	

* highly recurrent

One third of mutations are present in CpG dinucleotides, which represent ''hot spot'' mutation sites favouring the onset of recurrent mutations (Koeberl et al.,1989). However, identity by descent may be suspected in several cases, particularly in mild hemophilia.

MILD HEMOPHILIA A

The large size and the complex structure of the FVIII gene have hampered a detailed analysis and characterization of molecular lesions in hemophilia A (rewieved by Tuddenham et al., 1991). In addition spontaneous mutations are thought to account for a large number of cases of sporadic hemophilia A (Vogel and Rathenberg, 1975; Bernardi et al., 1987). Recent advances in molecular genetic techniques provide interesting insights in the pattern of mild hemophilia A mutations (Higuchi et al., 1991).

Table 2. Mutations in mild hemophilia A.

PATIENT	CLOTTING	MUTATION	COMMENTS
?	7-10	Dupl ex 13	
JH10	5.5	Del ex 22	
JH104	9-18	Leu1843->Leu	splicing
JH1	5-10	G->A IVS4	cryptic site?
JH107	?	G->A IVS12	splicing
H72	5	Val162->Met	A1
JH39	19	Lys166->Thr	A1
JH87	14-16	Thr295->Ala	A1
JH35	5	Arg372->His	activation
JH131	10	Leu412->Phe	A2
JH94	15	* Arg527->Trp	A2
JH97	6	Arg531->Cys	A2
JH144	9	Arg531->Gly	A2
JH123	7	Gln565->Lys	A2
JH82	?	* Arg593->Cys	A2
JH136	14	Ala644->Val	A2
JH40	10	Tyr1680->Phe	sulphation vWF binding
HP15	7	Arg1689->His	B
JH103	15	Pro1825->Ser	A3
TM	5	Arg1941->Gln	A3
JH133	11	Phe2101->Leu	C1
JH134	5-8	Ser2119->Tyr	C1
JH57	5-7	* Arg2150->His	C1
JH138	10	Arg2159->Cys	C1
JH75	7	Pro2300->Leu	C2
H104	10	Arg2307->Gln	C2

* recurrent

A1, A2, B, A3, C1, C2: FVIII domains

Some mutations provide examples of peculiar molecular mechanisms causing mild hemophilia A:

i) an in-frame deletion of exon 22 which removes 52 aminoacids from the C1 domain (Youssoufian et al., 1987);

ii) a duplication involving exon 13 (Murru et al., 1990);

iii) a point mutation in intron 4 which could activate a cryptic donor splice site (Youssoufian et al., 1988) and

iv) a missense mutation (Tyr 1680 to Phe) which suppresses a sulphated residue critical for interaction between FVIII and von Willebrand factor (vWF) (Leyte et al., 1991). No mutation in the promoter has been reported to date.

It is of great interest that the clinical phenotype in patients with the same mutation is not always the same.

Some of these mutations (372 and 1689) are located on proteolytic cleavage sites of FVIII (Arai et al.,1989; Schwaab et al., 1991).

We have described two unrelated patients (H1, H20) with a G to A transition at codon 2209 causing a severe phenotype (Bernardi et al., 1988; Bernardi et al., 1989). Moderate

Table 3 Variable phenotype with the same FVIII mutation.

PATIENT	MUTATION	CLOTTING	SEVERITY
H26	Val162->Met	8	Moderate
H72	" "	5	Mild
H44	Val326->Leu	?	Severe
JH30	" "	?	Moderate
JH35	Arg372->His	5	Mild
H453	" "	3	Moderate
J254	" Cys	3	Moderate
HP14	Arg1689->Cys	<1	Severe
ARC5	" "	2-5	Mild/Moderate
J242	" "	4-5	Moderate
HP15	" His	7	Mild
H1/H20	Arg2209->Gln	1-2	Severe
JH18/JH19	" "	<1	Severe
HP16	" "	7	Mild
H156	" Leu	3	Moderate
H6	Arg2307->Gln	2	Moderate
H104	" "	10	Mild

hemophilia with the same mutation has been reported (Levinson et al., 1990). "Positive" and additional FVIII mutations or possible epistatic effects have to be considered (discussed by Schwaab et al., 1990).

VON WILLEBRAND DISEASE

The study of gene lesions in von Willebrand disease (vWD) is hampered by the large size of the gene, the exon number (52), the presence of a partial pseudogene, the many protein polymorphisms, and by the autosomal localization. Moreover posttranslational processing of vWF is a particularly complex process that requires many different steps, the alteration of which may cause a partial reduction of vWF expression.

Gene lesions giving rise to type II vWD (qualitative defect) have been studied in detail by different groups. Missense mutations are the cause of type IIA and IIB phenotypes and most of them have been localized in the exon 28, which, given its size, does represent a large target for mutations (Cooney et al., 1991; Randi et al., 1991). A molecular mechanism that involves an enhanced affinity of mutated vWF for a platelet receptor appears to explain the observed type IIB phenotype.

We have described a type II vWD variant characterized by the presence of a partial heterozygous deletion (Bernardi et al., 1990). The deleted, in-frame mRNA, from which 820 codons are removed, has been isolated and characterized.

Mutations localized in the amino terminal portion of the molecule have been found associated with an impaired FVIII binding (Normandy variant, Cacheris et al., 1991; Jorieux et al., 1992).

PROSPECTS FOR THE FUTURE

New techniques have greatly improved the analysis of mutations in clotting factor genes. We can be optimistic about future developments in unravelling the molecular components of hemostatic diseases in virtually all patients. We hope that new insight into normal coagulation biology will be acquired, thus stimulating design of innovative strategies for treatment and prevention of diseases.

ACKNOWLEDGMENTS

This work was supported by P.F. Ingegneria Genetica CNR, and Ric Sanit Final Regioni Emilia Romagna and Veneto.

REFERENCES

Arai, M., Inaba, H., Higuchi, M., Antonarakis, S.E., Kazazian, H.H.Jr., Fujimaki, M.

Hoyer, L.W, 1989, Direct characterization of factor VIII in plasma: detection of a mutation altering a thrombin cleavage site (arginine 372 to histidine), Proc. Natl. Acad. Sci. USA 86:4277.

Bernardi, F., Marchetti, G., Bertagnolo, V., Faggioli, L., Volinia, S., Patracchini, P., Bartolai, S., Vannini, F., Felloni, L., Rossi, L., Panicucci, F., and Conconi F., 1987, RFLPs analysis in families with sporadic hemophilia A: stimate of the mutation rate in male and female gametes, Hum. Genet. 76:253.

Bernardi, F., Legnani, C., Patracchini, P., Rodorigo, G., De Rosa, V., and Marchetti, G., 1988, A Hind III RFLP and a gene lesion in the coagulation factor VIII gene, Hum. Genet. 78:359.

Bernardi, F., Volinia, S., Patracchini, P., Gemmati, D., Boninsegna S., Schwienbacher C, and Marchetti, G., 1989, A recurrent missense mutation (Arg->Gln) and a partial deletion in factor VIII gene causing severe Hemophilia A, Br. J. Haematol. 71:271.

Bernardi, F., Marchetti, G., Guerra, S., Casonato, A., .op Gemmati, D., Patracchini, P., Ballerini, G., and Conconi, F., 1990, A "de novo" and heterozygous gene deletion causing a variant of von Willebrand disease, Blood 75:677.

Cacheris, P.M., Nichols, W.C., and Ginsburg, D., 1991, Molecular characterization of a unique von Willebrand disease variant, J. Biol. Chem. 266:13499.

Cooney, K.A., Nichols, W.C., Bruck, M.E., Bahou, W.F., Shapiro, A.D., Bowie, E.J.W., Gralnick, H.R., and Ginsburg, D., 1991, The molecular defect in type IIB von Willebrand disease. Identification of four potential missense mutations within the putative GpIb binding domain, J.Clin.Invest. 87:1227.

Crossley, M., and Brownlee, G.G., 1990, Disruption of a C /EBP binding site in the factor IX promoter is associated with haemophilia B, Nature 345: 444.

Giannelli, F., Green, P.M., High, K.A., Lozier, J.N., Lillicrap, D.P., Ludwig, M., Olek, K., Reitsma, P.H., Goossens, M., Yoshioka, A., Sommer, S., and Brownlee, G.G., 1990, Haemophilia B: database of point mutations and short additions and deletions, Nucl. Acids Res.18:4053.

Jorieux, S., Tuley, E.A., Gaucher, C., Mazurier, C., and Sadler J.E., 1992, The mutation Arg(53)->Trp causes von Willebrand disease Normandy by abolishing binding to factor VIII. Studies with recombinant von Willebrand factor, Blood 79:563.

Higuchi, M., Antonarakis, S.E., Kasch, L., Oldenburg, J., Economou-Petersen, E., Olek, K., Arai, M., Inaba, H.,and Kazazian, Jr., H.H., 1991, Molecular characterization of mild-to-moderate hemophilia A: detection of the mutation in 25 of 29 patients by denaturing gradient gel electrophoresis, Proc. Natl. Acad. Sci. USA 58:8307.

Koeberl, D.D., Bottema, C.D.K., Buerstedde, J.M., and Sommer, S.S., 1989, Functionally important regions of the factor IX gene have a low rate of polymorphisms and a high rate of mutation in the dinucleotide CpG, Am. J. Hum. Genet.45:448.

Levinson, B., Lehesjoki, A.E., de la Chapelle, A., and Gitschier, J., 1990, Molecular analysis of hemophilia A in the Finnish population, Am. J. Hum. Genet. 46: 53.

Leyte, A., van Schijndel H.B., Niehrs, C., Huttner, W.B., Verbeet, M.P., Martens, K., and van Mourik, J.A., 1991, Sulfation of Tyr 1680 of human blood coagulation factor VIII is essential for the interaction of factor VIII with von Willebrand factor J. Biol. Chem. 266:740.

Murru, S., Casula, L., Pecorara, M., Mori, P., Cao, A., and Pirastu, M., 1990, Illegitimate recombination produced a duplication within FVIII gene in a patient with mild hemophilia A, Genomics 7:115.

Randi, A. M., Rabinowitz, I., Mancuso, D.J., Mannucci, P.M., and Sadler, J.E., 1991, Molecular basis of von Willebrand disease type IIB. Candidate mutations cluster in one disulfide loop between proposed platelet .op glycoprotein Ib binding sequences, J.Clin.Invest. 87:1220.

Reitsma, P.H., Mandalaki, T., Kasper,C.K., Bertina, R.M., and Briet, E., 1989, Two novel point mutations correlate with an altered developmental expression of blood coagulation factor IX (hemophilia B Leyden phenotypes), Blood 73: 743.

Schwaab, R., Ludwig, M., Oldenburg, J., Brackmann, H.H., Egli, H. Kochhan, L., and Olek, K., 1990, Identical point mutations in the factor VIII gene that have different clinical manifestations of hemophilia, Am. J. Hum. Genet 47:743.

Schwaab, R., Ludwig, M., Kochhan, L., Oldenburg, J., McVey, J.H., Egli, H., Brackmann, H.H., and Olek, K., 1991, Detection and characterization of two missense mutations at a cleavage site in the factor VIII light chain, Thromb. Res. 61:225.

Tuddenham, E.G.D., Cooper, D.N., Gitschier, J., Higuchi, M., Hoyer, L.W., Yoshioka, A., Peake, I.R., Schwaab, R., Olek, K., Kazazian, H.H., Lavergne, J.-M., and Antonarakis, S.E. 1991, Haemophilia A: database of nucleotide substitutions, deletions, insertions and rearrangements of the factor VIII gene, Nucleic Acids Res. 19:4821.

Vogel, F., and Rathenberg, R., 1975, Spontaneous mutation in men, in: "Advances in Human Genetics," H. Harris and K. Hirschhorn, eds., Plenum, New York.

Youssoufian, H., Antonarakis, S.E., Aronis, S., Tsiftis, G., Phillips, D.G., Kazazian, H.H., 1987, Characterization of five partial deletions of factor VIII gene, Proc. Natl. Acad. Sci. USA 84: 3772.

Youssoufian, H., Kazazian, Jr., H.H., Patel, A., Aronis, S., Tsiftis, G., Hoyer, L.W., and Antonarakis, S.E, 1988, Mild hemophilia A associated with a cryptic donor splice site mutation in intron 4 of the factor VIII gene, Genomics 2:32.

DISCUSSION

Bichet: With a deletion of 10 exons, could you use the PCR amplification for the detection of the lesion?
Bernardi: Yes, both at the DNA and MRNA level.

Bichet: In about half the haemophilia cases in a recent report, no gene alteration was found. Why?
Bernardi: It is not a technical problem. The lesions are not present in these cases in splicing junctions or exons, but are in other portions of the gene or outside the gene.

Bichet: Some techniques do not detect all abnormalities.
Bernardi: This is true. That is why we use more than one technique. With the denaturing technique we can detect 80-90% of the abnormalities.

Mayadas-Norton: Are there mutations in the propolypeptide which have been identified, since it is important in vitro in the multimerization and storage of vWf?
Bernardi: In vitro they have been produced, but I will have to check the literature about their existence in patients.

Mayadas-Norton: What happened to the vW multimerization in your Type 2 deletion mutant? Because D3 and Dprime domains are sufficient in vitro to promote vWf interdimer disulfide bonds.
Bernardi: The multimers are severely reduced, and the ristocetin co-factor activity is approximately 3%. A portion of the D3 domain involved in multimer formation is removed in our patient.

Mayadas-Norton: Have you found any mutations in the B domain that altered the FVIII activity or stability? There are plans to drop it in commercial preparations since the Factor VIII is more efficiently secreted and appears functional in heterologous cells transfected with the altered Factor VIII cDNA.
Bernardi: There is not a high mutation rate in the B domain. It does not appear to be important, but we have not examined this portion of the molecule in our patient.
Seremetis: The B domain has been removed in recombinant FVIII and it is still effective.

DDAVP - CLINICAL USE AND THERAPEUTIC LIMITATIONS IN PATIENTS WITH CONGENITAL BLEEDING DISORDERS: THE AUCKLAND EXPERIENCE

Elizabeth W. Berry

Haemophilia Centre
Auckland Hospital
Private Bag 29024
Auckland 1001
New Zealand

Paul R. Berry

Department of Anaesthesia
Greelane/National Womens Hospital
Private Bag
Auckland 1003
New Zealand

INTRODUCTION

Desmopressin (DDAVP) was first used to treat patients with inherited coagulation disorders by Mannucci et al (1977).Subsequently, mechanisms of drug action, different formulations and dosage schedules have been studied (Nilsson and Lethagen 1991). Responses to DDAVP have suggested differences in types of von Willebrand's disease (vWD) (Menon et al 1978), and this has been followed by greater understanding of vWD pathophysiology (Ruggeri and Zimmerman 1987). Administration of DDAVP reduces blood product consumption and the desire to decrease exposure where possible has led to attempts to expand the indications for its use. Its role in the treatment of disorders of haemostasis is in some instances well established, but in other situations its precise role is not defined (Mannucci 1988).

This paper will review and update the clinical use of DDAVP at the Auckland Hospital Haemophilia Centre in mild to moderate haemophilia and vWD including its perceived limitations (Berry 1990), as well as experience in the minimal bleeding disorders, (MBD) a heterogeneous group of patients who have considerable morbidity with many surgical procedures.

PATIENT POPULATION

The Auckland Haemophilia Centre has 80 individuals with mild to

Desmopressin in Bleeding Disorders, Edited by G. Mariani *et al.*
Plenum Press, New York, 1993

moderate haemophilia and 16 expressed carriers, 228 patients with vWD are registered, 25 type I with factor VIII (FVIII) less than 20% and 3 type I with FVIII less than 10%. The vWD population is completed with 6 type II, 2 of whom have been identified as type IID. The overall number in the community will be somewhat greater as registration depends on requests from primary physicians and/or patient. Thus, our numbers are comprised of those with positive individual or family bleeding histories or those where management has been required for haemostatic problems.

Similarly, only a small percentage of those with minimal bleeding disorders are registered (101), although from a survey done of all haemostasis screening in the area (1.3 million population) the frequency approximates to 50 new cases annually, about half of whom will have vWD and the other half defined platelet defects or isolated prolonged bleeding times. These figures are in keeping with Bachmann's estimates (Bachmann, 1980).

Table 1. DDAVP Use Auckland Haemophilia Centre 1978-1991

		Haemophilia		vWD		MBD
Surgical	- Dental	39	(9)	59	(2)	71
	- Other	18	(7)	21	(2)	11
Soft tissue injury		22	(4)	2	(2)	
Muscle haematoma		20	(7)	5	(2)	
Haemarthrosis		15	(6)	9	(1)	
Other		7	(0)	14	(0)	
Epistaxis		2	(0)	16	(0)	
Menorrhagia				2	(1)	

( ) Supplementary blood products.

TREATMENT RESULTS

Between 1978 and 1990, DDAVP has been used in 123 treatment episodes in individuals with mild to moderate haemophilia, 128 episodes in vWD and 82 in patients with MBD (Table 1). The bracketed figures denote the use of supplementary blood products to reach appropriate factor levels, to stop immediate or delayed haemorrhage or to promote wound healing. The majority of treatments have been for dental surgery, mainly the oral surgical removal of third molars which are often impacted.

Dental Regimen

Initially, DDAVP dosage was 0.4 μg/Kg in 50mls normal saline (less for children) over 30 minutes at one hour pre, and 12, 24, 36 hours post operatively, with an additional dose before suture removal. Antifibrinolytic agents were given preoperatively and continued for 7 - 14 days. Subsequently, DDAVP dosage has been decreased to 0.3 μg/Kg as has the frequency. Consistent use has been made of antifibrinolytic mouthwashes, usually epsilon aminocaproic acid (EACA) (Berry et al 1977).

Currently, for an uncomplicated pre molar extraction a single dose of DDAVP is used aiming for FVIII greater than 20%. For major oral surgery, the aim is for 50% FVIII. Antibiotics and systemic antifibrinolytic agents are given for five - 10 days together with EACA mouth washes three times daily until healing is complete. A pureed diet is advised.

For 10 years of the period covered all procedures were performed by two oral surgeons and one dentist who, in addition to the described regimen have, at various times, also used collagen, fibrin glue, topical thrombin, cyanoacrylate and mechanical splinting.

Dental - Mild Haemophilia

DDAVP produced a 1.5 - 7.2 fold rise in FVIII (average 3.6) giving levels of 35 - 72%. Results are summarised in Table 2. Bleeding, for which one further dose of DDAVP was given, occurred in two patients on days 4 and 5. Blood products have been used in 9 episodes (23%) - in 5 to further raise FVIII levels prior to extraction, in 4 (10%) for treatment of bleeding. This includes two patients whose FVIII levels were over 45%. Bleeding from a flap at day 6 in another patient, required blood products for several days to ensure healing after failure to respond to further DDAVP. Replacement therapy was also given for continuing bleeding in a patient whose diastolic BP rose 10mmHg, post DDAVP. No bleeding problems were seen in patients with FVIII levels over 50% preoperatively.

It is difficult to reconcile the lower levels of FVIII for successful dental surgery in some series with the Auckland Haemophilia Centre experience. Literature levels vary from 10% for all surgery (Ramstrom et al 1989, Sindet-Pedersen et al 1988) to 15 - 40% depending on type of challenge (Dal Bo Zanon et al 1986) and the standard texts which recommend 50% (Davies and Tuddenham 1987).

Precise correlation of FVIII levels and surgery is sparse. The emphasis on local antifibrinolytic therapy has consistently decreased the incidence of post operative bleeding, but there are bleeding episodes reported in the literature at FVIII levels similar to those described here (Mariani et al 1984).

Dental - Mild Haemophilia with Inhibitor

DDAVP has been useful in the management of patient 7 who has mild haemophilia and an inhibitor. This 68 year old had received on average 1 - 2 treatments annually with cryoprecipitate (cryo) and the inhibitor was detected following a poor response to therapy. DDAVP producing a FVIII rise from 10 - 31% and cryo (1500 FVIII units) were given prior to seven extractions when inhibitor levels were unmeasurable. There were difficulties with tooth fracture and hard bone as well as which a lip lesion was noted and excision biopsy performed. Radiotherapy given for this lesion, an incompletely excised adenoid cystic carcinoma, produced a deterioration in dental status. When the inhibitor level had fallen to 2.4 BU/ml nine months later, DDAVP and FVIII concentrate (total 15,500 FVIII units) were used for a dental clearance. FVIII concentrate was added to raise initial FVIII level above 50% in view of previous surgical problems and then alternated with DDAVP 12 hourly for three days because of known tachyphylaxis and age. Four weeks later the inhibitor measured 134 BU/ml to human FVIII. There was no cross reactivity with porcine FVIII.

DDAVP administration when the inhibitor was undetectable and again at 2.4 BU/ml showed equivalent FVIII rise with half lives of 5 and 6 hours respectively. After DDAVP there was neither immediate change in the inhibitor level nor an anamnestic response, indicating non reactivity to endogenous FVIII. The kinetic pattern was type I. The inhibitor is unusual in that its activity is immediate without progression and thus an initial

Table 2. Dental Surgery - Haemophilia A and Expressed Carriers

Total patients			39
A.	DDAVP alone		30
	Baseline FVIII	12 - 31%	
	DDAVP response	35 - 72%	
B.	DDAVP and prophylactic/therapeutic FVIII		9

Case	DDAVP (Day)	Level %	Bleeding	Treatment	Comment
1	0,0,1,6	10-47	Day 6	VIII	Impacted 8's
2	0	9-47	Immediate	VIII	Impacted 8's
3	0,1,2,6	9-45	3 hrs D6	Cryo	Impacted 8's
4	0	6-28	Immediate	Cryo	Infected molar
					BP rise
5	0,1,3,6	7-34	Nil	Cryo	Impacted 8's
6a	0	3-6	Nil	Cryo	6 teeth
6b	0	5-12	Nil	Cryo	Impacted molar
7a	0,1,2	10-31	Nil	Cryo	7 teeth
7b	0,1,2	12-31	Nil	VIII	Clearance
					FVIII inhibitor

screen test for inhibitors was negative. Investigations for possible lupus anticoagulant are negative. Molecular studies show no evidence of a major defect. DDAVP has shown a similar beneficial effect in two other reports of mild haemophiliacs with high titre FVIII inhibitors (Lowe et al 1977; Kesteven et al 1984).

Dental - von Willebrand's Disease

Only 2 of 59 patients needed blood products, one for co- existing FVII deficiency, the other in a patient with type I vWD with a non corrected bleeding time (BT) who responded quickly to cryo. Haemostasis was achieved in two patients with type IID although their bleeding times did not correct.

Non Dental Surgery - Haemophilia

Mainly external and minor surgical procedures have been performed (Table 3).

Table 3. Surgery Haemophilia A including Expressed Carriers

Patient	Surgery	FVIII Level % Pre		Post	DDAVP Doses	FVIII Units	Comment
la	Toenail avulsion	17	-	35	4		
lb	"	23	-	66	2		
2	"	16	-	44	3		
3	Vasectomy	14	-	75	2		
4	"	20	-	60	2		
5a	Tonsillectomy	17	-	43	8		
5b	Tendon repair	29	-	50	3		
6	Appendicectomy	36	-	52	3		
7	Mole removal	25	-	60	2		
8	Grommets	18	-	43	1		
9	Caesarian section	46	-	?	1		
10a	Plating of fracture	38	-	90	6	10,000	Arterial bleeding day 5
10b	Removal of plate	26	-	90	7	10,000	Infection day 4
11	Arthroscopy	14	-	64	4	1,000	Swelling day 2, FVIII 31%
12	Crushed finger	9	-	53	4	3,000	Skin graft not healing
13	Pyelolithotomy	17	-	35	3	7,000	Pre-operative supplement Severe headache with DDAVP
14	Angioplasty	17	-	50	1	2,000	Vessel reocclusion, angina
15	Nerve release	25	-	40	4	8,000	Staff anxiety

Post DDAVP FVIII levels were under 40% in one and 40 - 50% in 4 patients. Systemic antifibrinolytics were used with cutaneous and oral cavity surgery. Several patients warrant comment. Of those who had DDAVP alone, patient 5 who had 8 doses of DDAVP for a tonsillectomy would now be given 2 - 3 doses on a daily basis and if needed, for bleeding.

Patient 9, an expressed carrier with a history of excess bleeding and wound haematoma and a baseline of 25% was asymptomatic after DDAVP post delivery for repeat caesarean section.

For more extensive soft tissue and internal procedures, FVIII concentrates have been given as well as DDAVP to ensure levels of 50 - 60% FVIII at surgery. Patient 10 had surgical and infective problems following internal fixation of an unstable forearm fracture and subsequent removal of the plate. On each occasion good haemostasis was achieved by DDAVP alone for the first several days.

Patient 11 had his swollen knee post arthroscopic menisceal surgery treated on day 2 when FVIII levels post DDAVP were 31%. This may or may not have been a bleed.

The skin graft after a finger crush injury in patient 12 was in jeopardy with oozing, and FVIII concentrate was given alternating with DDAVP until healing took place. Severe headache restricted further use of DDAVP in patient 13.

DDAVP usage during angioplasty in patient 14 was associated with vessel occlusion and angina, a 5% complication of this procedure and FVIII was given to maintain levels during 24 hours of heparinisation (retrospectively, this was an inappropriate use of DDAVP).

Medical staff anxiety led to the final patient having FVIII concentrate alternating with DDAVP and achieving FVIII levels of 80 - 100% for four days post operatively.

Although reports of major surgery with DDAVP alone in mild and moderate haemophilia are few, success has been reported with levels as low as 25% for menisectomy and, 40% for bilateral herniorrhaphy (Mariani et al 1984) and 28% for appendicectomy (Ghirardini et al 1988). This experience has not been universal (Schulman 1991). Our data shows tachyphylaxis in most haemophiliacs with, on average, half the response by the third dose of DDAVP. With the availability of virally inactivated FVIII concentrates, a conservative approach has been adopted for non visible surgical sites raising the FVIII levels to 50 - 60% before surgery and maintaining the trough above 30% for several days by using FVIII concentrate at night and DDAVP by day when laboratory monitoring is more readily available.

Non Dental Surgery - von Willebrand's Disease

DDAVP as a sole agent (1 - 9 doses) was used for 19 surgical procedures when baseline FVIII was 18 - 50% (Table 4).

Bleeding time corrected in all but one type IID patient undergoing haemorrhoidectomy. Ristocetin cofactor (vWF:RCof) levels were frequently below 20% post DDAVP. The one patient who required blood products did so on day 6 post septoplasty, after failing to respond to a second dose of DDAVP, local antifibrinolytic agents and antibiotics, despite initial bleeding time correction with FVIII parameters above 80%. Four days of alternating blood products and DDAVP achieved wound healing. A wound haematoma developed after an hysterectomy in a patient with co-existent familial mild thrombocytopenia.

Table 4. Surgery - von Willebrand's Disease

	Cases	Days DDAVP	Comment
Skin lesions	4	2, 2, 2, 2	
Tonsillectomy	2	9,3	
Hysterectomy	2	7,3	
Pyelolithotomy	1	7	
Splenectomy	1	5	
Appendicectomy	1	4	
Haemorrhoidectomy	1	3	Type IID
Septoplasty	1	3	Cryo day 6
Laminectomy	1	4	Prophylactic cryo
Cholecystectomy	1	2	
Neurosurgery	1	2	
Eye surgery	1	2	
Tubal ligation	1	2	
Evacuation haematoma	1	2	
Arthroscopy	1	1	
Bunionectomy	1	1	

Planned use of combined DDAVP and blood products has been used in such situations as laminectomy and has raised vWF:RCof levels to 30%. Even so greater bleeding than expected was reported by the surgeons.

An adequate monitor for haemostasis is not readily apparent as although BT correction and adequate FVIII levels are usually considered satisfactory, raising vWF:RCof levels to 50% for major surgery is also recommended (Scharrer 1991). The results of a family with mild vWD (Table 5) show the discrepancy between BT and vWF:RCof levels and emphasise the difficulty of using laboratory results to predict successful surgical outcome. Similar patients have been described (Mariani 1984).

The importance of BT correction is also unclear as good haemostasis has been achieved in some type IIA variants as well as type IID without bleeding time correction (Rodeghiero et al 1991).

Successful limb surgery with low FVIII levels (Ghirardini et al 1988) may in part reflect the influence of tissue factor release associated with use of a tourniquet.

Haematomata and haemarthrosis

Although post DDAVP levels have ranged from 20 - 119%, the clinical results with DDAVP alone have been variable and often unsatisfactory.

Table 5. Type 1 vWD Kindred

	BT Min	FVIII:C %	vWF:Ag %	vWF:RiCof %	Surgery	Days of DDAVP	Comments
1	8	23	22	<10	Pyelolithotomy	0,0,1,2,4,6,8	
*	4	92	42	15			
11$_1$	>15	26	<10	<10	Laminectomy	0,1,2,4	Cryo
*	6	69	29	18			
11$_2$	>15	38	<10	15	Tubal ligation (L)	0,1	
*	5	56	25	22			
111$_1$	>15	34	<10	<10	Tonsillectomy	0,1,2	Amicar
*	6	72					
111$_4$	>15	38	15	<10	Traumatic Hyphaema	0,1	Rebleed
*	8	56	22	25			
					Surgical drainage		Cryo

* Value post DDAVP

Prompt treatment after minor trauma with 1 or 2 doses of DDAVP has given good results, but established bleeds have required aggressive and ongoing treatment with blood products. Ten thigh, 5 calf and 5 arm bleeds treated with DDAVP gave similar FVIII levels in those who responded and those who did not. The exception was a patient with a biceps bleed given blood products with a post DDAVP FVIII level of 9%. Four of 9 knee and 1 of 5 elbow haemorrhages failed to continue responding to DDAVP despite good initial FVIII levels of 35 - 53%. All followed significant trauma or occurred in a previously damaged joint.

Pain following DDAVP administration has recurred with FVIII levels over 40% acutely and in the rehabilitative phase for both haematomata and haemarthroses on four occasions post DDAVP suggesting further haemorrhage and raising the question of fibrinolysis as a causative factor. This phenomenon has also been noted by de la Fuente et al (1985) and the possible role of systemic antifibrinolytics needs clarification.

Additional problems include the severity of the injury and delay before receiving therapy.

The behaviour of some kindreds with mild haemophilia or vWD who repeatedly bleed at levels of FVIII which are usually satisfactory for therapy, whether these levels are produced in response to DDAVP or by exogenous FVIII, suggests that in some families, additional unidentified defects may be present. The same 5 haemophiliac patients including a sibling pair have accounted for 13 of the 25 episodes in which blood products were given to secure haemostasis.

Minimal Bleeding Disorders

Frequent consultations are sought about patients with a positive bleeding history where a persistently prolonged bleeding time is the only laboratory abnormality. Seventy one patients in this category have had dental surgery of all grades of difficulty. Initial bleeding times ranged from 9 to 30 minutes correcting to less than 8 minutes in 65, partial correction to 8 to 15 minutes in 4 and no change in two. One patient with a defined platelet storage pool deficiency and persistently prolonged bleeding time required a second dose of DDAVP which was clinically effective for prolonged oozing on day 2. Two others with post DDAVP bleeding times shortening to 17 and 18 minutes were haemostatic. One patient with Glanzmann's thrombasthenia and a partial defect shortened from 30 to 15 minutes, but a second with no platelet GpIIb/IIIa did not respond. These results are in keeping with the findings of others (Kobrinsky et al 1984, Schulman 1991).

The proven lack of platelet alpha granules and platelet vWF in a patient with gray platelet syndrome did not prevent bleeding time correction on two of three occasions, allowing dental and nasal surgery to be successfully performed. DDAVP in this situation at least cannot be acting via platelet vWF (Pfueller et al 1988).

Table 6. Significant Side Effects

- Severe angina following balloon angioplasty.
- Transient hemiparesis 24 hours.
- Myocardial infarction post ASD repair, normal coronary vessels.

Morbidity in the minimal bleeding disorders was virtually absent with the use of DDAVP enabling outpatient and office procedures as well as decreasing blood product exposure.

SIDE EFFECTS/ADVERSE EFFECTS

The side effects seen most commonly are flushing, mild headache and fatigue. Severe headache occurred on two occasions, mild hyponatremia was noted twice after a third infusion of DDAVP and there were two instances of a rise in diastolic blood pressure of more than 10 mmHg. The frequency of the less mild side effects approximates to 1 per 1,000 doses. More serious adverse effects have been noted in the later part of the time period from ours and other New Zealand institutions (Table 6). These are all significant cardiovascular complications and from calculated national usage data would approximate to 1:2,000 doses, a figure significantly higher than reported international experience (Mannucci and Lusher 1989). Since exclusion of patients with cardiovascular disease, there have been no further reports of such complications.

CONCLUSIONS

Administration of DDAVP results in sufficient rise in FVIII parameters for many patients with mild to moderate haemophilia and vWD to be treated for a wide variety of bleeding problems and for dental and other surgery to be performed without need for blood products with their attendant risks. Availability of a product suitable for self administration may allow early and continuing outpatient rather than hospital based treatment.

Successful use of DDAVP in haemophilia depends in general on the FVIII level achieved and the nature of the bleeding episode. Where not appropriate as a sole therapeutic agent, DDAVP can be used in association with blood products to conserve FVIII concentrates. It also has a role to play in management of mild haemophiliacs with factor VIII inhibitors. In haemophilia tachyphylaxis develops more quickly than in vWD, but responsiveness has usually returned within 48 hours. Routine use of antifibrinolytic agents in muscle and joint haemorrhages commencing prior to initial therapy through to rehabilitation, appears to decrease the incidence of rebleeding which could be due to increased fibrinolytic activity.

Some patients and kindreds appear to continue bleeding despite the attainment, whether by transfusion of blood products or DDAVP of levels that are usually haemostatic. Perhaps an additional unidentified defect is also present.

The precise FVIII level required for dental surgery is uncertain but use of a variety of ancillary local measures may decrease blood product usage even further. Reported results following this approach need further substantiation.

Successful use of DDAVP in vWD variants where BT may not be corrected and the rise in vWF:RCof transient and suboptimal draws attention to the inadequacies of measured parameters in predicting haemostasis. DDAVP also avoids morbidity in the minimal bleeding disorders.

The anecdotally reported New Zealand experience of adverse effects suggests rigorous exclusion of patients with cardiovascular disease.

Finally, in view of the ubiquity of MBD it can be speculated that use of DDAVP in a mass casualty situation could significantly conserve blood products when surgery is required.

ACKNOWLEDGEMENTS

Thanks to Ronnie Hedges, and Department of Medical Photography and Illustration, for secretarial and editorial assistance.

REFERENCES

Bachmann, F., 1980 Diagnostic approach to mild bleeding disorders. *Semin. in Hematol.* 17:292.

Berry, E,W., 1990. Use of DDAVP and cryoprecipitate in mild to moderate haemophilia a and von Willebrand's disease, *in* "Recent Advances in Hemophilia Care," C,K., Kasper, ed. Alan R.Liss, NewYork. 324:269.

Berry, P,R., Coster, A,B., Berry, E,W., 1977. Local use of epsilon aminocaproic acid in dental therapy. *Thromb. Haemost.* 38:373.

Dal Bo Zanon, R., Calzavara, M., Vicari., T., Miotti, A.,Girolami,

A., 1986, Dental extraction in congenital haemorrhagic patients, *Folia Haematol.* (Leipz) 113(6):799.

Davies, J.A., and Tuddenham, E,G,D., 1987. Haemostasis and Thrombosis, *in* "Oxford Textbook of Medicine'" Weatherall, D,J., Ledingham, J,G,G., Warrell, D,A., eds. Oxford University Press, Oxford. 19:215.

de La Fuente, B., Kasper, C.K., Rickles, F.R., Hoyer, L.W., 1985. Response of patients with mild and moderate haemophilia A and von Willebrand disease to treatment with desmopressin. *Ann.Intern.Med.* 103:6.

Ghirardini, A., Chistolini, A., Tirindelli, M,C., Di Paolantonio, T., Iacopino, G., Mariani, P., Chirletti, P., Agrestini, F., Mariani, G., 1988. Clinical evaluation of subcutaneously administered DDAVP. *Thromb. Res* 49:363.

Kesteven, P,J., Holland, L,J., Lawrie, A,S., Savidge, G,F., 1984. Inhibitor to factor VIII in mild haemophilia. *Thromb. Haemost.*, 52:50.

Kobrinsky, N.L., Israels E.D., Gerrard J.M., Cheang,M,S., Watson,C,M., Bishop, P, J., 1984. Shortening of the bleeding time by 1-deamino-8-Darginine vasopressin in various bleeding disorders. *Lancet* 1:1145-8.

Lowe, G., Pettigrew, A., Middleton, S., Forbes, C, D., Prentice, C,R,M., 1977. DDAVP in haemophilia. *Lancet* 11:614.

Mannucci, P, M., 1988. Desmopressin: a non transfusional form of treatment for congenital and acquired bleeding disorders. *Blood* 72;5:1449.

Mannucci, P,M., and Lusher, J,M., 1989 Desmopressin and thrombosis. *Lancet* 2:676.

Mariani, G., Ciavarella, N., Mazzucconi, M.G., Antonceachi, S., Solinas, S., Ranieri, P. et al, 1984. Evaluation of the effectiveness of DDAVP in surgery and in bleeding episodes in hemophilia and von Willebrand's disease. A study of 43 patients. *Clin.Lab Haematol* 6:229-238.

Menon, N, C., Berry, E, W., Ockelford, P,A., 1978. Beneficial effect of DDAVP on bleeding time in von Willebrand's disease (letter). *Lancet* 2:743.

Nilsson, I,M., and Lethagen, S., 1991. Current status of DDAVP formulations and their use, *in* "Hemophilia and von Willebrand's disease in the 1990's.'" J.M., Lusher and C.M.Kessler, eds. Elsevier Science Publishers B.V.

Pfueller, S.L., Howard, M.A., White, J,G., Menon, C., Berry, E,W., 1987. Shortening of the bleeding time by 1-deamino-8-arginine vasopressin (DDAVP) in the absence of platelet von Willebrand factor in gray platelet syndrome. *Thromb.Haemost.* 58:1060.

Ramstrom, G., Blomback, M., Egberg, N., Johnsson, H., Ljungberg, B., Schulman, S., 1989. Oral Surgery in patients with hereditary bleeding disorders. A survey of treatment in the Stockholm area (1974-1985). *Int. J Oral Maxillofac. Surg.* 18:130.

Rodeghiero, F., Castaman, G., Mannucci, P, M., 1991. Clinical indications for desmopressin (DDAVP) in congenital and acquired von Willebrand disease. *Blood Reviews* 5:155-161.

Ruggeri, Z,M., and Zimmerman, T.S., 1987, von Willebrand factor and von Willebrand disease. *Blood* 70:895.

Scharrer, I., 1991, The treatment of von willebrand's disease, *in* 'Hemophilia and von Willebrand's disease in the 1990's,' J,M., Lusher and C,M., Kessler, eds. Elsevier Science Publishers B.V. Amsterdam.

Schulman, S., 1991. DDAVP - the multipotent drug inpatients with coagulopathies. *Transfusion Med.Rev.* 5:132.

Sindet-Pedersen, S., Ingerlou, J, Ramstrom G., Blomback, M., 1988. Management of oral bleeding in haemophilia patients. *Lancet* (letter) 21:566.

DISCUSSION

Lusher: In patients with acquired inhibitors given DDAVP and Factor VIII concentrate, why choose human Factor VIII rather than porcine?

Berry: It is a question of availability and funding. We only have a small supply of porcine Factor VIII.

Lusher: What do you think is the mechanism in the two patients mentioned who had possible increased fibrinolysis after DDAVP treatment for muscle hemorrhage?

Berry: It could be the extent of the large mass of blood clot.

Kobrinsky: Does the increased symptomatology after DDAVP therapy not reflect ongoing bleeding but just inflammation after the incident?
Berry: Pain arose within hours of the DDAVP infusion and was sometimes associated with swelling.

Berry: has anyone else had problems with dental surgery?
Schulman: We had problems with a few hemophiliacs we thought could be managed by desmopressin and a Factor VIII level under 10%. They also continued to bleed after Factor VIII concentrate as well as after DDAVP. The DDAVP was not at fault: the problem lay with fibrinolysis, blood vessel contraction, or with some other factor.

Mariani: This needs considerable caution. First the selection of patients is important, because patients with Factor VIII levels above 20% and others with levels below 10% were treated with DDAVP. There are also variations in use of local measures, fibrin glue, antifibrinolytic drugs and so on. Some claim fibrin glue is enough, or that antifibrinolytics are enough. This report does not allow evaluation of any drug in this field.

Kobrinsky: Do you think that the ristocetin co-factor is important?
Berry: No.

Mariani: Should each patient be tested for response to DDAVP?
Berry: Ideally all patients should be tested except perhaps the very mild, but one is more confident if patients have a pattern of responsiveness. It is also desirable to monitor the platelet count in vW disease during one DDAVP treatment.

MULTICENTER EVALUATION OF A NEW CONCENTRATED DESMOPRESSIN PREPARATION (EMOSINT) ADMINISTERED INTRAVENOUSLY OR SUBCUTANEOUSLY: ANALYSIS OF BIOLOGICAL RESPONSES AND SIDE-EFFECTS IN 49 PATIENTS WITH HEMOPHILIA A AND VON WILLEBRAND'S DISEASE

Francesco Rodeghiero[1], Giancarlo Castaman[1], Rosario Giustolisi[2] and Guglielmo Mariani[3]

[1]Department of Hematology, Hemophilia and Thrombosis Center, San Bartolo Hospital, Vicenza;
[2]Chair of Physiopathology of Hemostasis, University of Catania;
[3]Department of Human Biopathology, Hematology Section, "La Sapienza" University, Rome, Italy

INTRODUCTION

After Köhler et al[1] first administered desmopressin subcutaneously, Köhler's[2] and Mariani's[3,4] groups proved that the subcutaneous (s.c.) and the intravenous (i.v.) route were pharmacologically and biologically equivalent. A minor difference was that the peak level of elicited factor VIII (VIII:C) was reached 60 minutes after s.c. injection compared to 30 minutes after the end of i.v. infusion. First clinical trials with s.c. administration were similarly successful[4,5]. With the availability of a more concentrated preparation of desmopressin the s.c. route was increasingly used for clinical reasons and this way of administration was confirmed as a simple, safe and effective alternative [5,6]. Furthermore, Mannucci et al.[7] provided experimental evidence suggesting that 0.3 μg/kg is a dose sufficient to elicit a maximal biological response, at least in terms of VIII/vWF increments and that the drug absorption after s.c. administration is less bound to intersubject variability. From the review of the above cited papers, more than one hundred cases are evaluable, including about 10 cases with von Willebrand disease, subcutaneously injected with desmopressin. Of them, at least 50 % received the concentrated formulation s.c., mostly for clinical reasons. In 30 cases the two routes of administration were examined in a cross-over design in the same subject[3,4,7] and proved strictly comparable in terms of VIII:C increment.

Desmopressin in Bleeding Disorders, Edited by G. Mariani *et al.*
Plenum Press, New York, 1993

In this multicenter study, a new concentrated formulation of desmopressin (EMOSINT, SCLAVO, SIENA, ITALY) has been evaluated in 49 patients with mild or moderate hemophilia A and von Willebrand disease.

PATIENTS AND METHODS

After informed consent, 49 patients with mild or moderate hemophilia A and von Willebrand disease were enrolled. Patients' characteristics and median basal VIII:C are summarized in table 1.

Table 1. Patient characteristics

Patients	Age (years) median	Age (years) (range)	VIII:C (U/dL) median	VIII:C (U/dL) (range)
von Willebrand (n = 23)	32	(10 - 70)	40	(19 - 87)
Hemophilia A (n = 26)	31.5	(9 - 64)	11.2	(2.8 - 37)

DESMOPRESSIN FORMULATION AND ADMINISTRATION

The agent was provided by the manufacturer in concentrated formulation, in vials of 4 μg/0.5 mL, 20 μg/mL and 40 μg/mL. The drug was subcutaneously injected in 12 patients (5 hemophilia A and 7 von Willebrand disease) whereas 37 (21 hemophilia A and 16 von Willebrand disease) received the drug intravenously. For the latter, the drug was diluted in 100 mL of isotonic saline and infused over 30 min at a dosage of 0.3 μg/kg.

Methods

Factor VIII procoagulant activity (VIII:C) was assayed by one-stage method, using factor VIII deficient plasma. Bleeding time (BT) was measured according to Ivy, using a Simplate II device (General Diagnostics, Morris Plains, USA).

RESULTS

Table 2 shows the median VIII:C increase (folds over basal level). In 6 patients intravenously injected (all von Willebrand disease patients), VIII:C was not evaluated. The time of VIII:C peak level showed that the peak was achieved at 30 or 60 minutes from starting infusion in 87% (27/31) of cases intravenously infused, whereas 84 % (10/12) of patients had no side effects, 17 (35%) had flushing, 5 60 minutes.

Table 2. Median VIII:C increment (folds over basal level) in 31 patients infused i.v. versus 12 patients injected s.c..

Time (min)	Intravenous Folds (range)	Subcutaneous Folds (range)
15	2.1 (1.2 - 7)	2.1 (1.3 - 4.2)
30	3.2 (1.6 - 7)	2.6 (1.3 - 5.9)
60	3.4 (1.6 - 6.3)	3.3 (2 - 7.8)
120	2.8 (1.4 - 5.2)	2.7 (2 - 4.8)

Table 3. Effect on the bleeding time in 23 patients with von Willebrand disease

Time (min)	Bleeding time (min) Median (range)	Normal/Total (%)
0	15 (5 - > 20)	5/23 (22 %)
60	8 (5 - 14.2)	18/23 (74 %)

Table 3 shows the effect on the BT in 23 patients with von Willebrand disease.

As can be seen, 75 % of patients had their BT normalized after desmopressin, with shortening being observed in the remaining cases.

As to the side effects, they were mild. Twenty-nine (59%) of patients had no side effects, 17 (35%) had flushing, 5 (8%) cardiopalmus, 3 (6%) headache and 2 nausea (4%). Seven patients had two of these symptoms. The urine output was evaluated in 10 patients before and 24 hours after desmopressin administration. There was a significant decrease, albeit not dramatic, of diuresis (1,565 ml vs 1,226 ml; $P < 0.001$).

Table 4. Cardiovascular side-effects

Center	Blood pressure: Systolic	Blood pressure: Diastolic	Heart rate
	Maximum Variation over basal (mean %)		Maximum Variation over basal (mean %)
A) CATANIA	+ 8.7	+ 14.7	+ 18.9
B) ROMA	+ 6.5	+ 8.9	+ 9.8
C) VICENZA	- 3.4	+ 8.3	+ 8.4

Table 4 shows the effects of the drug upon the cardiovascular system, divided by the center of treatment. Each measurement was recorded before, 15, 30, 60 and 120 minutes from drug administration. As can be seen, a costant increase of diastolic pressure and of heart rate (maximum increase was usually observed 15 to 30 minutes from drug administration) was observed, whereas the effect on the systolic pressure was less uniform.

Table 5 summarizes the clinical efficacy of desmopressin in 13 patients. A single infusion (plus tranexamic acid for dental extraction) was administered, with complete success.

DISCUSSION

Concentrated desmopressin intravenously administered at dosage of 0.3 μg/kg elicited an increase of VIII:C in

Table 5. Clinical efficacy of DDAVP in 13 patients

Disease	VIII:C (U/dL) Pre	VIII:C (U/dL) Peak	BT (minutes) Pre	BT (minutes) Peak	Clinical circumstance
vWD	---	---	18	8	Epistaxis
vWD	---	---	19	8	Dental extraction
H.A.	7.2	40	--	--	Dental extraction
H.A.	6.5	15	--	--	Epistaxis
vWD	---	---	15	7	Tonsillectomy
vWD	---	---	16	7	Abortion - Curettage
vWD	---	---	18	8	Phimosis
H.A.	6.9	16	--	--	Hemorrhoidectomy
vWD	---	---	15	8	Gum bleeding
H.A.	2.8	14	--	--	Hemarthrosis
H.A.*	18	58	--	--	Dental extraction
vWD *	87	232	5.5	7.5	Epistaxis
vWD *	70	166	7.7	5	Dental extraction

* Subcutaneous

hemophilia A and von Willebrand disease comparable to that previously reported in these patients with the standard formulation. Similarly, BT correction in von Willebrand disease was comparable to that observed with standard DDAVP. Similar magnitude of VIII:C and BT responses was observed in the 12 patients subcutaneously injected. Side effects were similar to those previously reported for intravenous standard DDAVP. The careful control of possible side effects in the present study provides for the first time an estimate of the effect of the agent upon the cardiovascular system and renal function. It appears that an increase of diastolic pressure and heart rate is a costant finding in treated patients, suggesting that the drug is best avoided in severe hypertension or heart failure. Moreover, in 10 patients it has been clearly demonstrated that desmopressin induces a significant decrease of diuresis during the 24 hours after desmopressin administration. Thus, fluid restriction is advisable on the day of desmopressin administration, especially if repeated infusions are anticipated.

In 13 cases minor surgery or spontaneous bleeding episodes were successfully treated with a single dose of concentrated desmopressin, either intravenously (10 cases) or subcutaneously (3 cases). In conclusion, this new concentrated formulation of desmopressin provided biological and clinical results similar to those previously reported for standard DDAVP or other concentrated formulations. Side effects were minimal or absent, but the drug is best avoided in severe hypertension or heart failure.

REFERENCES

1. M.Köhler, P.Hellstern, B.Reiter, G.von Blohn, E.Wenzel, The subcutaneous administration of the vasopressin analogue 1-deamino-8-D-arginine vasopressin in patients with von Willebrand's disease and haemophilia, Klin. Wschr. 62: 543 (1984).
2. L.De Sio, G.Mariani, M.G.Mazzucconi, A.Chistolini, M.C.Tirindelli, F.Mandelli, Comparison between subcutaneous and intravenous DDAVP in mild and moderate hemophilia A, Thromb. Haemostas. 54: 387 (1985).
3. A.Ghirardini, G.Mariani, G,Iacopino, M.C.Tirindelli, S.Solinas, T.Moretti, Concentrated DDAVP: further improvement in the management of mild factor VIII deficiencies, Thromb. Haemostas. 58: 896 (1987).
4. M.Köhler, P.Hellstern, C.Miyashita, G.von Blohn, E.Wenzel, Comparative study of intranasal, subcutaneous and intravenous administration of desamino-D-arginine vasopressin (DDAVP), Thromb. Haemostas. 55: 108 (1986).
5. A.Ghirardini, A.Chistolini, M.C.Tirindelli, T. Di Paolantonio, G.Iacopino, P.Mariani, P.Chirletti, F.Agrestini, G.Mariani, Clinical evaluation of sucutaneously administered DDAVP, Thromb. Res. 49: 363 (1988).
6. M.Köhler, P.Hellstern, H.Tarrach, R.Bambauer, E.Wenzel, G.A.Jutzler, Subcutaneous injection of desmopressin (DDAVP): evaluation of a new, more concentrated preparation, Haemostasis 1: 38 (1989).

7. P.M.Mannucci. V.Vicente, I.Alberca, E.Sacchi, G.Longo, A.S.Harris, A.Lindquist, Intravenous and subcutaneous administration of desmopressin (DDAVP) to hemophiliacs: pharmacokinetics and factor VIII responses, Thromb. Haemostas. 58: 1037 (1987).

MANAGEMENT OF SPONTANEOUS BLEEDING AND PREVENTION OF BLEEDING AFTER DENTAL EXTRACTIONS AND OTHER SURGICAL PROCEDURES IN MILD HEMOPHILIA A AND VON WILLEBRAND'S DISEASE: TEN YEARS OF EXPERIENCE AT THE VICENZA HEMOPHILIA AND THROMBOSIS CENTER

Giancarlo Castaman, Marco Ruggeri,
Eros Di Bona and Francesco Rodeghiero

Department of Hematology
Hemophilia and Thrombosis Centre
San Bortolo Hospital,
I-36100 Vicenza, Italy

INTRODUCTION

Desmopressin (DDAVP) is the treatment of first-choice for the management of patients with mild hemophilia A and von Willebrand disease[1,2]. This agent is cheap and safe and it is useful in about 80 % of cases. DDAVP has had a major impact in the therapeutic efforts for the prevention and treatment of bleeding in such patients. Since its introduction for clinical use[3], the large majority of patients with these disorders can safely avoid the use of blood products (cryoprecipitate, commercial factor VIII concentrates), that, although rendered almost completely safe by virucidal methods, still have a potential risk of transmitting blood-borne viruses[4,5].

In this paper, we report the experience with the use of DDAVP in the treatment of bleeding in patients with von Willebrand disease and hemophilia A at our Institution during a ten-year period (1982-1991).

PATIENTS AND METHODS

The records of all 378 patients with von Willebrand disease (vWD) and 17 with mild hemophilia A followed at our institution from 1982 to 1991 have been reviewed. All DDAVP infusions administered as test-infusions or for clinical reasons have been checked for biological responses in terms of factor VIII/von Willebrand factor measurements and bleeding time (BT) and their clinical outcome. Furthermore, all administrations of blood products have been reviewed in order to assess the global impact of DDAVP use in the treatment of bleeding in these patients.

Desmopressin in Bleeding Disorders, Edited by G. Mariani *et al.*
Plenum Press, New York, 1993

DDAVP Infusion

DDAVP (Minirin, Valeas, Milano) has been infused at 0.3 (0.4 till 1990) μg/kg b.w. diluted in 100 ml of isotonic saline over 30 minutes. Factor VIII/von Willebrand Factor measurements were carried out before, at the end of infusion, 60, 120 and 240 minutes from the starting of the infusion. Bleeding time was usually measured before, at the end of infusion and 120 min after starting the infusion. Platelet count was checked each time in a Coulter Counter IV Plus (Hialeah, Florida, USA).

In 12 patients concentrated formulation of desmopressin was administered subcutaneously for experimental purposes: these cases were not included in this analysis.

Methods

Factor VIII coagulant activity (VIII:C) was measured by one-stage method using F VIII-deficient plasma, von Willebrand Factor antigen (vWF:Ag) by Laurell electroimmunoassay until 1985 and thereafter by a commercial ELISA[6]. Ristocetin Cofactor activity (RiCof) of vWF was measured by an aggregometric method using formalin-fixed platelets[7] (9), with ristocetin at 1 mg/mL. Plasma to be tested was diluted with plasma from a patient with severe von Willebrand disease, with no measurable vWF:Ag and RiCof[8]. Ristocetin-induced platelet aggregation (RIPA) was determined by measuring the concentration of ristocetin able to induce 30% of aggregation 3 minutes later. BT was measured using a Simplate II device (General Diagnostics, Morris Plains, NJ, USA) by making two standardized vertical incisions on the volar surface of the forearm.

Platelets isolated by Ficoll-hypaque gradients were lysed after incubation with 1/40 v/v of 20 % Triton-X, as previously described[9]. The supernatants were removed and stored at - 80°C for no more than 2 weeks for vWF:Ag and RiCof measurements[10].

RESULTS AND DISCUSSION

A) Biological Evaluation

Table 1 shows the median VIII:C response to DDAVP in 70 patients with vWD (median basal VIII:C level 19 %; range 7 - 80%) and in 13 patients with mild hemophilia A (median basal VIII:C 18 %; range 8 - 45%). As can be seen, median VIII:C post-infusion was higher for type I vWD in comparison both to type II and hemophilia A. It is noteworthy that almost all cases showed a peak VIII:C level higher than 50 %.

When grouping type I vWD patients according to platelet vWF content, the magnitude of VIII:C response in terms of folds over basal level appeared to be higher in type 1A platelet normal and Vicenza, both with normal vWF structure and content in platelets[11,12], in comparison to type I platelet low or type I platelet discordant subtype, with reduced or abnormal vWF in platelets[11] (table 2).

Table 1. Median VIII:C response to DDAVP (folds over basal level and range) in patients with von Willebrand's disease and mild hemophilia A.

von Willebrand disease				Mild Hemophilia A	
Type I (n = 63)		Type II (n = 7)		(n = 13)	
Peak	N°>50%*	Peak	N°>50%*	Peak	N°>50%*
5.6	99/101	3.7	11/11	2.9	21/34
(1.3 - 20)		(1.4 - 11.9)		(1.5 - 12.7)	

* number of infusions achieving VIII:C levels > 50% post-DDAVP

As to the disappearance time of autologous VIII:C elicited by DDAVP in patients with von Willebrand's disease, De La Fuente et al.[13] analyzed 13 patients (8 type I, 4 II A and 1 IIB) and found a rapid return to baseline values within 5 hrs after infusion in 5 (4 type I and 1 IIA) and a slower decrease with more than twice the basal level up to 5 hrs in 8 (4 type I, 3 IIA and 1 IIB).

Mannucci et al.[14] in 11 type I vWD found a mean half-life of 5 hrs ± 1, but probably these authors calculated their figure on the slower, second part of the disappearance curve (pharmacological half-life). In a subsequent study, in 7 type I, a mean biological half-life of 76 min ± 8 was demonstrated[15]. We evaluated 14 patients with type I platelet normal subtype. The mean biological half-life was 72 min ± 11[9]. These data were recently confirmed in 6 patients with

Table 2. Median VIII:C response to DDAVP (folds over basal level and range) in patients with type I von Willebrand disease according to platelet von Willebrand factor content

Platelet normal (n = 25)		Vicenza (n = 8)		Discordant - Low (n = 6)	
Peak	N°>50%	Peak	N°>50%	Peak	N°>50%
5.5	40/40	7.6	17/17	2.4	10/12
(2 - 20)		(4.5 - 20)		(1.3 - 4)	

vWD Vicenza (normal platelet vWF content) and 7 patients with type I platelet normal[12]. The mean biological half-lives were 76 min ± 8 and 68 min ± 13[12].

In a recent paper, we reported the consistency in time of responses to DDAVP in vWD and hemophilia A[16]. In that study, we have demonstrated that in about 80 % of patients the magnitude of departure from average peak level between the two or more infusions was less than 20 %[16]. Similar findings were observed examining the BTs of the separate infusions. A similar figure was observed for hemophilia A patients. Table 3 shows the consistency in patients with vWD evaluated during the ten-year period of study.

Table 4 shows the effect of DDAVP upon the BT. It can be observed that a favourable effect was always observed in type I whereas about 30 % of patients with type II had no minimal effect on their BT.

Table 3. Analysis of 88 separate DDAVP infusions given to 38 patients with von Willebrand disease.

Magnitude of departure from average peak level (%)	Number of instances (%)	
	VIII:C	Bleeding Time
0 - 10	50/88 (57)	23/53 (43)
11 - 20	20/88 (23)	16/53 (30)
21 - 30	10/88 (11)	10/53 (19)
31 - 40	8/88 (9)	4/53 (8)

Table 4. Effect on the bleeding time in 70 patients with von Willebrand disease.

Bleeding time	Type I	Type II
A) Correction[1]	62 (82 %)	3 (27 %)
B) Shortening[2]	14 (18 %)	5 (46 %)
C) No effect	- -	3 (27 %)

[1] < 7.5 min; [2] from infinite to finite time or shortening of at least 30 % of basal time

B) Clinical Evaluation

DDAVP was used for spontaneous or traumatic bleedings in 16 patients with von Willebrand's disease. Most of these episodes were epistaxis and muscle hematomata. In about 40% of case basal VIII:C was less than 15 %. In all cases a favourable effect was observed after a single DDAVP infusion and no further treatment was required. All these patients had a full correction of BT post-infusion.

Dental extractions were carried out in 44 patients with von Willebrand disease (including 1 type II I, 2 type I low with BT not normalized and 8 type Vicenza with BT not normalized in 2). Among the patients with type I normal, BT was not normalized in 3 patients. Our protocol consisted of a single DDAVP administration plus tranexamic acid (45 mg/kg/day) for 6 days after extraction, starting the day before. In about 60 % of cases basal VIII:C was ≤ 15 %, but in all cases peak level was above 50 %. Bleeding complication was observed in 3 patients (1 type I platelet normal and 2 type Vicenza; BT was normal after DDAVP): in 2 bleeding was of minor importance and promptly subsided after a second DDAVP administration. In the third patient, HEMATE P was required for the control of bleeding. Fifteen patients underwent more than one dental extraction. In 23 patients, 2 or more teeth were extracted: in only 3 instances DDAVP was repeated after 8-12 hours as a precaution. It appears that full correction of BT is not required for the prevention of bleeding during dental extraction.

Table 5 shows surgical precedures carried out in patients with von Willebrand disease (including 1 type II B with BT not shortened, 1 type II I, 5 type I Vicenza with BT not normalized in 1).

Two patients had bleeding (1 type I normal and 1 type

Table 5. Surgery with DDAVP in 26 patients with vWd. Cases divided according to basal and peak VIII:C (20 minor, 5 major, 1 tonsillectomy).

Basal VIII:C (%)	Peak VIII:C (%) < 50	Peak VIII:C (%) > 50	Bleeding
6-10		2	
11-15		7	1 thyroidectomy, cryoprecipitate 1 knee surgery, new intervention
16-30		13	
>30		4	

Vicenza) despite a normal BT after DDAVP infusion. The patient with type IIB was infused before the occurrence of post-DDAVP thrombocytopenia was known[17]. Nevertheless, despite BT remained markedly prolonged (> 25 min) post-infusion, a single DDAVP infusion proved effective and no bleeding was observed. A patient with type I Vicenza underwent thyroidectomy. BT was corrected post-infusion and VIII:C approached 100%. Three additional DDAVP infusions during the following 44 hours were administered, with VIII:C reaching always 50 %. No bleeding was observed. An additional patient with type I platelet normal, despite VIII:C and BT normalization post-infusion, had a severe bleeding 36 hours post-intervention and cryoprecipitate was required, despite a further DDAVP infusion 12 hours after intervention. A patient with type I Vicenza underwent major orthopedic surgery for the reconstruction of knee ligaments and bled severely, despite two additional DDAVP infusions. Subsequently, it was possible to demonstrate that bleeding derived from a vessel injured near the bone. A new intervention after DDAVP infusion led to the stopping of the bleeding. Another patient underwent laparotomy for hemoperitoneum due to rupture of an ovaric cyst: three DDAVP infusions were administered during a 36-hour period with BT normalization and successful VIII:C increase. Table 6 summarizes the type of surgery carried out in vWD patients.

A total of 10 patients with mild hemophilia A received DDAVP for clinical use: dental extractions (n = 3), curettage (n = 5), gum bleeding (n = 1), muscle hematoma (n = 3), arthrocentesis (n = 3), minor surgery (n = 2) (phimosis

Table 6. Type of surgery in von Willebrand disease

Type of surgery	n
- Cholecistectomy	n = 1
- Thyroidectomy	n = 2
- Laparotomy for hemoperitoneum with ovariectomy-appendectomy	n = 1
- Major orthopedic	n = 1
- Ankle surgery	n = 1
- Abortion and curettage	n = 3
- Arthroscopy	n = 2
- Emorrhoidectomy	n = 2
- Nasal sept repair	n = 2
- Tonsillectomy	n = 1
- Appendectomy	n = 2
- Meniscectomy	n = 1
- Saphenectomy	n = 2
- Tendineous cyst	n = 1
- Colon polip resection	n = 1
- Arthrocentesis	n = 2
- Arteriography	n = 1

Table 7. Reasons for treatment with blood products in von Willebrand disease at the Hemophilia and Thrombosis Center of Vicenza (1982-1991)

A) TYPE III

- epistaxis, dental extraction, gum bleeding, hemarthrosis

B) TYPE II A

- post-partum bleeding

C) TYPE II B

- Rettorrhagia, gum bleeding, osteotomy femur fracture

D) TYPE II I

- Total hip replacement

E) TYPE I

- Total hip replacement, tongue cancer in elderly patient, failure DDAVP for dental extraction, large hematoma in mechanic heart valve carrier, failure DDAVP for thyroidectomy, surgery for colon cancer, clinical trial for a new concentrate, partial abruptio placentae at 6th month of pregnancy

correction, excision of cutaneous tumor). No bleeding was observed. DDAVP was repeated 36 hours after phimosis correction as a precaution.

In summary, it appears that DDAVP allowed the safe management of a large majority of cases of spontaneous bleeding, dental extraction and surgical procedures in vWD and mild hemophilia A. For the same time interval, DDAVP was administered in 70 patients with vWD as test-infusion and for clinical reasons in 62 of them. Blood products (cryoprecipitate and/or commercial factor VIII concentrate were used in 17 patients (4 type III, 3 type IIB, 1 type IIA, 1 type II I and 8 type I). Table 7 summarizes the reasons for treatment in these patients.

A total of 107 infusions were administered. It appears that blood products were needed for the management of peculiar instances in type I, whereas in type III they represent the mainstay of treatment. Needless to say that the advent of DDAVP in the clinical management of these patients has had a major impact.

CONCLUSIONS

In almost all cases of type I and II vWD a peak level > 50 % can be achieved by DDAVP. The high consistency of the responsiveness in terms of VIII:C and BT after separate DDAVP infusion makes a test-infusion useful for subsequent patient management especially when the correction of BT is required, such as in the case of mucosal bleeding.

More than 90 % of bleeding episodes in a large group of patients with vWD of type I and II could be safely treated. Despite in some cases BT not being normalized, hemostasis was effective and the rink of blood-borne viruses could be completely avoided in these patients.

REFERENCES

1. P.M.Mannucci, Desmopressin: a nontransfusional form of treatment for congenital and acquired bleeding disorders, Blood 72: 1449 (1988).
2. F.Rodeghiero, G.Castaman, P.M.Mannucci, Clinical indications for desmopressin (DDAVP) in congenital and acquired von Willebrand disease, Blood Reviews 5: 155 (1991).
3. P.M.Mannucci, Z.M.Ruggeri, F.I.Pareti, A.Capitanio, DDAVP: a new pharmacological approach to the management of haemophilia and von Willebrand's disease. Lancet 1: 689 (1977).
4. P.M.Mannucci, M.Colombo, Virucidal treatment of clotting concentrates, Lancet 2: 782 (1988).
5. F.Rodeghiero, G.Castaman, D.Meyer, P.M.Mannucci, Replacement therapy with virus-inactivated plasma concentrates in von Willebrand disease, Vox Sanguinis, in press.
6. F.Rodeghiero, G.Castaman, A.Tosetto, von Willebrand factor antigen is less sensitive than ristocetin cofactor for the diagnosis of type I von Willebrand disease - Results based on an epidemiological investigation, Thromb. Haemostas. 64: 349 (1990).
7. F.Rodeghiero, G.Castaman, E.Dini, Epidemiological investigation of the prevalence of von Willebrand's disease, Blood 69: 454 (1987).
8. F.Rodeghiero, G.Castaman, Calibration of lyophilized standards for ristocetin cofactor activity of von Willebrand factor (vWF) requires vWF-deficient plasma as diluent for dose-response curves, Thromb. Haemostas. 58:978 (1987).
9. F.Rodeghiero, G.Castaman, E.Di Bona, M.Ruggeri, R.Lombardi, P.M.Mannucci, Hyper-responsiveness to DDAVP for patients with type I von Willebrand's disease and normal intra-platelet von Willebrand factor, Eur. J. Haematol. 40: 163 (1988).
10. F.Rodeghiero, G.Castaman, A.Tosetto, A.Lattuada, P.M.Mannucci, Platelet von Willebrand factor assay:results using two methods for platelet lysis, Thromb. Res. 59: 259 (1990).
11. P.M.Mannucci, R.Lombardi, R.Bader, L.Vianello,

A.B.Federici, S.Solinas, M.G.Mazzucconi, G.Mariani, Heterogeneity of type I von Willebrand disease: evidence for a subgroup with an abnormal von Willebrand factor, Blood 66: 796 (1985).
12. P.M.Mannucci, R.Lombardi, G.Castaman, J.A.Dent, A.Lattuada A, F.Rodeghiero, T.S.Zimmerman. von Willebrand disease "Vicenza" with larger-than-normal (supranormal) von Willebrand factor multimers, Blood 71: 65 (1988).
13. B.De La Fuente, C.K.Kasper, F.R.Rickles, L.W.Hoyer, Response of patients with mild and moderate hemophilia A and von Willebrand's disease to treatment with desmopressin, Ann. Intern. Med. 103: 6 (1985).
14. P.M.Mannucci, M.T.Canciani, L.Rota, B.S.Donovan, Response of factor VIII/von Willebrand factor to DDAVP in healthy subjects and patients with haemophilia A and von Willebrand's disease, Br. J. Haematol. 47: 283 (1981).
15. P.M.Mannucci, R.Lombardi, R.Bader, G.Finazzi, C.Besana, J.Conard, M.Samama, Studies of the pathophysiology of acquired von Willebrand's disease in seven patients with lymphoproliferative disorders or benign monoclonal gammopathies, Blood 64: 614 (1984).
16. F.Rodeghiero, G.Castaman, E.Di Bona, M.Ruggeri, Consistency of responses to repeated DDAVP infusions in patients with von Willebrand's disease and hemophilia A, Blood 74: 1997 (1989).
17. L.Holmberg, I.M.Nilsson, L.Borge, M.Gunnarsson, E.Sjorin, Platelet aggregation induced by 1-desamino-8-D -arginine vasopressin (DDAVP) in type IIB von Willebrand's disease, N. Engl. J. Med. 309: 816 (1983).

MULTICENTER ITALIAN STUDY ON SUBCUTANEOUS CONCENTRATED DESMOPRESSIN (EMOSINT) FOR THE IN-HOSPITAL AND HOME TREATMENT OF PATIENTS WITH VON WILLEBRAND DISEASE AND MILD OR MODERATE HEMOPHILIA A: OUTLINE OF THE PROJECT

Francesco Rodeghiero and Giancarlo Castaman
on behalf of the Scientific Committee
of the National Hemophilia Foundation

Department of Hematology
Hemophilia and Thrombosis Centre
San Bortolo Hospital
I-36100 Vicenza, Italy

INTRODUCTION

In the last 15 years desmopressin has been increasingly used for the management of patients with von Willebrand disease (vWD) and mild or moderate hemophilia A[1-3]. More recently, this agent proved also successful in the management of patients with platelet function defects[4] or for the correction of bleeding diathesis of uremia[5]. In most cases, this synthetic drug allows the avoidance of any blood products resulting in a safe and cheap treatment. Several hundred patients have already been treated all around the world, but due to the initial limitation posed by the unavailability of the concentrated form of this agent, most treatment was administered intravenously and for this reason was reserved to in-hospital patients.

The side effects of this treatment were invariably mild and transitory and any causal relationship with major disabling side effects remains unproven. Recent studies have clearly demonstrated that the intravenous and subcutaneous routes of administration are bioequivalent in terms of pharmacokinetics and clinical efficacy[6-8]. The availability of a concentrated form of desmopressin makes the subcutaneous the preferred route of administration without the need for hospitalization or of physician supervised treatment. The potential usefulness and limitation of subcutaneous desmopressin as a form of home therapy in patients with congenital and acquired bleeding disorders responsive to this treatment remains unsettled.

Desmopressin in Bleeding Disorders, Edited by G. Mariani *et al.*
Plenum Press, New York, 1993

AIM OF THE PROJECT

Clinical evaluation of the use of concentrated desmopressin (Emosint, Sclavo, Siena, Italy) administered subcutaneously for the treatment of in-hospital and out-patient (home-therapy) patients with von Willebrand disease and mild or moderate hemophilia A and symptomatic hemophilia A carriers. Treatment with Emosint will be reserved for spontaneous bleedings, dental extractions and minor surgery. The participating centers are all Italian hemophilia centers able to enroll at least 5 cases.

Patient Eligibility

Patients with von Willebrand disease and mild or moderate hemophilia A aged 10-65, responsive to a dose test of desmopressin. Patients with type II B von Willebrand disease are excluded. Patients with hemophilia A should have a basal level of VIII:C of at least 5 %. Patients enrollement is scheduled till 30 october 1992.

Exclusion Criteria

A) Relative: bronchial asthma; hypo- or hypertension requiring treatment.

B) Absolute: type II B von Willebrand disease; advanced atherosclerotic disease; epilepsy; heart failure; pregnancy.

Route of Administration and Dosage

0.3 μg/kg s.c. with an insulin syringe into deltoidal or lateral abdominal wall regions. Biological responsiveness to desmopressin test infusion will be assessed according to the following:

Patients	VIII:C		Bleeding time	
von Willebrand	Basal	1 hr after	Basal	1 hr after
Hemophilia A or symptomatic carriers	Basal	1 hr after	Basal*	1 hr after*

* facultative

Methods

Factor VIII procoagulant activity (VIII:C) will be measured by a one-stage method at each participating center. The bleeding time (BT) will be measured using a Simplate II device, making 2, vertical incisions in the volar surface of the forearm: the mean between the two incisions will be recorded.

Criteria of responsiveness

Patients with von Willebrand disease are considered responsive if post-infusion VIII:C level is ≥ 50 %, irrespective of BT. Patients with hemophilia A are considered responsive if post-infusion level is ≥ 50 % for dental extraction and minor surgery or ≥ 20 % for spontaneous bleeding.

IN-HOSPITAL TREATMENT (reasons and schedule of treatment)

Responsive patients should be treated and evaluated for:

A) Spontaneous bleeding (hematomata, menorrhagia, gum bleeding, epistaxis)

   - Single Emosint injection; further injections every 12 hours to a maximum of 5, as required.

B) Minor surgery (including tonsillectomy)

   - Emosint before, 8-12 hours and 24 hours subsequently (24 hours injection facultative).

C) Dental extractions

   - Emosint before and 8-12 hours later (8-12 hours injection facultative). Tranexamic acid (45 mg/kg/die) is facultative.

VIII:C level (and BT whenever possible) should be assessed after each infusion of Emosint.

Home-Treatment

Self-evaluation of clinical efficacy by the patient. Candidate patients should be instructed by the physician responsible for the study (preferably at the time of test-infusion) on:

- reasons for treatment
- possible side effects
- conduct to follow for any specific bleeding situation
- dosage and route of administration
- how to record clinical efficacy

Evaluation of the Use and Clinical Efficacy of Emosint for Home-Treatment

Every patient will receive 10 vials containing 1 ml of Emosint (20 μg/vial or 40 μg/vial depending on body weight < 70 kg or ≥ 70 kg) plus 10 insulin syringes. Individual dosage will be communicated to the patients.

Record forms specific for the different bleeding episodes should be completed by the patient. Patients will be provided with specific record forms for epistaxis, menorrhagia and for all other spontaneous or traumatic bleedings, including dental extraction carried out at the office of the patients dentist. Patient is required to register the reason and the time of first desmopressin injection and to classify the clinical efficacy after 1 hour from injection as "poor" (totally uneffective), "good" (reduction of bleeding for external hemorrhages or reduction of pain otherwise), "excellent" (stopping of external bleeding or disappearance of pain). A maximum of 3 injections for epistaxis and menorrhagia and of 4 injections for other bleedings (spaced every 8-12 hours) will be allowed. For menorrhagia, the patient will be required to judge the clinical efficacy on the basis of the pads required compared to consumption in the previous untreated menstrual bleeding. On the basis of the registered pads consumption, the clinical efficacy of desmopressin will be classified as "very effective" (50 % reduction), "not effective" and "effective" (reduction between 0 and 50 %). Follow-up interviews at 3,6,12 months are scheduled and further furnishment of vials will be provided if required.

Evaluation of results and conclusions

At least 50 patients for in-hospital and 100 patients for home-treatment are expected to be evaluable at the end of the study. The results should be based on the examination of the in-hospital and home-treatment self-evaluation forms. The relationship between the degree of biological response (in terms of VIII:C and BT) and clinical efficacy will be determined (in-hospital treatment). Tachyphylaxis will be monitored in cases treated repeatedly.

The monitoring of vials used by the single patient during 1 year of home-treatment and for every treated episode will give an estimation of the efficacy and of the impact of self-treatment in mild or moderate hemophilia A and von Willebrand disease. The examination of record forms (along with the necessity or not for patients to in-hospital treatment during the period of study) will give an estimation of the clinical usefulness of home-treatment with concentrated desmopressin.

REFERENCES

1. P.M.Mannucci, Z.M.Ruggeri, F.I.Pareti, A.Capitanio, DDAVP: a new pharmacological approach to the management of haemophilia and von Willebrand's disease, Lancet 1: 869 (1977).
2. P.M.Mannucci, Desmopressin (DDAVP) for the treatment of disorders of hemostasis, Prog. Hemostas. Thromb. 8:19 (1986).
3. F.Rodeghiero, G.Castaman, P.M.Mannucci, Clinical indications for desmopressin (DDAVP) in congenital and acquired von Willebrand disease, Blood Reviews 5: 155 (1991).
4. P.M.Mannucci, Desmopressin: a nontransfusional form of treatment for congenital and acquired bleeding disorders, Blood 72: 1449 (1988).
5. P.M.Mannucci, G.Remuzzi, F.Pusineri, R.Lombardi, C.Valsecchi, G.Mecca, T.S.Zimmerman, Deamino-8-D -arginine vasopressin shortens the bleeding time in uremia, N. Engl. J. Med. 308: 8 (1983).

6. A.Ghirardini, G.Mariani, G,Iacopino, M.C.Tirindelli, S.Solinas, T.Moretti, Concentrated DDAVP: further improvement in the management of mild factor VIII deficiencies. Thromb. Haemostas. 58: 896 (1987).
7. A.Ghirardini, A.Chistolini, M.C.Tirindelli, T. Di Paolantonio, G.Iacopino, P.Mariani, P.Chirletti, F.Agrestini, G.Mariani, Clinical evaluation of sucutaneously administered DDAVP, Thromb. Res. 49: 363 (1988).
8. P.M.Mannucci, V.Vicente, I.Alberca, E.Sacchi, G.Longo, A.S.Harris, A.Lindquist, Intravenous and subcutaneous administration of desmopressin (DDAVP) to hemophiliacs: pharmacokinetics and factor VIII responses, Thromb. Haemostas. 58: 1037 (1987).

DISCUSSION

Kobrinsky: Young adults in North America may abuse this formulation of DDAVP, as it gives a "high" when given intravenously.

DESMOPRESSIN: AN OVERVIEW OF PRESENT AND FUTURE INDICATIONS WITH A REVIEW OF INVESTIGATIONS PERFORMED AT THE UNIVERSITY OF MANITOBA 1981-1989

Nathan L. Kobrinsky

Pediatric Hematology/Oncology
Roger Maris Cancer Center
Fargo, North Dakota, U.S.A.

INTRODUCTION

In 1976 Mannucci et al reported that desmopressin produced a marked though transient increase in FVIIIc and vWAg after intravenous infusion in healthy subjects. In patients with mild hemophilia (> 5% FVIIIc) a blunted but proportionate increase in FVIIIc was also observed. In patients with severe hemophilia (< 5% FVIIIc), the FVIIIc response was virtually absent. In contrast, the vWAg response was normal in both groups[1,2,3].

Since that time, desmopressin has been the treatment of choice for patients with mild hemophilia. The therapy is immediately effective after intravenous or subcutaneous administration and in most instances completely eliminates the need for blood products. In many centers, the "directed self-care" model developed for treatment of moderate and severe hemophiliacs with factor concentrates has been applied to the treatment of mild hemophiliacs with desmopressin. Patients may self-administer prior to dental or surgical procedures or with trauma prior to medical assessment.

CARRIER DETECTION OF HEMOPHILIA A

Desmopressin has been used diagnostically as well as therapeutically for patients with hemophilia and their families. Based on the blunted FVIIIc but normal vWAg responses in patients with hemophilia, in 1984 we proposed that carriers of hemophilia may similarly demonstrate a limited FVIIIc but an intact vWAg response to desmopressin and that this discordant response may improve hemophilia carrier detection[4].

Currently available molecular techniques have markedly increased the accuracy of hemophilia carrier detection;

Desmopressin in Bleeding Disorders, Edited by G. Mariani *et al.*
Plenum Press, New York, 1993

however, these techniques are not informative in all families. Furthermore, they are very costly and not generally available.

"Standard" non-molecular carrier detection methods for hemophilia A rely on the discordance between FVIIIc and vWAg as assessed by the FVIIIc/vWAg ratio. Using this methodology to classify carriers, 86.7% correct assignments with 7.7% false positives and 25.0% false negatives have been reported. A more accurate method of carrier detection not relying on molecular techniques would be of considerable value.

To evaluate the role of desmopressin in hemophilia carrier detection, 20 obligate carriers and 20 female controls were studied. Desmopressin was infused at a dose of 0.3 ug/kg. Blood samples before and 1 hour after the start of the drug infusion were collected for FVIIIc and vWAg determinations.

Before desmopressin infusion, FVIIIc was lower in carriers than in controls (59.5 $\pm$ 23.1% vs. 98.0 $\pm$ 20.7%, $p<.001$). After infusion, although FVIIIc increased in both groups ($p<.001$), the level achieved by carriers was lower than that in controls by 47.1% (137.5 $\pm$ 45.9% vs. 259.9 $\pm$ 57.4%, $p<.001$). The absolute increase in FVIIIc in carriers was less than that in controls by 51.9% (78.0 $\pm$ 36.6% vs. 162.0 $\pm$ 50.1%, $p<.001$).

Pre (105.2 $\pm$ 30.4% vs. 92.1 $\pm$ 33.0%) and post (171.9 $\pm$ 25.4% vs. 165.2 $\pm$ 25.6%) desmopressin vWAg levels were comparable in carriers and controls. The absolute increases (66.6 $\pm$ 17.8% vs. 73.2 $\pm$ 17.6%) were similarly comparable.

A discriminant function was derived based on the "standard" FVIIIc/vWAg ratio. Individual discriminant scores were calculated and subjects assigned to either carrier or control groups based on their distance from the group centroids. A similar function was calculated using the post-desmopressin FVIIIc/vWAg ratio.

Using the "standard" FVIIIc/vWAg ratio, control subjects were correctly assigned in 18/20 cases and carrier subjects were correctly assigned in 16/20 cases. Thus there were 10% false + and 20% false - assignments with an overall correct assignment of 85%. Using the post-desmopressin FVIIIc/vWAg ratio, control subjects were correctly assigned in 19/20 cases and carrier subjects were correctly assigned in 19/20 cases. Thus there were 5% false + and 5% false - assignments or an overall correct assignment of 95%.

In summary, obligate hemophilia carriers demonstrated a limited increase in FVIIIc (approximately 50% of control) but a normal increase in vWAg after desmopressin infusion. This discordant response, reflected by the post desmopressin FVIIIc/vWAg ratio, improved carrier detection from 85% to 95%.

It is likely that desmopressin improves carrier detection by identifying those individuals with a "normal" FVIIIc level but limited total FVIIIc stores. The post desmopressin FVIIIc may reflect total body FVIIIc stores more accurately than ambient FVIIIc determinations which may be affected by exercise or stress.

NEPHROGENIC DIABETES INSIPIDUS (NDI)

NDI is an X-linked recessive disorder characterized by polyuria and polydipsia despite an otherwise normal renal and metabolic status. It is due to inherent resistance of the renal tubules to the actions of vasopressin.

In 1985 we proposed that if this resistance was due to a generalized defect of the vasopressin receptor, other end organ responses may be absent[5]. vWAg and FVIIIc responses to intravenous desmopressin in 2 patients with NDI, 3 obligate NDI carriers and 35 control subjects were evaluated. vWAg and FVIIIc responses are summarized in Tables 1 and 2. Responses were absent in NDI patients and decreased by approximately 50% in obligate NDI carriers. These findings suggest that the receptor defect in NDI is not confined to the distal nephron, but is expressed equally, although asymptomatically in other

Table 1. vWAg Responses to desmopressin (des) in nephrogenic diabetes insipidus patients and carriers

Subjects	Before Des	After Des	Change	p*
NDI patients				
#1	145	135	-10	<.00001
#2	140	125	-15	<.00001
NDI carriers				
#1	180	240	60	.227
#2	87	125	38	.023
#3	99	118	19	.001
Controls (20)	92.1 ± 33.0	165.2 ± 20.6	73.2 ± 17.6	-

* Probabilty of control membership

tissues including vascular endothelium (the site of vWAG and prostacyclin production) and hepatic sinusoids and other unidentified tissues (the sites of FVIIIc production). Further, the blunted response observed in NDI carriers may be of value in NDI carrier detection.

There are at least two classes of vasopressin receptors - V_1 and V_2. The V_1 receptor mediates pressor effects and glycogenolysis. The V_2 receptor mediates antidiuretic effects. Desmopressin is a potent, long-acting V_2 agonist, essentially devoid of V_1 activity. It follows that vWAg and FVIIIc release are V_2 mediated and that the defect in NDI involves the V_2 receptor.

Table 2. FVIIIc Responses to desmopressin (des) in nephrogenic diabetes insipidus patients and carriers

Subjects	Before Des	After Des	Change	p*
NDI patients				
#1	117	103	-14	.0002
#2	128	126	- 2	.0005
NDI carriers				
#1	106	174	68	.030
#2	72	144	72	.036
#3	113	253	140	.330
Controls (20)	98.0 ± 20.7	259.9 ± 57.4	161.9 ± 50.1	-

* Probabilty of control membership

TREATMENT OF VON WILLEBRAND DISEASE

A number of early studies performed by Mannucci, Menon, Nilsson et al demonstrated that desmopressin produced a significant increase in FVIIIc and vWAg and a shortening of the template bleeding time in many but not all patients with von Willebrand disease[1,2,3,6]. Subsequent studies have confirmed that effects on the bleeding time in particular are related to the release of high molecular weight (HMW) multimers of vWAg necessary for platelet adhesion at sites of tissue injury. This effect varies in the different subtypes of von Willebrand disease[7].

In the pre-desmopressin era, cryoprecipitate was the treatment of choice for patients with von Willebrand disease and for other bleeding disorders. For example, in 1978, Gerristsen et al reported that cryoprecipitate was effective in correcting the bleeding time in patients with platelet storage pool deficiency[8]. In 1980, Janson et al reported that cryoprecipitate was effective in correcting the bleeding time in patients with uremia[9]. In all of these circumstances, cryoprecipitate was thought to improve hemostasis by increasing the concentration of vWAg.

TREATMENT OF PLATELET DISORDERS

Based on these observations, in the 1980's investigators began to evaluate the effect of desmopressin on the bleeding time in a wide range of congenital and acquired bleeding disorders. In 1983, Mannucci et al reported that desmopressin was effective in correcting the bleeding time in patients with uremia[10]. In 1984, we reported the drug's efficacy in a wide range of disorders characterized by a long bleeding time[11].

Thirty-eight subjects with primary bleeding disorders were evaluated, including 5 subjects with isolated prolongation of the bleeding time, 13 subjects with von Willebrand disease, 12 subjects with congenital platelet disorders and 8 subjects with combined von Willebrand/platelet function disorders. The mean age for the group was 9.0 ± 1.2 years. In addition, 2 subjects with acetylsalicylate induced platelet dysfunction and 2 normal subjects were studied.

All subjects received desmopressin at a dose of 10 ug/M^2 infused intravenously over 20 min. Before and 1 hour after the beginning of the drug infusion, platelet studies, plasma studies and a template bleeding time were performed.

Before desmopressin infusion, the bleeding time was prolonged in all groups with a mean of 15.4 ± 6.1 min. After desmopressin, the bleeding time shortened to 8.7 ± 3.4 min. The magnitude of the bleeding time correction was similar in all groups with a mean decrease of -7.2 ± 3.9 min (p=.0001). The bleeding time also shortened in 2 subjects with acetylsalicylate induced platelet dysfunction from 14.2 ± 0.4 to 7.0 ± 1.4 min. The magnitude of the decrease, -7.2 ± 1.8 min, was similar to that observed in subjects with primary bleeding disorders (p=.001). Shortening of the bleeding time from 7.5 ± 0.5 to 5.0 ± 0.0 min was also noted in the normal subjects studied (p=.001).

Desmopressin administration was associated with a decrease in the platelet count from 276 ± 73 to 258 ± 74 x 10^9/l (p=.02) and in the platelet volume from 9.9 ± 1.1 to 9.7 ± 1.1 fl (p=.006). An increase in glass bead platelet retention from 27 ± 19 to 62 ± 21% (p=.0001) was also noted. Effects on platelet factor 3 and on platelet aggregation were not observed.

Desmopressin administration was also associated with a decrease in the PTT from 109 ± 14 to 88 ± 15% of control (p=.0001). A change in the PT was not observed. Increases were noted in FVIIIc (98 ± 38 to 243 ± 88%, p=.0001), vWAg (82 ± 23 to 150 ± 52%, p=.0001) and vWF (66 ± 42 to 180 ± 95%, p=.0001).

Based on these studies, desmopressin was administered to patients with various bleeding disorders undergoing minor and major surgical procedures. In all cases, normal hemostasis was achieved and blood products were not required.

To define possible predictors of desmopressin induced bleeding time correction, baseline platelet and plasma factors were related to the absolute change in the bleeding time. Correction of the bleeding time correlated positively with the pre-desmopressin bleeding time (R=0.85, p=.0001) but not with any of the platelet or plasma factors in the whole group or in any of the subgroups. To define possible mechanisms of desmopressin induced bleeding time correction, changes in the platelet and plasma factors were related to the absolute change in the bleeding time. No correlations were found in the whole group or in any subgroup.

In summary, desmopressin corrected the bleeding time in a wide range of disorders including isolated bleeding time prolongation, von Willebrand disease, congenital and acetylsalicylate induced platelet disorders and combined von Willebrand/platelet function disorders. The bleeding time also shortened in normal subjects.

These effects, particularly the increase in vWAg, vWF and glass bead platelet retention, lend support to the notion that desmopressin induced bleeding time correction is due to the release of high molecular weight forms of vWAg necessary for adhesion of platelets to subendothelial connective tissue.

Despite the importance of this mechanism, it is likely that other factors play a role. Bleeding time correction was not restricted to patients with qualitative or quantitative abnormalities of vWAg. Further, neither the baseline concentration nor the magnitude of the rise in vWAg correlated with desmopressin induced bleeding time correction.

SHORTENING OF THE BLEEDING TIME IN CIRRHOSIS OF THE LIVER

Regardless of the mechanisms involved, it was clear by the mid 1980's that desmopressin was a powerful hemostatic agent effective in a wide range of congenital and acquired disorders characterized by a long bleeding time. These observations were extended with the report by Mannucci et al in 1986 that desmopressin corrected the bleeding time in patients with cirrhosis of the liver[12].

TREATMENT OF THROMBOCYTOPENIC BLEEDING

In 1988, we reported that desmopressin was also effective in the treatment of refractory thrombocytopenic bleeding[13]. Six patients aged 7 to 16 years were studied. Two were male and 4 female. The platelet count ranged from 10 to 34 x 10^9/l. Causes of thrombocytopenia included Fanconi anemia, aplastic anemia, acute myelogenous leukemia in relapse, acute lymphocytic leukemia in relapse (2) and chronic immune thrombocytopenic purpura. Types of bleeding included epistaxis (5), menorrhagia (2) and gingival bleeding (1). Whereas numerous other therapies had been ineffective, administration of desmopressin in standard doses resulted in cessation or clinically significant reduction of bleeding in all 6 patients. Based on this observation, the use of desmopressin should be considered in the emergency management of patients with thrombocytopenic bleeding when other "standard" measures have failed.

DECREASED BLOOD LOSS IN SPINAL FUSION SURGERY

In 1987, based on the observation that desmopressin shortened the bleeding time in normal subjects, we proposed that desmopressin may be effective in reducing operative blood loss in hemostatically normal patients undergoing extensive operative procedures.

To test this hypothesis, we conducted a randomized, double-blind, placebo controlled trial of desmopressin in patients with scoliosis undergoing spinal fusion surgery with Harrington Rod instrumentation. Operative blood loss and transfusion requirements were evaluated[14].

Thirty-five patients with scoliosis between the ages of 7 and 20 (mean 15.0 $\pm$ 2.6 years) were studied. Fifteen patients were male and 20 female. Scoliosis was idiopathic in 21 patients, secondary to cerebral palsy in 9 patients and secondary to neuromuscular disorders in 5 patients. Patients with a history of a bleeding diathesis as determined by a standardized questionnaire or with a history of acetylsalicylate ingestion within the preceding 14 days were excluded from study. Patients with a prolonged template bleeding time (> 9 minutes) were also excluded.

Three days prior to surgery, desmopressin was administered intravenously over 20 minutes to all subjects using a standard dose of 10 ug/M^2 and effects on hemostasis were evaluated. Plasma factors, platelet factors and the bleeding time were measured before and 1 hour after administering the drug.

Following the administration of desmopressin, the PTT shortened from 98 to 85%. The PT was unchanged. FVIIIc increased from 116 to 267%. vWAg increased from 106 to 183%. Desmopressin administration was associated with a decrease in the platelet count from 314 to 303 x 10^9/l. The mean platelet volume decreased from 9.3 to 8.9 fl. Glass-bead platelet retention increased from 43 to 79%. Desmopressin administration was also associated with a shortening of the bleeding time from 5.8 to 4.5 min. Prothrombin consumption increased from 82 to 91%. The hematocrit decreased from 0.40 to 0.38 l/l.

Patients were randomly assigned to receive desmopressin (10 ug/M^2; maximum dose 20 ug) or placebo at the time of surgery. The medication was administered immediately after the induction of anesthesia. Intraoperative blood loss was determined by weighing sponges and measuring suction drainage.

Patients in the 2 groups were comparable with regard to age, sex, physical characteristics, hemostatic characteristics and the number of vertebrae fused; however, the degree of scoliosis was more severe in the desmopressin group (Cobb angle 63 $\pm$ 17 vs. 51 $\pm$ 17°, p=.04). It was felt that this difference would not adversely affect the comparative analysis since if anything, this difference would increase the risk of surgical bleeding in those patients receiving desmopressin compared to placebo.

During surgery, overall blood loss was decreased by 547 ml (32.5%), blood loss per fused vertebra by 41 ml (28.8%) and concentrated red cell transfusions by 0.86 units (26.5%). Of the 12 patients who lost less than 1 litre of blood, 10 received desmopressin; conversely, of the 3 who lost more than 3 litres of blood, none received desmopressin (p=.035).

Overall, the reduction in blood loss was similar in patients with idiopathic scoliosis and with scoliosis secondary to cerebral palsy; however, patients with scoliosis secondary to neuromuscular disorders showed the greatest benefit. In these patients, blood loss was decreased by 2150 ml (p=.001); blood loss per fused vertebra by 162 ml (p=.003) and the need for red cell transfusions by 3.8 units (p=.0009).

By multivariate analysis, the main predictors of operative blood loss and transfusion requirements were glass bead platelet retention and the use of desmopressin. Of note, the pre-op bleeding time was not predictive.

Post-operatively, the serum sodium concentration was slightly but significantly lower in patients who had received desmopressin. The duration of analgesic treatment was 34 hours shorter in patients who received desmopressin than in those who received placebo (p=.014). This effect may reflect decreased bleeding into the surgical wound in the desmopressin group.

In summary, desmopressin decreased intra-operative blood loss by approximately 500 ml (32.5%) and the need for red cell transfusions by approximately 0.9 units in hemostatically normal patients undergoing spinal fusion surgery. Desmopressin also decreased the duration of treatment with analgesics by approximately 1.5 days. These effects were particularly noted in patients with neuromuscular disorders. Whether patients with neuromuscular disorders undergoing other operative procedures would similarly benefit is unknown.

DECREASED BLOOD LOSS IN CARDIAC SURGERY

The efficacy of desmopressin in decreasing blood loss has been demonstrated in other surgical settings. In 1985, Czer et al reported decreased blood loss after cardiopulmonary bipass[15]. In 1986, Salzman et al also reported decreased blood loss after cardiac surgery[16].

The role of desmopressin in adults undergoing coronary artery bipass surgery is somewhat unclear. Concern has been raised that these patients may be at risk of thrombotic complications from desmopressin therapy - specifically, that desmopressin may precipitate complete occlusion of severely narrowed coronary vessels. Certainly caution should be used in this setting e.g. restricting desmopressin use to patients with a prolonged bleeding time until more specific selection criteria can be defined.

SHORTENING OF THE BLEEDING TIME IN ACYANOTIC HEART DISEASE

To evaluate the role of desmopressin in pediatric cardiac surgery, children aged 2 to 20 years scheduled to undergo correction of various acyanotic congenital heart lesions were studied from May 1984 to December 1987[17].

All subjects had a CBC, PT, PTT and template bleeding time performed at the time of their pre-operative cardiac catheterization. If these studies were normal, no further coagulation tests were performed. If the bleeding time was prolonged, FVIIIc, vWAg, vWF and platelet aggregation studies were performed and repeated an hour following desmopressin infusion. Patients with a prolonged bleeding time received desmopressin at the time of cardiac surgery. For "closed" cases, the drug was administered prior to thoracotomy. For "open" cases, the drug was administered at the time of coming off cardiopulmonary bipass. Intraoperative assessment of blood loss in patients receiving and not receiving desmopressin was not performed in this study. Repeat coagulation studies were performed 6 months post-operatively in patients who had demonstrated an abnormal coagulation profile initially.

A total of 94 subjects were studied. The coagulation screening tests in these subjects were compared to a group of 35 orthopedic controls. The mean bleeding time was significantly longer in the cardiac surgery group than in the orthopedic control group (8.9 ± 1.0 vs. 5.8 ± 1.4 min, $p<.01$). Furthermore, 26/94 (28%) in the cardiac group had a prolonged bleeding time compared to 0/35 in the control group ($p<.01$).

Coagulation disorders identified in the patients with acyanotic heart disease and a long bleeding time included isolated prologation of the bleeding time (5), von Willebrand disease (13), platelet function disorders (7) and an acetylsalicylate induced platelet disorder (1).

Following the administration of desmopressin in patients with acyanotic heart disease, the bleeding time shortened from 17.2 ± 6.7 to 9.3 ± 3.8 min (p<.001). Complete correction of the bleeding time was observed in 10/14 (71%) patients. FVIIIc increased from 98 ± 29 to 207 ± 89% (p<.01). vWAg increased from 78 ± 32 to 149 ± 38% (p<.01). vWF increased from 51 ± 12 to 132 ± 40% (p<.01). The magnitude of the bleeding time correction, -7.9 min, was comparable to that observed in other patient groups. The FVIIIc, vWAg and vWF responses were also comparable.

Six months following surgery, the bleeding time had corrected from 15.8 ± 6.6 to 10.3 ± 3.4 min (p<.01). vWAg had increased from 86 ± 29 to 104 ± 41% (p<.05). vWF had increased from 56 ± 19 to 77 ± 21% (p<.01). FVIIIc was unchanged.

Based on the results of this study, one would predict that desmopressin would decrease operative blood loss in children undergoing cardiac surgery; however, a recently conducted randomized trial did not demonstrate benefit with the use of this therapy. Accordingly, it would seem appropriate to restrict the use of desmopressin to the 1/3 of children undergoing corrective cardiac surgery who demonstrate a prolonged bleeding time.

For children with cyanotic congenital heart disease, desmopressin should not be used. We recently reported that desmopressin precipitated a severe, life threatening cyanotic ("Tet") spell in a child with Tetralogy of Fallot. Desmopressin is a systemic vasodilator. When administered to patients with right heart outflow obstruction, blood may be shunted away from the lungs precipitating a cyanotic spell[18].

FUTURE INDICATIONS AND AVENUES OF RESEARCH

Desmopressin is of clear benefit in the medical and surgical management of patients with prolonged bleeding times and in orthopedic and cardiac surgery. Other surgical areas require further study. Gynecologic and oncologic surgery - areas where considerable blood loss may occur - are particularly important areas to explore. For example, vasopressin has been found to decrease blood loss from second trimester dilatation and evacuation abortion[19]. A similar trial with desmopressin should be considered.

Desmopressin should also be evaluated in surgical specialties where extremely delicate technique is required. Examples would include neurosurgery, ophthalmologic surgery and microvascular surgery (e.g. with organ grafts). The formation of scar tissue is directly related to surgical bleeding. Plastic surgery would therefore be another area where the drug should be evaluated. In these latter categories, decreased blood loss would not necessarily be the mark of the drug's success. Length of surgery, post-op complications, the adequacy of the surgical result, etc. would be more appropriate measures of success in these areas.

Drug combinations to enhance hemostasis should also be explored. For example, the combination of desmopressin and the related peptide oxytocin may be synergistic in the treatment of post-partum hemorrhage. By using the two together, a potentially lower dose of oxytocin may be required. Pain from oxytocin induced uterine cramping may thereby be decreased.

We have evaluated the combination of desmopressin with another hemostatic agent, ethamsylate, with considerable success[20]. Ethamsylate has been found to prevent periventricular hemorrhage in premature newborns, decrease excessive menstrual bleeding and reduce surgical blood loss in patients undergoing prostatic surgery or tonsillectomy. Whereas desmopressin enhances hemostasis by releasing vWAg from vascular endothelium, ethamsylate inhibits the production of prostacyclin by the blood vessel wall, thereby enhancing platelet activation. Since the mechanisms of action are different, we proposed that desmopressin and ethamsylate may produce a synergistic shortening of the bleeding time.

Desmopressin and ethamsylate were administered individually and together to 12 patients with markedly prolonged bleeding times known to be relatively or absolutely unresponsive to desmopressin alone. The bleeding disorders studied included Glanzmann's thrombesthenia (1), other platelet disorders (4), pseudo-von Willebrand disease (1), and von Willebrand disease type I (3), II (2) and III (1).

Desmopressin shortened the bleeding time from 23.9 $\pm$ 1.5 to 19.5 $\pm$ 2.3 min ($p=.03$). Ethamsylate alone was without effect. Desmopressin and ethamsylate together shortened the bleeding time to 11.2 $\pm$ 1.4 min ($p<.01$ compared with baseline; $p=.02$ compared with desmopressin alone). Toxic effects were not observed.

Five patients received desmopressin and ethamsylate prior to dental work with mandibular block (1), heart surgery requiring cardiopulmonary bipass (2) and adenotonsillectomy (2). Normal hemostasis was achieved in each case.

In summary, a synergistic shortening of the bleeding time was observed with the combination of desmopressin and ethamsylate in a wide range of bleeding disorders. Toxic effects were not observed. The use of the combination to decrease blood loss in hemostatically normal subjects merits future study.

DESMOPRESSIN - INDICATIONS NOT RELATED TO HEMOSTASIS

Desmopessin is known to influence a wide range of cell membrane related events including the transport of free water across the nephron, release of vWAg, prostacyclin and plasminogen activator from vascular endothelium and FVIIIc from hepatic sinusoids and tightening of endothelial cell junctions.

In view of these observations, the effects of desmopressin on membrane transport of various alkylating agents and amino acids were evaluated in L5178Y lymphoblasts _in vitro_[21]. Desmopressin stimulated melphalan uptake but conversely inhibited uptake of nitrogen mustard, choline (the natural substrate for the nitrogen mustard carrier), and leucine. No effect on the uptake of cyclophosphamide or glutamine was observed. Thus, desmopressin induced diverse but apparently specific effects on membrane transport of several alkylating agents and amino acids. Since the accumulation of alkylating agents such as melphalan within tumor cells is a major determinant of cytotoxicity, desmopressin may have a role as a biological response modifier in the treatment of malignant diseases.

Clearly, the future for this novel synthetic peptide is most promising.

REFERENCES

1. Manucci PM, Pareti FI, Homberg L, Nilsson IM, Ruggeri ZM. Studies on the prolonged bleeding time in von Willebrand's disease. J Lab Clin Med 88:662, 1976.

2. Mannucci PM, Ruggeri ZM, Pareti FI, Capitanio A: 1-Desamino-8-D-arginine vasopressin: A new pharmacological approach to the management of hemophilia and von Willebrand's disease. Lancet 1:869, 1977.

3. Mannucci PM, Canciani MT, Rota L, Donovan BS: Response of factor VIII/von Willebrand factor to DDAVP in healthy subjects and patients with hemophilia A and von Willebrand's disease. Br J Haematol 47:283, 1981.

4. Kobrinsky NL, Watson CM, Cheang MS, Bishop AJ, Israels ED. Improved hemophilia A carrier detection by DDAVP stimulation of Factor VIII. J Pediatr 104:718, 1984.

5. Kobrinsky NL, Doyle JJ, Israels ED, Winter JSD, Cheang MS, Walker RD, Bishop AJ. Absent factor VIII response to synthetic vasopressin analogue (DDAVP) in nephrogenic diabetes insipidus. Lancet 1:1293, 1985.

6. Menon C, Berry EW, Ockelford P. Beneficial effects of DDAVP on bleeding time in von Willebrand's disease [Correspondence]. Lancet 2:743, 1978.

7. Ruggeri ZM, Manucci PM, Lombardi R, Federici AB, Zimmerman TS. Multimeric composition of factor VIII/von Willebrand factor following administration of DDAVP: implications for pathophysiology and therapy of von Willebrand's disease subtypes. Blood 59:1272, 1982.

8. Gerritsen SW, Akkerman J-WN, Sixma JJ. Correction of the bleeding time in patients with storage pool deficiency by infusion of cryoprecipitate. Br J Haematol 40:153, 1978.

9. Janson PA, Jubeliver SJ, Weinstein MS, Deykin D. Treatment of bleeding tendency in uremia with cryoprecipitate. N Engl J Med 303:1318, 1983.

10. Manucci PM, Remuzzi G, Pusineri F, et al. Desamino-8-D-arginine vasopressin shortens the bleeding time in uremia. N Engl J Med 308:8, 1983.

11. Kobrinsky NL, Israels ED, Gerrard JM, Cheang MS, Watson CM, Bishop AJ, Schroeder ML. Shortening of the bleeding time by 1-deamino-8-D-arginine vasopressin in various bleeding disorders. Lancet 1:1145, 1984.

12. Manucci PM, Vicente V, Vianello L, et al. Controlled trial of desmopressin in liver cirrhosis and other conditions associated with a prolonged bleeding time. Blood 67:1148, 1986.

13. Kobrinsky NL, Tulloch H. Treatment of refractory thrombocytopenic bleeding with 1-desamino-8-D-arginine vasopressin (desmopressin). J Pediatr 112:993, 1988.

14. Kobrinsky NL, Letts M, Patel LR, Israels ED, Monson RC, Schwetz N, Cheang MS. 1-Desamino-8-D-arginine vasopressin (desmopressin) decreases operative blood loss in patients having Harrington rod spinal fusion surgery. Ann Int Med 107:446, 1987.

15. Czer L, Gray R et al. Prospective trial of DDAVP in treatment of severe platelet dysfunction and hemorrhage after cardiopulmonary bypass. Circulation 72 (suppl 3): 111, 1985.

16. Salzman EW, Weinstein MJ, Weintraub RM, et al. Treatment with desmopressin acetate to reduce blood loss after cardiac surgery: a double-blind randomized trial. N Engl J Med 314:1402, 1986.

17. Pelech AN, Levin M, Duncan KF, Barwinsky J, Giddins NG, Kobrinsky NL, O'Shaughnessy E., Hawkins L, Collins GF. Bleeding time prolongation in children with acyanotic congenital heart disease (submitted).

18. Israels SJ, Kobrinsky NL. Serious reaction to desmopressin in a child with cyanotic heart disease. N Engl J Med 320:1563 [Correspondence], 1989.

19. Schulz KF, Grimes DA. Vasopressin reduces blood loss from second-trimester dilatation and evacuation abortion. Lancet 2:353, 1985.

20. Kobrinsky NL, Israels ED, Bickis MG. Synergistic shortening of the bleeding time by desmopressin and ethamsylate in patients with various constitutional bleeding disorders. Am J Pediatr Hematol Oncol 13:437, 1991.

21. Miller L, Kobrinsky NL, Goldenberg GJ. Modulation of membrane transport of alkylating agents and amino acids by an analog of vasopressin in murine L5178Y lymphoblasts in vitro. Biochem Pharmacol 36:169, 1987.

DISCUSSION

Lusher: I am not familiar with this drug. It has been subjected to trial in infants, so does it not have side effects?

Kobrinsky: The original trial in children has been supplemented by another. After 5 years the neurological outcome of the children who received the drug was superior. we are now thinking of using it in mothers approaching term. It is available in the United Kingdom, but not in North America.

Stuart: How long did the bleeding time correction last?
Kobrinsky: We did not study this except in one patient, in whom the effect was gone in 2 hours.

Cattaneo: As ethamsylate is a prostacycline inhibitor, did you lose synergy in aspirin-taking patients?
Kobrinsky: No - and it can be given orally, intravenously, and subcutaneously.

Nilsson: Did it have any effect on the single vW patient?
Kobrinsky: No.

DISCUSSION

Lusher: Were the acyanotic children who corrected their defects several months after surgery in a particular group?
Kobrinsky: Those who did not correct hemostatically had an incomplete surgical correction, although there was no correlation with flow across the lesion. I think the origin was in turbulence. Atrial septal defects had the least hemostatic disturbance.

Cattaneo (Italy): We see a definite effect of desmopressin in patients who are hemostatically normal (in spinal fusion surgery) but not in those with acquired defects like cardiopulmonary bypass surgery. Can you explain this?
Kobrinsky: We need to analyze many more cases. Cardiac surgery has so many variables, we must look at it in more detail. Scoliosis is associated with platelet aggregation defects (according to an Israeli report), thought to be due to contraction of the platelet, in a defect similar to that in the muscles that causes the scoliosis.

Schulman: You made a cost analysis of your treatments. How did you explain the fall in costs with DDAVP?
Kobrinsky: The days in hospital among the DDAVP cases. This made the difference.

Rao: We have seen an adult patient with severe aortic stenosis with no high molecular weight multimers and a fall in vWf that reversed after surgery.

Weinstein: We have studied neonates and children in a randomized, placebo controlled trial, and DDAVP did not have a harmful or beneficial effect.

DESMOPRESSIN IN ACQUIRED HEMOPHILIA

Yvette Sultan

Centre des Hemophiles
Hopital Cochin
Paris - France

Development in non hemophilic patients of an inhibitor to factor VIII (F VIII) is a rare condition which causes severe bleeding problems. These inhibitors are considered as autoantibodies occurring during autoimmune diseases such as lupus erythematosus, rhumatoid polyarthritis, after drug reaction, in the post partum and in 45% of cases in otherwise healthy individuals (1). Bleeding episodes are currently treated with massive doses of human or porcine factor VIII concentrates and in some cases autoantibodies to f VIII respond to intravenous immunoglobulins (2) or immunosuppressive therapy.

The difference between hemophiliacs with an inhibitor to F VIII and patients with spontaneous inhibitors is that patients with acquired hemophilia have a normal synthesis of factor VIII and von Willebrand factor. The decreased level of F VIII activity in the circulation is the consequence of specific antibodies against factor VIII. In these patients neutralization of the procoagulant activity occurs as soon as F VIII is released from the liver cells. An important increase in factor VIII and vW factor after administration of DDAVP in normal volunteers is usually observed suggesting that an endogenous source of F VIII might also be available in patients with spontaneous inhibitor to factor VIII. This endogenous release of F VIII might contribute to form an inhibitor-factor VIII complex and decrease the inhibitor titer. In low titer inhibitors formation of these complexes might result in the presence of free factor VIII in circulation and contribute to significant improvement of hemostasis.

The efficacy of DDAVP is therefore dependent on the degree of vWf-F VIII complex released in the circulation and the number of specific molecules of IgG directed against F VIII.

In 1985, De La Fuenté and colleagues (3) reported the treatment of a 47-year-old patient with an antifactor VIII inhibitor using DDAVP. The inhibitor had type II kinetic properties. The titer had risen to 120 BU when oral cyclophosphamide therapy was started (150 mg/d). The inhibitor titer gradually fell to 1.9 BU over an 18 month period.

The inhibitor titer was 1.8 BU and the circulating factor VIII level was between 13 and 18 U/dl.

DDAVP was administered intravenously at a dose of 0.3 µg/ml in saline and was associated to epsilon aminocaproic acid.

Results are summarized in Table 1.

Desmopressin in Bleeding Disorders, Edited by G. Mariani *et al.*
Plenum Press, New York, 1993

Table 1. Desmopressin and factor VIII-related properties

De La Fuente, 1985	Before DDAVP	After DDAVP
Inhibitor titer BU	1) 1.9 2) 1	0.5 <0.3
F VIII U/dl	1) 13 2) 18	80 80
F VII C Ag	1) 43 2) 55	200 150
vWf Ag	1) 120 2) 150	200 200

F VIII remained elevated for 3 hours then returned to the baseline level. Dental extraction was carried out on both occasions without complications.

In the literature, four additional examples of patients with spontaneous inhibitors to F VIII treated with desmopressin have been reported. The first case was reported by Chistolini et al in 1987 (4). The patient was 60 years old when he developed a spontaneous inhibitor to F VIII. In this patient immuno-suppressive therapy had been partially successful, decreasing the inhibitor titer to 1 Bethesda Unit associated to a factor VIII activity of 6.7 U/dl. Subcutaneous administration of 0.3 µg.Kg bw resulted in an important increase in F VIII level from 6.7 U/dl to 110 U/dl with a peak of activity 3 hours after injection associated to the total disappearance of the inhibitor. The delayed response was attributed to the competition between endogenous F VIII and the inhibitory immunoglobulins. The rise in F VIII activity did not persist for more than 4 to 5 hours.

Three other cases were described by Naorosi-Abidi from St. George's Hospital in London (Table 2) in 1988 (5). The first case was a 75 year old with a 10 BU inhibitor to F VIII which did not respond to a six week treatment with cyclophosphamid. Factor VIII level was 7 U/dl when intravenous desmopressin was administered at a dose of 0.3 µg/Kg. An increase of F VIII to 140 U/dl was observed after infusion. 24 hours later the F VIII level was still 40 U/dl. The two other patients were two women of 20 and 27 years of age respectively who had developed an inhibitor to F VIII in the post partum period. As shown in Table 1, after intravenous administration of desmopressin the inhibitor titer fell from 4 to 2 BU in the first patient. The rate for the second patient is not given. Increase in F VIII was observed from 1 to 18 U/dl in the first case and from 2 to 27 U/dl in the second one. Desmopressin infusion was associated in both patients to significant clinical improvement. In one patient the hemostasis level was sufficient to cover dental extraction. The authors suggest that repeated doses of desmopressin should be administered to intervals of 6 hours to achieve more complete neutralization.

Table 2. Inhibitor titer and F VIII level before and after DDAVP administration in patients with acquired hemophilia.

	Inhibitor in BU		F VIII levels in U/dl	
	Before DDAVP	After	Before	After
Chistolini et al 1987				
1) 60 years old	1	und	6.7	110
Naorosi Abidi et al, 1988				
2) 75 years old	10		7	140
3) 20 years old	4	2	1	18
4) 27 years old			2	27
			48 h later 1	18

REFERENCES

1. Green D. Lechner K : A survey of 215 non-haemophilic patients with inhibitors to factor VIII. Thromb Haemost 1981, 45:200-203.
2. Sultan Y, Kazatchkine M, Maisonneuve P, Nydegger U: Anti-idiotypic suppression of auto antibodies to factor VIII (Antihemophilic factor) by high dose intravenous gammaglobulin. Lancet 1984, ii:765-768.
3. De La Fuente B, Panek S and Hoyer LW: The effect of 1-deamino-8-D-arginine vasopressin (DDAVP) in a nonhemophilic patient with an acquired type II factor VIII inhibitor. Br J Haematol 1985, 59:127-131.
4. Chistolini A, Ghirardini A, Tirindelli MC, Moretti T, Mancini F, Di Paolantonio T and Mariani G: Inhibitor to factor VIII in a nonhaemophilic patient: evaluation of the response to DDAVP and the vitro kinetics of factor VIII. A case report. Nouv Rev Fr Haematol 1987, 29:221-224.
5. Naorosi Abidi SM, Bond LR, Chitolie A, Bevan DH: Desmopressin therapy in patients with acquired factor VIII inhibitors. Lancet 1988, 13, 366.

DISCUSSION

Lusher: What about the patient with low titre inhibition who did not respond? Was there anything unusual about this patient, such as D.I.C. or a large hematoma?
Sultan: He had a large hematoma, and later responded to Factor VIII concentrate.

Nilsson: On our 11 patients with acquired haemophilia, six responded to DDAVP treatment, but the remaining five with no Factor VIII and high inhibitor levels did not respond.

Seremetis: Was there an anamnestic response?
Mariani: We did not find one.
Sultan: I cannot comment.
Nilsson: We saw no anamnestic response in 10 patients.

INTRAVENOUS AND SUBCUTANEOUS DESMOPRESSIN: CLINICAL RESULTS

Michael Köhler[1] and Guglielmo Mariani[2]

[1]Department of Transfusion Medicine
University of Göttingen
3400 Göttingen
Germany

[2]Department of Human Biopathology
University of Rome
00161 Rome
Italy

INTRODUCTION

Within the last several years, desmopressin (DDAVP) has become the medication of choice for the prevention or treatment of bleeding in patients with mild forms of haemophilia A or von Willebrand disease (vWd). In addition, DDAVP has proven to be effective in the treatment of several other disorders of haemostasis, such as platelet function defects, uraemic bleeding and liver cirrhosis (for a review see Mannucci, 1988). In contrast to diabetes insipidus centralis, the standard route of administration in cases of bleeding disorders was short-time (10 to 30 min) intravenous infusion. At least three dosages were recommended: 0.2 µg/kg body weight (b.w.)in Sweden, 0.3 µg/kg b.w. in Italy and 0.4 µg/kg b.w. in Germany. In Italy, DDAVP was frequently used in combination with inhibitors of fibrinolysis, in Germany without these drugs. When other routes of administration and different preparations (concentrated solutions) became available, we began to investigate subcutaneous (s.c.) injection of DDAVP for the treatment of bleeding disorders. The main question being whether s.c. injection is as efficaceous as i.v. infusion.

Here we report on more than 10 years of experience gathered in two haemophilia centers (Rome and Homburg/Saar) with special attention to the efficacy of s.c. administered DDAVP.

METHODS

Most of the data presented here have been described in detail elsewhere (Köhler et al., 1984; 1989, Mariani et al., 1984; DeSio et al., 1985; Ghirardini et al, 1987, Köhler 1987, Girardini et al., 1988, Mörsdorf et al., 1988). The patients suffered from mild and moderate forms of haemophilia or von Willebrand disease, predominantly type I.

Desmopressin in Bleeding Disorders, Edited by G. Mariani *et al.*
Plenum Press, New York, 1993

Treatment protocols differed significantly. At Rome, the standard dosage was 0.3 µg/kg b.w., and DDAVP was only administered for a limited number of days with a total of 1 to 5 infusions. When DDAVP was administered during and after surgery, tranexamic acid was given. At Homburg/Saar, the standard dosage was 0.4 µg/kg b.w. administered at 12 to 24 h intervals until wound healing was present (up to 10 days after surgery). No antifibrinolytic drugs were given. Initially, in both centers, the standard preparation with 4 µg DDAVP/ml was utilized, and later the more concentrated solution with 40 µg DDAVP/ml.

The factor VIII (FVIII) and von Willebrand factor (vWF) determinations were performed using standard procedures. The effects of desmopressin on haemostasis are also expressed as a ratio, i.e. peak level divided by basal level, in order to allow for a better comparison of the data.

RESULTS

Haemophilia A

When the conventional preparation (4 µg/ml DDAVP) was s.c. injected at a dosage of 0.4 µg/kg or 0.3 µg/kg, in haemophilia A patients, a 2.4 -fold increase (n=9, from 13.4 U/dl to 34 U/dl after 3h) and a 3.2-fold increase (n=16, from 11.6 U/dl to 37.1 U/dl after 60 min.) of FVIII:C was observed respectively (Köhler et al., 1984, DeSio et al., 1985). In 8 haemophilia patients, the response to i.v. and s.c. DDAVP was compared. A 3.1 -fold and 3.6-fold increase of FVIII:C levels was found 1 hour after s.c. injection or infusion, respectively (DeSio et al., 1985).

Peak levels were observed 1 h after injection when using the more concentrated compound (40 µg/ml DDAVP), and FVIII:C increases were approximately 3.5-times basal levels (n=25) and 3.0-times basal levels (n=11) following administration of 0.3 µg DDAVP/kg b.w. and 0.4 µg DDAVP/kg b.w., respectively (Ghirardini et al., 1987; Köhler et al., 1989). The FVIII:C levels in patients are shown in fig. 1.

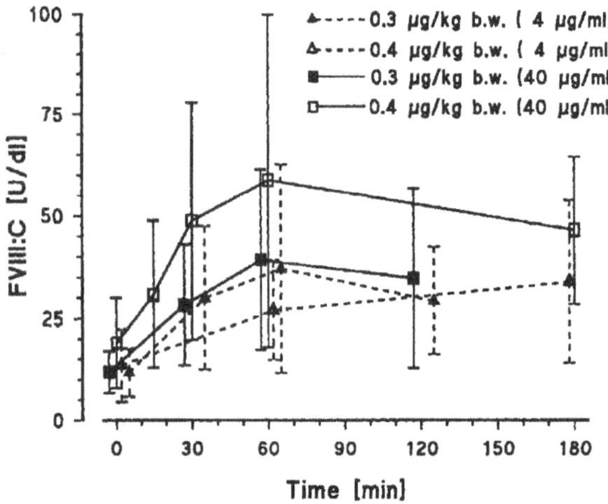

Figure 1: Factor VIII:C levels after s.c DDAVP in haemophilia A patients. Mean values and standard deviation (Ghirardini et al. 1987, Köhler et al. 1984, 1989)

Dental extractions were performed on 16 haemophilia A patients who had received 1 to 3 i.v. infusions of DDAVP at a dose of 0.3 or 0.4 µg/kg b.w. In one patient (basal FVIII:C level 8 U/dl), haemorrhaging occurred and FVIII concentrate had to be administered. Two late bleeding complications, which could be treated with DDAVP again, were observed. Additionally, in 4 patients, spontaneous bleeding episodes were successfully treated (Mariani et al., 1984).

Subcutaneously administered desmopressin was used in 7 patients on several occasions for the treatment and prevention of haemorrhagic complications during surgery. In one patient (basal FVIII:C level 17 U/dl) DDAVP was used in combination with FVIII-concentrate (orthopaedic surgery). In another patient wound haemotoma developed after herniotomia despite DDAVP, and FVIII-concentrate being given (Köhler, 1987). In 16 patients, Ghirardini et al. (1988) used 0.3 µ/kg b.w. during 6 operations for dental extractions, and 6 cases of spontaneous bleeding with good success.

von Willebrand disease

In our first study, 21 patients with type I vWd receiving desmopressin were compared with 22 patients receiving the drug by i.v. infusion. The increase of vWF:Ag was 1.9-fold vs. 2.1-fold, and that of FVIII:C was 3.4-fold vs. 2.7-fold, as measured 30 min after i.v. infusion or s.c. injection, respectively (Köhler et al., 1984). Also, a significant shortening of bleeding time was observed.

Later, a total of 52 patients suffering from type I vWd were evaluated. A 2.7-fold increase (prior to injection 47 ± 12.5 U/dl, 60 min after injection 122 ± 22.9 U/dl) of vWF:Ag levels was observed (Mörsdorf et al., 1988). The individual increase is shown in fig 3. No correlation between the basal vWF:Ag level and the amount of increase was apparent.

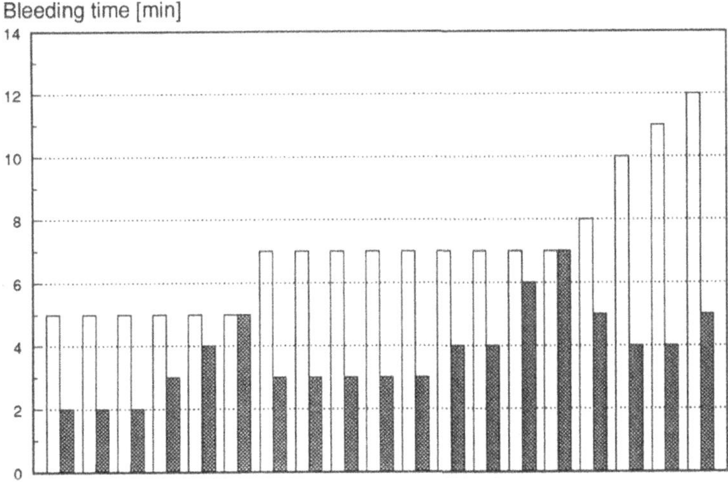

Figure 2: Bleeding time determinations in patients with von Willebrand disease type I. (Normal value : < 5 min)

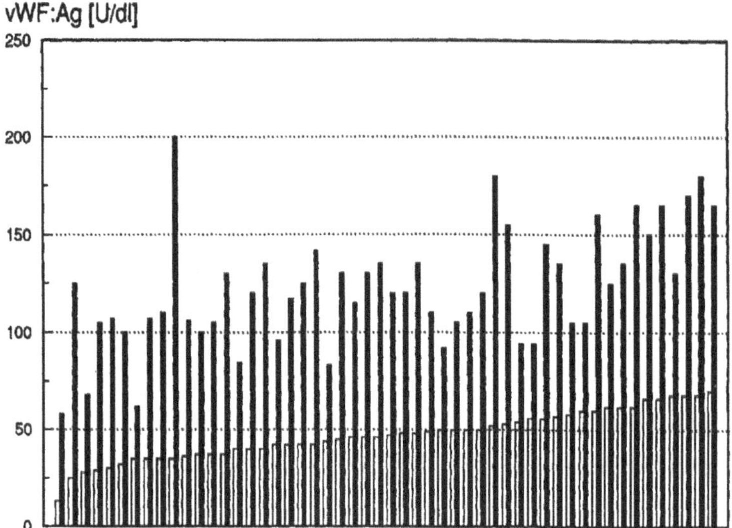

Figure 3: von Willebrand factor antigen levels before and after s.c DDAVP (4 µg/ml). Open bars represent basal levels, closed bars levels after 60 min.

The concentrated preparation was investigated in 4 patients with type I vWd. Reduction of bleeding times and an increase of FVIII/vWF was observed (Ghirardini et al., 1988). In 9 patients with type I and II vWd, dental extractions were performed without bleeding complications when i.v. DDAVP was given (Mariani et al., 1984).

In patients with mild von Willebrand disease type I, 0.4 µg/ml s.c. DDAVP was used to prevent bleeding during and after surgery. Ten tonsillectomies, and 8 other surgical procedures (4 abdominal operations) were performed without bleeding (Mörsdorf et al., 1988). Ghirardini et al. (1988) used s.c. 0.3 µg/kg DDAVP in 6 patients with vWd during 4 operations and 4 spontaneous bleeding episodes with good results. No difference in efficacy between the two different preparations (4 and 40 µg/ml) was observed. The clinical results are summarized in Table 1.

Table 1: Number of patients, in whom DDAVP was used to prevent or to treat spontaneous bleeding episodes.

The number in parentheses shows failure of DDAVP, or when FVIII concentrate had to be given. Surgery includes also dental extractions.

	0.3 µg/kg b.w. i.v.	**0.3 µg/kg b.w. s.c.**	**0.4 µg/kg b.w. s.c.**
Haemophilia A			
Surgery	16 (3*)	7 (0)	7 (2)
Bleeding	4 (0)	6 (0)	2 (0)
vWd			
Surgery	9 (0)	4 (0)	20 (0)
Bleeding	5 (0)	4 (0)	

* 2 late bleedings, which could be terminated with DDAVP alone

Uraemic bleeding

In a prospective study, 8 patients with prolonged bleeding times and chronic renal failure received 0.4 µg/kg b.w. of the concentrated compound via s.c. injection (Köhler et al., 1989). The bleeding was significantly reduced (median values before DDAVP: >15 min, after DDAVP 6 min). Platelets retention also increased (before DDAVP 19 %, after 44 %, see fig.4).

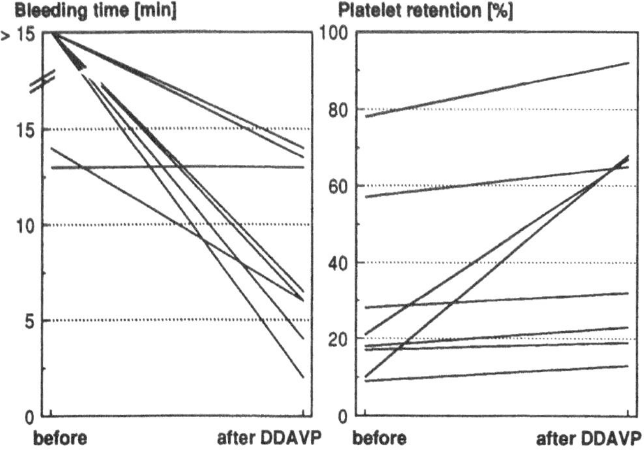

Figure 4: Bleeding time determinations and platelet retention in patients with uraemia before and 90 min after 0.4 µg/kg b.w. DDAVP (40 µg/ml).

CONCLUSION

The data presented in this paper describe a portion of our more than 10 years of experience with desmopressin, with special attention to s.c. administration. Despite the different test systems applied, different study populations and different treatment protocols, several conclusions can be drawn.

1. The combination of desmopressin with antifibrinolytic drugs seems not to be necessary, since DDAVP alone can prevent bleeding complications during and after surgery. Indeed, it was recently recommended that the concomitant use of antifibrinolytic drugs with DDAVP should be avoided, in order to prevent thrombo-embolic events (Mannucci and Lusher, 1989).

2. Both i.v. and s.c. administration of DDAVP are equally efficiacious in preventing bleeding complications in patients with bleeding disorders. Even in disorders of primary haemostasis, s.c. administration appears to be clinically effective (Cattaneo et al., 1990; Vigano et al., 1989).

3. At Rome and Homburg/Saar the number of injections/infusions differed significantly. Although we observed no severe adverse efects during long-term administration, it remains to be studied whether the number (and duration) of injections after surgery can be reduced in the absence of antifibrinolytic drugs.

4. Two dosages and two different solutions (4 and 40 µg/ml) were studied.

The more concentrated solution appears to be superior in terms of its small injection volumes, and a better resorption and effect. The higher dosage of 0.4 µg/kg b.w. DDAVP was not superior in terms of clinical effect or FVIII increase. It may even be that the lower dosage exerts higher FVIII increases, which may be apparent from dose response studies in patients and healthy volunteers. Although some of these results are not statistically significant, it may well be that the maximum of FVIII-increase is reached with 0.3 µg/kg b.w. and a further increase of dosage leads to a lesser increase of FVIII (Mannucci et al., 1981, 1987; Lethagen et al., 1987).

REFERENCES

1. Cattaneo, M., P. M. Tenconi, I. Alberca, V. V. Garcia, and P. M. Mannucci. 1990. Subcutaneous desmopressin (DDAVP) shortens the prolonged bleeding time in patients with liver cirrhosis. Thromb Haemostas 64:358-360.
2. De-Sio, L., G. Mariani, M. G. Muzzucconi, A. Chistolini, M. C. Tirindelli, and F. Mandelli. 1985. Comparison between subcutaneous and intravenous DDAVP in mild and moderate hemophilia A. Thromb. Haemost. 54:387-389.
3. Ghirardini, A., A. Christolini, M. C. Tirindelli, T. DiPaolantonio, G. Iacopino, P. Mariani, P. Chirletti, F. Agrestini, and G. Mariani. 1988. Clinical evaluation of subcutaneously administered DDAVP. Thromb. Res. 49:363-372.
4. Ghirardini, A., G. Mariani, G. Iacopino, M. C. Tirindelli, S. Solinas, and T. Moretti. 1987. Concentrated DDAVP: Further improvement in the management of mild factor VIII deficiencies. Thromb Haemostas 58:896-898.
5. Köhler, M. 1987. Grundlagen und Bedeutung der Anwendung von Desmopressin in der Transfusionsmedizin. Habilitationsschrift, Homburg/Saar.
6. Köhler, M. and A. Harris. 1988. Pharmacokinetics and haematological effects of desmopressin. Eur. J. Clin. Pharmacol. 35:281-285.
7. Köhler, M., P. Hellstern, C. Miyashita, G. von-Blohn, and E. Wenzel. 1986. Comparative study of intranasal, subcutaneous and intravenous administration of desamino-D-arginine vasopressin (DDAVP). Thromb. Haemost. 55:108-111.
8. Köhler, M., P. Hellstern, B. Reiter, G. von Blohn, and E. Wenzel. 1984. The subcutaneous administration of the vasopressin analogue 1-desamino-8-D-arginine vasopressin in patients with von Willebrand's disease and hemophilia. Klin Wschr 63:543-548.
9. Köhler, M., P. Hellstern, H. Tarrach, R. Bambauer, E. Wenzel, and G. A. Jutzler. 1989. Subcutaneous injection of desmopressin (DDAVP): Evaluation of a new, more concentrated preparation. Haemostas 19:38-44.
10. Lethagen, S., A. S. Harris, E. Sjörin, and I. M. Nilsson. 1987. Intranasal and intravenous administration of desmopressin: Effect on FVIII/vWF, pharmacokinetics and reproducibility. Thromb Haemostas 58:1033-1036.
11. Mannucci, P. M., M. T. Canciani, L. Rota, and B. S. Donovan. 1981. Response of factor VIII/von Willebrand factor to DDAVP in healthy subjects and patients with haemophilia A and von Willebrand's disease. Br. J. Haematol. 47:283-293.
12. Mannucci, P. M. and J. M. Lusher. 1989. Desmopressin and thrombosis [letter]. Lancet 2:675-676.
13. Mannucci, P. M., V. Vicente, I. Alberca, E. Sacchi, G. Longo, A. S. Harris, and A. Lindquist. 1987. Intravenous and subcutaneous administration of desmopressin (DDAVP) to haemophiliacs: Pharmacokinetics and factor VIII responses. Thromb Haemostas 58:1037-1039.
14. Mariani, G., N. Ciavarella, M. G. Mazzucconi, S. Antoncecchi, S. Solinas, P. Ranieri, P. Pettini, F. Agrestini, and F. Mandelli. 1984. Evaluation of the effectiveness of DDAVP in surgery and in bleeding episodes in haemophilia and von Willebrand's disease. A study on 43 patients. Clin. Lab. Haematol. 6:229-238.
15. Mörsdorf, S., M. Köhler, G. Leipnitz, and E. Wenzel. 1988. The clinical significance of diffent routes of desmopressin (DDAVP) administration in various bleeding disorders. Folia Haematol. (Leipz.) 4:503-507.
16. Vigano, G. M., P. M. Mannucci, A. Lattuada, A. H. Harris, and G. Remuzzi. 1989. Subcutaneous desmopressin (DDAVP) shortens the bleeding time in uremia. Am. J. Hematol. 31:32-35.

DISCUSSION

Rao: How would you recommend managing patients with major surgery?
Kohler: We divide the types of surgery into 3:
- 1 Dental extraction, if bleeding occurs, there is no great harm, and it can be readily seen. One injection alone is usually enough, and is without risk.
- 2 Abdominal surgery. Dr Flordal addressed these points: we do not rely on drainage measurement for our decision. Instead we apply the standard treatment - antifibrinolytics and successive doses of DDAVP - until wound healing is seen or expected. Repeated doses are not dangerous in terms of water retention and hyponatremia.
- 3 Neurosurgery or ophthalmic surgery when minor bleeding can spoil the operation or even cause death. In such operations care must be taken with desmopressin, as the problem of tachyphylaxis must be faced, and 3 days of treatment is not enough.

Mannucci: You gave a dose of 0.4 mcg/kg DDAVP every 12 hours for 7 days - treatment on a heroic scale. Did you monitor Factor VIII and osmolarity and sodium levels?
Kohler: Two patients were begun on this dose, then changed to a 24-hour scheme, so that they had two injections in the first day, then one injection daily afterwards. There were severe problems with hyponatremia only in one patient with liver disease. We were astonished at the high DDAVP levels after 12 hours after 30 - 50 pcg/ml, a dose which is surely antidiuretic. The vWf Type 1 patients responded in the same way at the beginning of treatment. There was tachyphylaxis in patients with hemophilia A.

Harris: You showed equivalence in efficacy between intravenous and subcutaneous therapy. What was the experience of tachyphylaxis and adverse effects with them?
Kohler: There were no side effects, apart from the patient with cirrhosis and hyponatremia, and the expected flushing.

Schulman: Patients who undergo major surgery with different anesthetics, different intravenous solutions, different liver and renal function can run into salt and fluid balance problems, with or without DDAVP, so that monitoring is essential.
Kohler: I agree completely.
Schulman: The optimal dose of DDAVP is 0.3 mcg: this causes maximal shortening of bleeding times. On 0.4 mcg the effect is less.

INTRANASAL APPLICATION OF DDAVP - BIOLOGICAL FUNCTION, PHARMACOKINETICS AND REPRODUCIBILITY

Inga Marie Nilsson and Stefan Lethagen

Department for Coagulation Disorders
University of Lund
Malmö General Hospital
S-214 01, Malmö, Sweden

INTRODUCTION

In recent years, more and more interest has been focused on the intranasal route for administration of DDAVP. Intranasal administration of DDAVP makes self-treatment possible for patients with mild hemophilia A, von Willebrand's disease or various platelet disorders. One important aim in the introduction of intranasal DDAVP was that it could be used in blood donors before blood collection in order to obtain higher yields of factor VIII in concentrates manufactured from their plasma.

In the early studies, DDAVP was administered by blowing into the nasal cavity drops of a 1300 µg/ml DDAVP solution by means of a plastic rhinyle catheter or a single dose nasal pipette. Kobayashi (1979), Mannucci and coworkers (1981) and our group in Malmö (Nilsson et al., 1982) were the first to explore the intranasal route of administration in healthy volunteers. Figure 1 (from Nilsson et al., 1982) shows the results of such a study where DDAVP was administered in 20 normal persons, by means of a calibrated catheter in two doses of a solution containing 1300 µg/ml. Dose-dependent increases were obtained of factor VIII activity (VIII:C), von Willebrand factor antigen (vWF:Ag) and plasminogen activator activity (PA), with peak concentrations about 1 h after instillation. After the largest dose, 390 µg (0.3 ml DDAVP solution), the VIII:C concentration was almost trebled and that of vWF:Ag almost doubled, results comparable with those of an intravenous administration of 0.2 µg/kg. This means that the dose of DDAVP required for intranasal application is more than 20 times greater than the intravenous dose.

Desmopressin in Bleeding Disorders, Edited by G. Mariani *et al.*
Plenum Press, New York, 1993

However, further development of intranasal application of DDAVP in drop form by rhinyle catheter or single-dose pipette was hampered by reports of poor reproducibility and unpredictable clinical response (Köhler et al., 1986; Streit et al., 1984; Mikaelsson et al., 1984). Obviously, a poor response will be obtained if a substantial portion of the volume of DDAVP delivered with the rhinyle catheter or pipette escapes down the posterior part of the pharynx and is not adsorbed.

Since 1986, Ferring Pharmaceuticals in Malmö, Sweden, has made available a precompression, metered-dose spray for the intranasal administration of DDAVP (Harris et al., 1986).

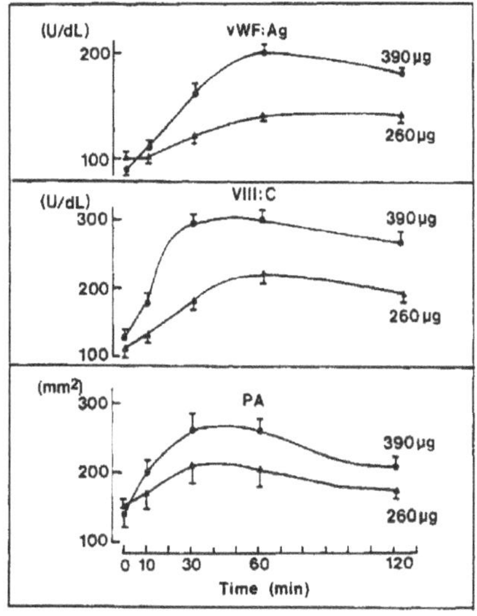

Figure 1. Effect of i.n. administration of two doses of a solution of DDAVP (1300µg/ml) by rhinyle catheter in 20 normal persons (mean ± s.e.m.).

In 1986, Harris and our group (Harris et al.,1986) compared intranasal deposition of DDAVP in healthy volunteers as administered by rhinyle catheter, single-dose pipette and two different sprays. The deposition and clearance of DDAVP in the nasal cavity was measured with gamma scintigraphy, and systemic absorption of DDAVP with a specific radioimmunoassay. The effect on circulating concentrations of VIII:C was also determined. Each device also contained human serum albumin radiolabeled with 99mTc. The rhinyle catheter and the pipette deposited the solution toward the rear of the nasal cavity at the site of the nasopharynx, whereas the sprays deposited it in the anterior nasal cavity. The bulk of the DDAVP deposited by the rhinyle catheter and the pipette was eliminated very rapidly, whereas the drug deposited by the sprays cleared at a much slower rate. Peak plasma concentrations both of DDAVP and VIII:C were significantly higher after spray administration than after drop administration. The spray giving 300 µg of DDAVP in 100 μl manifested a somewhat better effect than the spray giving 300 μg DDAVP in 200 μl. The importance of the dose volume on nasal bioavailability and biological effect has been confirmed in further studies (Harris et al., 1988 a, b).

From these studies it is clear that intranasal administration of DDAVP by spray is strikingly superior to the intranasal single-dose pipette or rhinyle cathether delivery systems. Thus, the sprays produce a clear enhancement in absorption and bioavailability.

The spray pump now used (Octostim, Ferring AB, Malmö, Sweden) delivers 100 μl of a DDAVP solution containing 1500 μg/ml. The normal dose of 300 μg is obtained by giving one squirt of the spray in each nostril.

COMPARISON OF INTRAVENOUS AND INTRANASAL ADMINISTRATION OF DDAVP IN HEALTHY VOLUNTEERS

Lethagen and co-workers (1987) compared intravenous and intranasal administration of DDAVP by spray in 10 volunteers with regard to VIII:C, vWF and t-PA response and

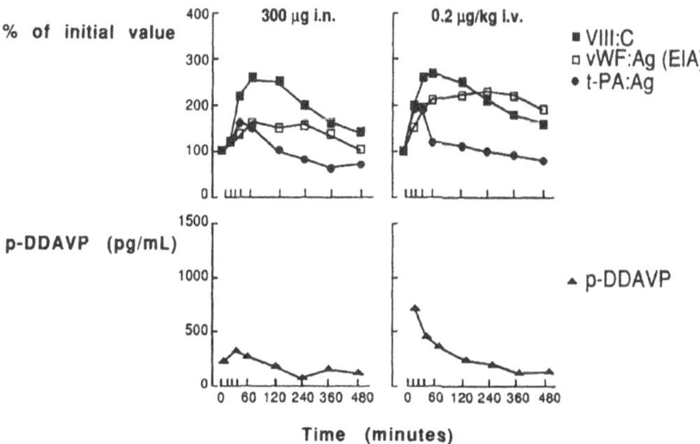

Figure 2. Response to DDAVP in normal volunteers.

pharmacokinetics (Fig. 2). The VIII:C concentration was almost trebled, that of vWF:Ag doubled, and that of t-PA 2.5 times its baseline level, an effect comparable with an intravenous administration of 0.2 μg/kg. Peak concentrations were reached after 60 min. The half-life values of VIII:C and vWF were 5 h and 7 h, respectively, both after intranasal and intravenous administration. In the same study, we measured the plasma concentration of DDAVP by a radioimmunoassay. Remarkably, the intranasal route gave very low concentrations of DDAVP in plasma, despite the VIII:C and vWF concentrations being increased to levels comparable with those obtained after an intravenous injection of 0.2 μg/kg. We have no explanation for this.

REPRODUCIBILITY OF RESPONSE TO INTRANASAL DDAVP

To study the reproducibility of the spray effect, 300 µg DDAVP was given by the spray pump to 10 volunteers on five different occasions with an interval of at least one week (Lethagen et al .,1987). Intra-individual variation in the spray effect on VIII:C was 21 ± 10%, and inter-individual variation 27 ± 5%. This compares favourably with the inter-individual variation after intravenous administration, 32% at a dosage of 0.2 µg/kg, 28% at 0.3 µg/kg and 23% at a dosage of 0.4 µg/kg. Thus, the spray is as good as the intravenous route in terms of reproducibility.

TACHYPHYLAXIS

Repeated dosage of DDAVP at short intervals is known to cause rapidly decreasing response (tachyphylaxis) in hemophilic patients (Nilsson et al., 1982; Mannucci, 1986). The cause of this is not known. Five healthy volunteers were studied to ascertain whether tachyphylaxis also occurs in healthy subjects, and whether the tendency for tachyphylaxis to develop varies with dosage or mode of administration. DDAVP was given at three different dosages: 0.2 and 0.4 µg/kg intravenously, and 300 µg by spray, each dose being given repeatedly with an interval of 12 hours for five days, and a wash-out period of at least one week between the different dose regimens. As shown in Figure 3, there were no differences between the modes of administration. A progressive decrease in response for VIII:C was seen during the first 3 to 4 administrations, after which response leveled out. VIII:C concentrations did not decrease below the baseline level.

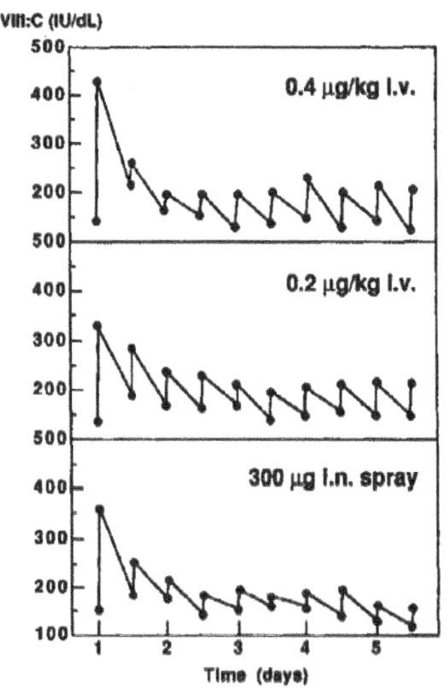

Figure 3. Repeated dosage of DDAVP with 12 hours interval for 5 days. Mean values from five volunteers.

EXPERIENCE WITH INTRANASAL ADMINISTRATION OF DDAVP BY SPRAY IN HEMOPHILIA A AND VON WILLEBRAND'S DISEASE

In a recent study (Lethagen et al., 1990) we compared the effect of DDAVP administered intranasally by spray in a dose of 300 μg with that of DDAVP given intravenously at dosages of 0.3-0.4 μg/kg in 8 patients with mild hemophilia A. DDAVP given by spray induced a significant increase in VIII:C from 9 ± 2 IU/dl to 22 ± 4 IU/dl. This compared favourably with intravenous infusion which increased the VIII:C concentration from 8 ± 2 IU/dl to 20 + 6 IU/dl. Baseline concentrations of VIII:C in the hemophilia A patients ranged from 3 IU/dl to 16 IU/dl, and all patients showed a 2-4-fold increase in VIII:C, both after intranasal spray and intravenous injection of DDAVP. Response in a given patient on different occasions was found to be reasonably consistent.

In a study of 22 patients with von Willebrand's disease type IA (Lethagen et al., 1990), we tested and compared the effect of intravenous injection of 0.3-0.4 μg DDAVP/kg with that of 300 μg DDAVP administered by nasal spray. Plasma concentrations of VIII:C and vWF:Ag increased significantly after both methods of administration, but more so after intravenous administration. Thus, VIII:C increased from 39 ± 4 to 113 ± 19 IU/dl after intranasal spray, and from 46 ± 5 to 170 ± 15 IU/dl after intravenous injection. The vWF:Ag increased from 25 ± 3 to 63 ± 11 IU/dl after intranasal spray, and from 23 ± 3 to 82 ± 16 IU/dl after intravenous injection. However, both modes of administration were equally effective in reducing Simplate-II bleeding times, which shortened significantly from 1232 ± 91 to 560 ± 47 seconds after intranasal spray, and from 1431 ± 88 to 570 ± 54 seconds after intravenous injection. In some of these patients with von Willebrand's disease type IA, the effect on VIII:C and vWF:Ag concentrations of DDAVP administered by nasal spray was followed for 24 h. The VIII:C and vWF concentrations peaked after about 1.5 h, and after 12 h the mean concentrations were about 1.5 times their baseline levels.

From these studies it was concluded that intranasal delivery of DDAVP by spray is a convenient and accurate form of administration, suitable for self-treatment in patients with mild hemophilia A and mild von Willebrand's disease type I.

At the center in Malmö hitherto 78 patients with mild hemophilia A, with von Willebrand's disease or a platelet disorder, have received the spray for home treatment. The spray has mainly been used to deal with nose bleeding, profuse menstrual bleeding and in connection with trauma or such minor surgery as dental extraction (Table 1). One male patient with von Willebrand's disease type I used the spray successfully against recurrent hematuria. We recommend that our patients use tranexamic acid in combination with the spray, especially in connection with bleedings from the oral mucosa or menstrual bleedings, and in connection with tooth extractions, where local fibrinolysis is known to contribute to the bleedings (Nilsson, 1975). If repeated doses are required, our patients using the spray at home are recommended to observe an interval of 8-12 h between doses. If the treatment is prolonged for more than 3 or 4 days, plasma concentrations of

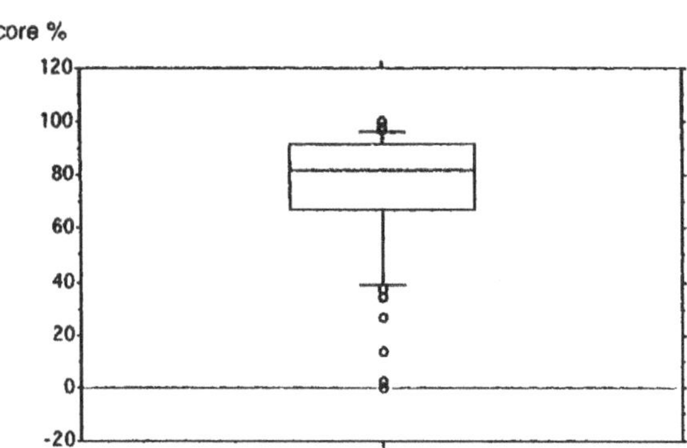

Figure 4. Effect of desmopressin (DDAVP) nasal spray. Box Plot of scores by 75 patients (46 F, 29 M) aged 4-59 years. Score represents efficacy on bleeding symptoms. 0 = No effect; 100 = Very good effect (median 82%, range 0-100%).

Table 1. DDAVP nasal spray for home treatment.

Disorder	No. of pat.	Indications for spray administration: Nose bleed-ings	Menor-rhagia	Trauma, muscle bleedings	Tooth extrac-tions	Minor surgery
vWD	45	31	15	8	5	1
Hemophilia A (1 carrier)	12	4	1	8		
Platelet disorders	19	10	13	4	2	
Others	2	1		1		
Total	78	46	29	21	7	1

VIII:C and vWF must be monitored because of the risk of tachyphylaxis. The patients who had received the spray were asked about their experience in using it. They rated the efficacy of the spray to reduce bleedings by marking an analogue scale where 0 represented 'no effect' and 100 'very good effect'. The Box Plot (Fig 4) shows the results of the inquiry. The median score was 82, and the range 0-100.

Before surgery and in connection with severe bleeding when a prompt response is required, we still recommend the use of intravenous DDAVP. For home treatment and before minor surgical procedures, the currently available spray is now recommended for patients with mild hemophilia A, mild von Willebrand's disease, and in some forms of platelet defects. A test dose of intranasal DDAVP is recommended in each case to ensure that the patient's response in terms of factor VIII and von Willebrand factor and reduction of bleeding time is sufficient to achieve hemostasis.

ACKNOWLEDGEMENT

This investigation was supported by grants from the Swedish Medical Research Council (00087).

REFERENCES

Harris, A.S., Nilsson, I.M., Wagner, Z.G., and Alkner, U., 1986, Intranasal administration of peptides: Nasal deposition, biological response, and absorption of desmopressin. *J. Pharm. Sci.* 75:1085.

Harris, A.S., Ohlin, M., Lethagen, S., and Nilsson, I.M., 1988a, Effects of concentration and volume on nasal bioavailability and biological response to desmopressin. *J. Pharm Sci.* 77:337.

Harris, A.S., Svensson, E., Wagner, Z.G., Lethagen, S., and Nilsson, I.M., 1988b, Effect of viscosity on particle size, deposition, and clearance of nasal delivery systems containing desmopressin. *J. Pharm. Sci.* 77:405.

Köhler, M., Hellstern, P., Miyashita, C., von Blohm, G., and Wenzel, E., 1986, Comparative study of intranasal, subcutaneous and intravenous administration of desamino-D-arginine vasopressin (DDAVP). *Thromb. Haemostas.* 55:108.

Kobayashi, I.,1979, Treatment of hemophilia A and von Willebrand's disease patients with an intranasal dripping of DDAVP. *Thromb. Res.* 16:775.

Lethagen, S, Harris, A.D, and Nilsson, I.M., 1990, Intranasal desmopressin (DDAVP) by spray in mild hemophilia A and von Willebrand's disease type I. *Blut* 60:187.

Lethagen, S., Harris, A.S., Sjörin, E., and Nilsson, I.M., 1987, Intranasal and intravenous administration of desmopressin: Effect on F VIII/vWF, pharmacokinetics and reproducibility. *Thromb. Haemostas.* 58:1033.

Mannucci, P.M., 1986, Desmopressin (DDAVP) for treatment of disorders of hemostasis. *Prog. Hemost. Thromb.* 8:19.

Mannucci, P.M., Canciano, M.T., Rota, L., and Donovan, B.S., 1981, Response of factor VIII/von Willebrand factor to DDAVP in healthy subjects and patients with hemophilia A and von Willebrand's disease. *Br. J. Haematol.* 47:283.

Mikaelsson, M., Nilsson, I.M.,Cedergren, B., Jonsson, S., Rydberg, L., and Wiechel, B., 1984, The use of desmopressin (DDAVP) in the preparation of improved factor VIII concentrate. *Scand. J. Haematol.* Suppl. 40, 33:93.

Nilsson, I.M., 1975, Local fibrinolysis as a mechanism for haemorrhage. *Thromb. Diath. Haemorrh.* 34:623.

Nilsson, I.M.,Vilhardt, H., Holmberg, L., and Åstedt, B., 1982, Association between factor VIII related antigen and plasminogen activator. *Acta Med. Scand.* 211:105.

Streit, A., Furlan, M., and Beck, E.A., 1984, Desamino-8-D-arginin vasopressin-Nasentropfen zur Behandlung der milden Hämophilie A und des morbus von Willebrand. *Schw. Med. Wschr* 114:1389.

DISCUSSION

Harris: What dose do you use in children?
Nilsson: Half the adult dose - one ''squirt''.

Kohler: You gave repeated doses over several days: were there signs of water retention?
Nilsson: The patients only had 1 - 3 doses. However, in the normal volunteers, who received repeated doses at intervals of 12 hours, there were gains of several kilos in weight.

USE OF A HIGHLY CONCENTRATED INTRANASAL SPRAY FORMULATION OF DESMOPRESSIN IN PERSONS WITH CONGENITAL BLEEDING DISORDERS

Jeanne M. Lusher, Erin Miller, Carol H. Wiseman, Madonna Draughn and Indira Warrier

Division of Hematology-Oncology
The Children's Hospital of Michigan and
Wayne State University School of Medicine
Detroit, Michigan 48201

INTRODUCTION

For the past three decades, plasma-derived factor VIII concentrates have been the mainstay of treatment for patients with hemophilia A and for those with severe or moderately severe von Willebrand disease (vWD). However, for persons with classic (Type I) vWD or mild and moderate hemophilia A (characterized by FVIII coagulant activity (F VIII:C) levels of 0.06-0.30U/dl and 0.01-0.05U/dl respectively, desmopressin (1-desamino-8-d-arginine vasopressin; DDAVP) is considered the treatment of choice. When given intravenously (IV) or subcutaneously, DDAVP effects a short-term rise in all components of the F VIII system as well as in plasminogen activator (PA).[1-4] The major advantage of DDAVP is that it is a synthetic agent which makes it possible to avoid the risk of transfusion-transmitted viral diseases such as hepatitis B, C, HIV/AIDS and parvovirus B19.

Although the precise mechanism of action by which DDAVP raises the F VIII complex has not been elucidated, it has been postulated that the drug effects the release of a second messenger from the CNS which in turn stimulates the release of vWF and PA from endothelial cell storage sites.[2,4] Endogenous release is a more probable mechanism rather than increased synthesis because the rise in F VIII/vWF following DDAVP is quite rapid, and a diminishing response (tachyphylaxis) is often seen when DDAVP is given on consecutive days, presumably due to depletion of endothelial cell stores.[3,4] There is also some evidence to suggest that DDAVP may have a direct effect on the vessel wall itself, resulting in increased platelet adhesion and enhanced platelet spreading at sites of injury.[5]

Currently in the United States (U.S.) the only form of DDAVP which is licensed, commercially available and effective for hemostatic indications is the

Desmopressin in Bleeding Disorders, Edited by G. Mariani *et al.*
Plenum Press, New York, 1993

parenteral form (4 mcg/ml). Because patients with mild hemophilia or vWD do not need frequent treatment for bleeding they are seldom started on home treatment programs with IV DDAVP. An intranasal (IN) route of administration would seem ideal, making self-treatment for occasional bleeding episodes much simpler and without delay. However, the dilute (0.1 mgm/ml) IN formulation (produced for use in patients with diabetes insipidus) has been shown to be ineffective for hemostatic indications, where 10-15 times as much DDAVP is needed. This formulation of DDAVP is so dilute that a large volume of nasal drops had to be given and much of the drug was swallowed rather than being absorbed.[6] Additionally, it has been shown that the IN drop mode of administration deposits solution more posteriorly in the nasal cavity where the drug is cleared rapidly due to ciliary transport to the nasopharynx. These factors resulted in unpredictable results but generally quite poor responses.[7-9] In response to the need for an IN formulation which would be more suitable for hemostatic purposes, scientists at Ferring Pharmaceutical Co., Malmo, developed a highly concentrated IN spray form of DDAVP (1.5 mg/ml).[8-10] This IN spray has been shown to result in a significantly increased nasal absorption and decreased clearance after administration as compared to the nasal drops.[7,8] This corresponds to a 2- to 3-fold greater bioavailability and therefore a significantly higher maximum biological response.[7-10] Unfortunately, this highly concentrated IN spray formulation of DDAVP is not licensed for use the U.S., and has even been difficult to obtain for clinical research studies.

The aims of the current study were 1) to determine whether or not the new, not yet licensed IN spray form of DDAVP is an effective drug for hemostatic purposes, resulting in predictable and reproducible increases in F VIII components; 2) to determine whether the F VIII responses are comparable to those seen following IV DDAVP; 3) to determine whether in the IN spray formulation effected a shortening of the bleeding time in persons with vWD; and 4) to assess home use of the IN spray. We hoped that the demonstration of efficacy, reproducibility, and safety of the IN spray form of DDAVP in a group of patients studied in the U.S. might lead to earlier licensure by the U.S. Food and Drug Administration (FDA) and thus widespread availability of this formulation of DDAVP for use in treatment of persons with vWD, mild and moderate hemophilia A and perhaps other hereditary hemostatic disorders as well.

SUBJECTS, MATERIALS AND METHODS

Subjects

Two groups of subjects were studied on three separate occasions each, at the Hemophilia Center at Children's Hospital of Michigan. The first group consisted of fifteen patients with Type I vWD, characterized by a decreased amount of functionally normal F VIII/vWF and an autosomal dominant pattern of inheritance. The second group consisted of four patients with mild hemophilia A. In the latter four subjects baseline F VIII:C values were 0.06-0.19 U/d (normal range 0.60-1.50 U/dl).

At a later date (Fall 1991) eight subjects with either Type I vWD (6) or moderate hemophilia A (2) were started on home treatment with the IN spray formulation of DDAVP.

Materials

The two test preparations were 1) the commercially available parenteral form of DDAVP (which contains 4 mcg DDAVP/dl), and 2) the highly concentrated IN spray form of DDAVP (1.5 mg/dl). The latter formulation, which is not licensed for use in the U.S.,was obtained from Ferring Pharmaceutical Co., Malmo, Sweden, and more recently from Rohrer Central Research (of Rhone - Poulenc Rohrer), Collegeville, Pennsylvania.

Methods

Each subject was given DDAVP on three separate occasions, at least 10 days apart. Initially each was given a single dose of IV DDAVP, 0.3 mcg/kg body weight. After being mixed with 50ml isotonic saline solution the drug was infused slowly over a period of 15 minutes using an infusion pump. On each of two subsequent occasions, each subject received the concentrated IN spray DDAVP. The IN spray was administered at a dose of 300 mcg (or 150 mcg for smaller patients), giving a 0.1 ml solution (1.5 mg/ml) in each nostril, with the patient sitting in an upright position. Ferring's precompression, metered dose spray pumps were used, which give 150 mcg per actuation. The pump was primed 5 times before use. If the patient was over 50 kg, two doses of 150 mcg were dispensed during normal inhalation, with the contralateral nostril open. If under 50kg, the subject received only one spray. The only post-DDAVP restriction was a limited fluid intake over the subsequent 24 hour period in very small children, in view of the drug's potent antidiuretic effects.

Blood Collection and Assay Methods

Blood samples were collected by venipuncture (23-gauge butterfly needles) into vacutainer tubes containing 0.105 M sodium citrate (blood: anticoagulant ration, 9:1). Platelet-poor plasma was obtained after centrifugation at 3000 x g for 15 minutes at 4°. Samples were then stored in aliquots at -80°C until assayed.

Assays of F VIII:C, F VIII-related antigen (vWf:Ag) and ristocetin cofactor activity (R Cof) were performed at the following intervals: baseline, 1/2 hour and three hours post-DDAVP. F VIII:C was assayed by one-stage method[11] based on a modification of the activated partial thromboplastin time (APTT). In this technique, the percent factor VIII activity in the test sample is measured by determining the degree of correction obtained when the test plasma is added to a F VIII deficient plasma (obtained from George King Bio-Medical, Inc., Overland Park, Kansas). A comparison is then made to the degree of correction from a commercial reference plasma (also obtained from George King Bio-Medical, Inc.) which has been calibrated against the WHO International Standard.

The concentration of vWf:Ag was measured by an enzyme immunoassay method (ELISA).[12] Antiserum to vWf:Ag (Dako Corp., Santa Barbara, California) was attached to a microtitre plate. vWf:Ag present in the test or reference plasma was then bound to the antibody. The third layer added was a peroxidase-labeled anti-vWf:Ag (Dako Corp., Santa Barbara, California). Upon subsequent addition of 0-phenylenediamine (Sigma Chemical Co.; St. Louis, Missouri), an enzymatic reaction yields a colored product. The intensity of the color is proportional to the vWAg concentration in the sample.

Although no in vitro test completely reflects vWf activity, the R Cof assay[13] is often used. In this assay, the antibiotic Ristocetin is added to washed formalin-fixed normal platelets in a platelet aggregometer. An aliquot of the patient's plasma is then added and the rate of platelet agglutination is proportional to the amount of vWf present in the plasma sample.

Other tests performed at baseline, 1/2 hour and 3 hours post-DDAVP included measurements of blood pressure, pulse rate, and template bleeding time. Bleeding times were performed on the vWD subjects only, using a modified Ivy technique with the Simplate-II bleeding time device (General Diagnostics, Morris Plains, New Jersey). Because DDAVP has antidiuretic properties, serum sodium was measured at baseline and at 3 hours post-DDAVP.

For subjects using the IN spray formulation of DDAVP at home, no laboratory tests were performed. However, each subject was given instructions for filling out a form each time they used the DDAVP IN spray, each was asked to call in the hemophilia center after using the spray, and to send in the reporting form (see table 1 below). Each was also advised to limit fluid intake for 24 hours after DDAVP, and to immediately report any adverse effects to hemophilia personnel.

These studies were approved by the Institutional Review Board of the Children's Hospital of Michigan and informed consent was obtained from each subject and/or their parents.

Table 1. Information Requested on Form for Home Use of IN Spray Formulation of DDAVP

1. Subject identification (name, birth date).
2. Type of bleeding disorder (e.g., von Willebrand disease, mild hemophilia).
3. Site/type of bleeding.
4. Time, date of onset of bleeding.
5. Time, date of use of IN spray.
6. Dosage (1 spray, 2 sprays).
7. Immediate side effects, if any.
8. Any problems encountered in use of spray? (If yes, please describe).
9. Response:
   Did bleeding stop? If so, when (time, date).
   Did bleeding recur? If so, when (time, date).
10. Was any other form of treatment used? If yes, please give date time, dosage.
    Amicar
    Cyclokapron
    Other
11. What was your overall impression of the ease of use, effectiveness of the IN spray form of DDAVP?

Note: Please remember to avoid drinking large amounts of fluid over the next 24 hours. Also, please call the Hemophilia Center after each use of the IN spray.

RESULTS

In subjects with vWD, the concentrated IN spray formulation of DDAVP was effective in elevating the levels of F VIII:C, vWf:Ag and R Cof to well within the normal ranges. As shown in Table 2, responses to the IN spray formulation compared quite favorably with those seen following administration of IV DDAVP. With a paired t-test analysis, it was noted that all values from pre- to post-DDAVP were significantly different ($p < .02$). The values for F VIII:C showed a greater increase than the values for vWf:Ag and R Cof which is consistent with previous studies with IV administration of DDAVP.[3,11] The bleeding time was shortened in 71% of vWD subjects following IV DDAVP, and in 67% and 71% of subjects following the first and second trial of the IN spray, respectively. Using a two-way analysis of variance, we found no significant difference in any laboratory parameters between the first and second IN spray trials, thus demonstrating reproducibility. With an interval of ten days or more between consecutive doses of the IN spray, no tachyphylaxis was observed.

Table 2. Comparison of Response to DDAVP Given IV and by Intranasal Spray1 in 15 Subjects with Type I vWD

Assay	Mode of treatment	Pre-DDAVP[2]	Post-DDAVP[2]	Fold Increase
F VIII:C	IV	0.78 (26)	2.56 (.83)*	3.3
(normal	IN-1	0.73 (24)	1.40 (.58)**	1.9
0.60-1.50U/ml)	IN-2	0.64 (35)	1.34 (.52)**	1.8
vWf:Ag	IV	0.59 (0.23)	1.24 (.36)*	2.1
(normal	IN-1	0.54 (0.21)	0.88 (.27)**	1.6
0.5-1.77U/ml)	IN-2	0.45 (0.20)	0.76 (.23)**	1.4
R Cof	IV	0.61 (26)	1.23 (.43)*	2.0
(normal	IN-1	0.57 (26)	0.88 (.39)***	1.5
0.64-1.63U/ml)	IN-2	0.50 (26)	0.78 (.37)***	1.6

[1]Each subject received doses of 3 DDAVP, given at intervals of 10 days or greater. One dose was given IV and the other two were given by IN spray (designated IN-1 and IN-2).

[2]Values are expressed as mean (SD).
* p <.001
** p <.005
*** p <.02

In subjects with mild hemophilia A, the F VIII:C values increased to a hemostatic level (>30%) in all (see Table 3 below). Paired t-test analysis showed the pre- to post-DDAVP values for IV and the first IN dose (IN-1) to be significantly different with $p < .001$and $p < .01$respectively. Due to a small sample size (n), the second IN dose (IN-2) did not show significance. However, by increasing n by 2, significance is achieved ($p < 0.5$).

Table 3. Responses of F VIII:C in 4 Patients with Mild Hemophilia A following IV Infusion and 2 Intranasal Spray Trials (Designated IN-1 and IN-2) of DDAVP

Assay	Mode of treatment	Pre-DDAVP[1]	Post-DDAVP[1]	Fold Increase
F VIII:C	IV	0.15 (.10)	0.52 (.24)*	3.6
(normal	IN-1	0.20 (.11)	0.41 (.20)**	2.0
0.60-1.50U/ml)	IN-2	0.15 (.12)	0.49 (.35)***	3.3

[1] Values are expressed as mean (SD).
* $p<.001$
** $p<.01$
*** NS, (using 2n, $p<.05$)

The side effects associated with this new, highly concentrated IN spray form of DDAVP were minimal. The most common observation was slight facial flushing and facial warmth following administration of DDAVP. Changes in blood pressure or pulse rate were not observed in any subject. Serum sodium did not change significantly over the brief time of observation (3 hours) following either the IV or IN spray administration of DDAVP.

In subjects using the concentrated IN spray of DDAVP at home, response has been reported as good to excellent. Subjects with vWD Type I have used the spray pump at home without difficulty, for epistaxis and for menorrhagia.

CONCLUSION

Our results confirm those of others[10,14] in documenting that the highly concentrated IN spray formulation of DDAVP is an effective mode of administration for elevating levels of F VIII:C, vWf:Ag, and R Cof in persons with vWD Type I and in persons with mild hemophilia A, and in shortening the bleeding time in vWD Type I. Results approached (but did not equal) those achieved by IV administration of the drug. We found that with minimal instruction subjects could easily use the spray pump device effectively. Thus, it would appear that the IN spray will be very useful in allowing subjects with vWD or mild-moderate hemophilia A to treat bleeding episodes promptly, without having to travel to a medical facility. While our subjects have not yet used the IN spray prophylactically in such situations as prior to office surgical procedures, dental extractions or contact sports, from a theoretical standpoint it should be effective for such situations.

As is done with patients receiving IV DDAVP, each patient should receive a test dose[15] of the IN spray in the office or clinic prior to relying on it for bleeding episodes, in order to ensure the effectiveness of the product in that individual, as well as to make sure that the subject knows how to use the spray pump.

While DDAVP, whether given by IN spray or IV, is a potent antidiuretic agent, persons with normal water metabolism rarely develop water intoxication unless they are being given large amounts of IV fluids, as post-operatively. In the latter situation, dilutional hyponatremia can become severe if this potential complication is overlooked.[16] Persons who are very young[17] or very elderly may also be at risk if there is not some fluid restriction for 24 hours post-DDAVP. The possibility of water overload should be discussed with each subject who will be using DDAVP at home, in order to avoid such complications.

In conclusion, our results indicate the IN spray formulation of DDAVP provides an effective and very convenient means for self-treatment for person with Type I vWD and mild-moderate hemophilia A.

ACKNOWLEDGEMENTS

This work was supported by a grant from the Hemophilia Foundation of Michigan. Medical student, Erin Miller's participation was supported by the Alumni Association of Wayne State University School of Medicine. The IN spray formulation of DDAVP for these studies was provided to us by Ferring Pharmaceutical Co., Malmö, and more recently by Rohrer Central Research (of Rhone-Poulenc-Rohrer), Collegeville, Pennsylvania.

REFERENCES

1. P.M. Mannucci, M. Aberg, I.M. Nilsson and B. Robertson. Mechanism of plasminogen activator and factor VIII increase after vasoactive drugs, *Br J Haematol*, 30:81-93(1975).

2. P.M. Mannucci, Z.M. Ruggeri, F.I. Pareti and A. Capitanio, 1-deamino-8-D-arginine vasopressin: A new pharmacologic approach to the management of hemophilia and von Willebrand's disease. *Lancet*, 1:869-872(1977).

3. P.M. Mannucci, M.T. Canciana, L. Rota and B.S. Donovan, Responses of factor FIII/von Willebrand factor in healthy subjects and patients with hemophilia A and von Willebrand's disease. *Br J Haematol*, 47:283-293(1981).

4. P.M. Mannucci, Desmopressin (DDAVP) for treatment of disorders of hemostasis. *ProgrHemostas Thrombos*, 8:19-45(1986).

5. M.I. Barnhart, S. Chen, and J.M. Lusher, DDAVP: Does the drug have a direct effect on the vessel wall? *Thromb Res*, 31:239-253(1983).

6. I. Warrier and J.M. Lusher, DDAVP: a useful alternative to blood components in moderate hemophilia A and von Willebrand's disease. *J Pediatric*, 102:228-233(1983).

7. A.S. Harris, I.M. Nilsson, Z.G. Wagner and U. Alkner, Intranasal administration of peptides, nasal deposition, biological response and absorption of desmopressin. *J Pharm Sci*, 75:1085-1088 (1986).

8. A.S. Harris, M. Ohlin, S. Lethagen and I.M. Nilsson, Effects of concentration volume of nasal bioavailability and biological response to desmopressin. *J Pharm Sci*, 77:337-339(1988).

9. J.M. Lusher, Pharmacology and pharmacokinetics of desmopressin in haemostatic disorders. *Drug Investigation* 2(suppl. 5):25-31, 1990.

10. I.M. Nilsson and S. Lethagen, Current status of DDAVP formulations and their use, in: "Hemophilia and von Willebrand's disease in the 1990s,"J.M. Lusher and C. Kessler, eds, *Elsevier Sci Publ*, Amsterdam, pp. 443-453 (1991).

11. J.V. Simone, J. Venderhelden and C.F. Abilgarrd, A semi-automatic one-stage factor VIII assay with a commercially prepared standard. *J Lab Clin Med*, 69:706 (1967).

12. J. Cejka, Enzyme immunoassay for F VIII related antigen. *Clin Chem* 28:1356-1358(1982).

13. D.A. Triplett and C.S. Harms, Ristocetin cofactor assay in: "Procedures for the coagulation laboratory," *Am Soc Clin Pathol*, Publ, Chicago (1981).

14. E.H. Rose and L.M. Aledort, Nasal spray desmopressin (DDAVP)--a simple technique for treatment of mild hemophilia A and von Willebrand disease. *Ann Intern Med*, 114:563-568 (1991).

15. J.M. Lusher, Desmopressin acetate: an alternative to the use of blood products for maintaining surgical hemostasis in mild hemophilia and von Willebrand's disease, *Excerpta Medica*, 1-15 (1985).

16. L. Shepherd, R. Hutchinson, E. Worden, C. Koopman and A. Coran, Hyponatremia and seizures after intravenous administration of desmopressin acetate for surgical hemostasis. *J Pediatr*, 114:470-472(1989).

NASAL SPRAY DESMOPRESSIN: LABORATORY AND CLINICAL IMPLICATIONS

Stephanie V. Seremetis and Louis M. Aledort

Department of Medicine, Mount Sinai School of Medicine
New York, New York 10029

INTRODUCTION

Desmopressin (DDAVP), a synthetic analogue of vasopressin used as replacement therapy in diabetes insipidus, was shown in 1977 to be clinically effective in preventing bleeding in patients with mild or moderate hemophilia A or von Willebrand disease (vWD)(1). Subsequent investigations confirmed these initial findings (2-4). Intravenous (IV) infusion of 0.3 ug/kg DDAVP typically causes 3- to 5-fold rises of Factor VIII activity (FVIII:C), von Willebrand antigen (vWAg) and Ristocetin cofactor activity (vWF) over baseline levels and can correct the Bleeding Time (BT). An individual patient's responses to DDAVP are usually consistent on different occasions, although there may be substantial variations among patients; a test infusion is recommended to assess effectiveness prior to elective treatment. The endogenously released FVIII:C and vWF are hemostatically and pharmacokinetically as effective as those obtained from exogenous infusion of plasma concentrates. Some patients treated with repeated doses of DDAVP more frequently than every 12 hrs over several days may develop tachyphylaxis with reduced responsiveness in factor levels, although the response can be restored after several days rest.

Since its approval for use in the U.S. in 1983, DDAVP has been used to treat bleeding episodes and for surgical prophylaxis in numerous hemophilia and vWD patients. In many cases, the need for blood products has been obviated, thus reducing the risk of transfusion acquired diseases such as hepatitis and HIV infections. Applications of DDAVP have been extended to include use in treatment of other platelet dysfunctions (5), uremia (6) and cirrhosis (7,8). DDAVP has also been used in hemostatically normal individuals undergoing procedures where substantial loss of blood is expected (9) or patients undergoing cardiopulmonary bypass (10-12). Subcutaneous (SC) administration has been shown to be as effective as IV-DDAVP (13-15) and can be adapted for self treatment. However, patients must inject as much as 4 to 6 ml of fluid using the present 4 ug/ml formulation.

Attempts to develop a more easily administered form of DDAVP which could be used at home have focused on intranasal (IN) administration. Initial attempts using a rhinyle catheter

Desmopressin in Bleeding Disorders, Edited by G. Mariani *et al.*
Plenum Press, New York, 1993

or pipette to deliver DDAVP as nasal drops gave erratic and unsatisfactory results (16). The development of an atomizer capable of delivering a measured amount of DDAVP as a nasal spray has made possible better absorption and more reproducible elevations of hemostatic factors. Lethagen and colleagues found that administration of 300 ug IN (150 ug to each nostril) by spray gave 2- to 3-fold rises in FVIII:C and vWF, which was equivalent to that obtained following an IV infusion of 0.2 ug/kg (17). Maximum activity levels were obtained 60 min following IN administration, in contrast to 30 min following IV infusion. The effects were reproducible, and the route of administration did not effect plasma half-lives of desmopressin of the factors.

We studied a group of mild hemophiliacs, symptomatic hemophilia A carriers and patients with vWD with both IV-DDAVP and nasal spray DDAVP and compared their biologic responses to assess the relative efficacy of the two methods of administration (18). Patients whose baseline testing showed favorable results were given the nasal spray for home-care use for bleeding episodes and prior to minor surgical procedures

MATERIALS AND METHODS

Patients

All patients had a previous, well-established laboratory diagnosis of either von Willebrand disease or hemophilia A or they were symptomatic carriers of hemophilia A. All had a history of bleeding and were already known to respond favorably to IV-DDAVP. There were 8 patients with mild hemophilia A, 3 symptomatic hemophilia carriers and 11 patients with vWD. All patients gave signed informed consent (approved by our institutional review board) prior to administration of the nasal spray and were free of respiratory infections at the time of testing. Patients whose baseline testing showed results comparable to those achieved with IV-DDAVP were allowed to take the spray home and self administer for bleeding episodes. They were instructed to report their observations to the investigators. In addition, these paients were offerred the option to use IN DDAVP for surgical prophylaxis.

Administration of Desmopressin

IV infusions were carried out using 0.3 ug/kg DDAVP (Stimate, Rorer), 4 ug/ml, diluted with normal saline to a total volume of 50 ml and infused over 20 min. DDAVP nasal spray was provided by Ferring Pharmaceuticals at a concentration of 1.5 mg/ml with a spray that delivers 0.1 ml per actuation. The standard dose for adult patients was 300 ug, or one actuation per nostril. The dose for children would be a single spray, or 150 ug.

Specimens and Collection

Blood was obtained by venipuncture prior to DDAVP administration and anticoagulated with 3.8% sodium citrate (1:9). Bleeding times in vWD patients were measured by the Ivy technique, using a template (Simplate, General Diagnostics). Post-treatment specimens were obtained at 30 min following the end of an IV infusion or 60 min following IN administration. BT were repeated at the same times, if indicated. Specimens were centrifuged at 4 C (2000g x 15 min) and plasma frozen at -70 C until analyzed. An individual patient's pre- and post-treatment specimens for a particular method of administration were analyzed together.

Assays

Factor VIII activity was measured by a one-stage method using commercially available human factor VIII deficient plasma (George King Bio-Medical, Inc., Overland Park, Kansas. Von Willebrand antigen was measured by Laurell rocket electroimmunoassay using a commercially available kit (Helena Laboratories, Beaumont, Texas). Ristocetin cofactor activity was measured using a platelet aggregation test with commercially available lyophilized platelets (Biodata Corporation, Hatboro, Pennsylvania).

Statistical Methods

Results are expressed as mean $\pm$ 1SD. Comparisons of pre- and post-treatment values were done using a paired t-test, with P values shown (see figures). In comparing different methods of administration, a paired t-test was applied to the relative increment in factor levels over baseline.

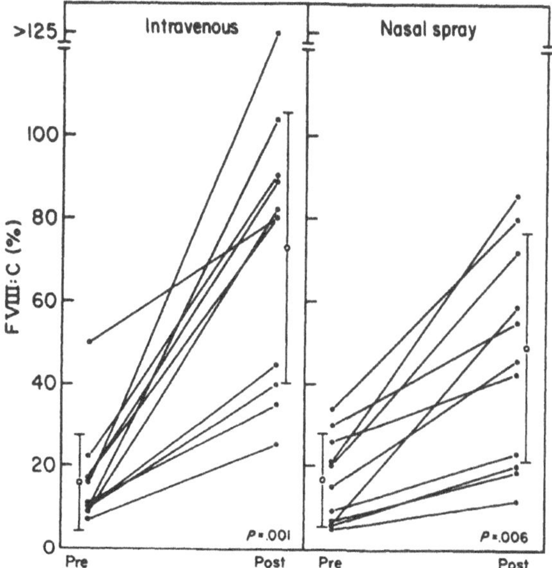

Figure 1: Individual (●) and mean (o) responses in FVIII:C obtained following IV and IN administration of DDAVP to mild hemophilia A patients and hemophilia A carriers

RESULTS

The results obtained for mild hemophilia A patients and symptomatic carriers are shown in Figure 1. Baseline levels of FVIII:C ranged from 5 to 50%. Both methods gave statistically significant rises in FVIII:C. For IN administration, FVIII:C increased from 17% + 11% to 50% + 28% (P=0.006). The relative rise in FVIII:C with the nasal spray ranged from 2- to 10-fold. This compared well with results obtained with IV infusion, where FVIII:C rose from 16% + 12% to 72% + 33% (P=0.001). Several patients were tested on more than one occasion, with comparable results.

In vWD patients, Statistically significant rises in FVIII:C, vWF and vWAg over baseline were seen following either IV or IN administration (Table 1). Both methods of administration

Table 1. Responses in FVIII:C. vWF and vWAg in patients with von Willebrand Disease after the intravenous or intranasal administration of DDAVP.

	Intravenous (%)			Intranasal (%)		
FACTOR	PRE	POST	P VALUE	PRE	POST	P VALUE
FVIII:C	39 ± 18	143 ± 51	0.0004	45 ± 22	115 ± 59	0.002
vWF	64 ± 47	143 ± 116	0.005	30 ± 29	77 ± 61	0.002
vWAg	46 ± 31	133 ± 58	0.0006	39 ± 35	94 ± 91	0.031

were equally effective at improving BT. Of 8 patients whose BT was prolonged, 5 were corrected with either method.

The side effects most frequently reported by patients were facial flushing and transient headache, noted by about half the patients. No adverse reactions were noted.

Selected patients whose baseline testing showed favorable results were allowed to take the spray home to self-administer during bleeding episodes and prior to minor surgical procedures. Excellent hemostasis was reported by 2 hemophilia carriers, one of whom underwent a mole excision and one of whom had a tooth extracted. Epsilon amino caproic acid (Amicar) was used in the latter case as an antifibrinolytic agent. Two hemophiliacs experienced traumatic hemarthroses and reported clinical improvement (decreased pain and improved range of motion in the affected joint) after using the spray. 1 hemophiliac succesfully used the IN-DDAVP for surgical prophylaxis.

In the vWD patients, 3 episodes of epistaxis were controlled and 5 women with menorrhagia who took the spray reported a significant decrease in bleeding. A patient who required extensive dental work took the spray prophylactically and the dentist reported excellent hemostasis.

Hand surgery for carpal tunnel release was required in one of the vWD patients. Baseline nasal spray testing in this patient, done 10 days prior to surgery, compared well with IV infusions done previously. She had already undergone several elective surgical procedures using IV-DDAVP and maintained excellent hemostasis. The patient self administered the nasal spray one hour before the procedure and the surgeon noted excellent hemostasis. The spray was then repeated every 24 hrs for 7 days and once more before suture removal. There was no significant bleeding post operatively. She did not develop tachyphylaxis to the spray, nor was hyponatremia or any sign. of fluid overload observed.

DISCUSSION

Previous studies have demonstrated the superiority of the DDAVP nasal spray to other methods of IN administration such as the rhinyle catheter or pipette. Harris, Nilsson and colleagues compared a single dose of the nasal spray to drops (17) and demonstrated that the nasal spray was deposited anteriorly in the nasal atrium and slowly absorbed across the mucosa. the drops tended to disperse along the length of the nasal cavity and were cleared much more rapidly. Peak plasma levels of DDAVP were significantly higher after nasal spray than after nasal drops and there was also significantly better biological response in FVIII and vWF levels following nasal spray. Administering a divided dose to both nostrils increased the area available for absorption and further enhanced the biological response (19).

We evaluated the effectiveness of a DDAVP nasal spray preparation in raising FVIII:C levels in a group of 11 hemophilia A carriers and patients with mild hemophilia A and found it to be effective in elevating FVIII:C levels over baseline. When compared with IV infusion, the difference between methods is not statistically significant, although IV administration tends to give higher levels. With IV-DDAVP, all subjects achieved levels adequate for surgical hemostasis; with nasal spray, 73% of them achieved such levels. Favorable clinical experiences were reported by 4 patients, of whom 2 used the spray for pre-surgical prophylaxis. The other 2 treated themselves for traumatic hemarthroses and reported subjective improvement after taking the spray.

For patients with vWD, 62% were able to correct their prolonged BT with DDAVP nasal spray, which is the same as the number whose BT corrected with IV-DDAVP. Levels of FVIII:C adequate for surgical hemostasis were achieved in all patients with either nasal spray or with IV-DDAVP. Significant elevations in vWF and vWAg over baseline were obtained with both methods. Although the IV method gave somewhat higher levels than the nasal spray, the differences did not achieve statistical significance. Clinical experiences were reported by 5 patients and included control of epistaxis (3 episodes in 2 patients), menorrhagia (2 patients), prophylaxis before dental work (1 patient) and pre-surgical prophylaxis for minor hand surgery (1 patient).

Our results compare well with those of Lethagen (20), who tested the same spray on a group of mild hemophilia A and vWD patients in Sweden. Significant rises in FVIII:C and vWAg were seen in both groups of patients, although the IV route gave larger increases than the IN route. The FVIII:C levels remained elevated (average 3-fold increase) for several hrs and after 12 hrs were still 1.4 times the baseline level.

Among our patients, side effects were limited to mild facial flushing and transient headaches, noted in about 50% of the patients. Hyponatremia has recently been reported in some patients receiving multiple doses of IV-DDAVP (21,22). Because most of our patients received no more than 2 successive doses of the spray, it is difficult to assess the risk for hyponatremia in this population. The one surgical patient who took DDAVP spray daily for a week did not develop hyponatremia.

Presently approved methods of administration of DDAVP are IV and SC injection. This new method is convenient, easy to learn, does not require the use of needles, and can effectively improve FVIII:C and von Willebrand factors in mild hemophilia A and vWD patients. It is adaptable for home use and will be a welcome addition the the treatment armamentarium for these hereditary coagulopathies.

REFERENCES

1. Mannucci PM, Reggeri ZM, Pareti FI, Capitano A. DDAVP: A new pharmacological approach to the management of hemophilia and von Willebrand disease. Lancet 1977; 1: 869-72.

2. Warrier I, Lusher JM. DDAVP: A useful alternative to blood components in moderate hemophilia Aand von Willebrnd's disease. J Pediatr 1983; 102: 228-33.

3. Mariani G, Ciavarella N, Mazzuconi MG, et al. Evaluation of the effectiveness of DDAVP in surgery and bleeding episodes in hemophilia and von Willebrand's disease. a study of 43 patients. Clin Lab Haematol 1984; 6: 229.

4. De La Fuente B Kasper CK, Rickles FR, Hoyer LW. Response of patients with mild and moderate hemophilia A and von Willebrand disease to treatment with desmopressin. Ann Intern Med 1985; 103: 6-14.

5. Kobrinsky NL, Isreal ED, Gerrard JM, et al. Shortening of bleeding time by 1-deamino-8-D-arginine vasopressin in various bleeding disorders. Lancet 184; 1: 1145-8.

6. Mannucci PM, Remuzzi G, Pusineri F, et al. Deamino-8-D-arginine vasopressin shortens bleeding time in uremia. N Engl J Med 1983; 308: 8-12.

7. Burroughs AK, Matthews K, Qadiri M, et al. Desmopressin and bleeding time in patients with cirrhosis. Br Med J 1985; 291: 1377.

8. Mannucci PM, Vicente V, Vianello L, et al. Controlled trial of desmopressin (DDAVP) in liver cirrhosis and other conditions associated with a prolonged bleeding time. Blood 1986; 67: 1148.

9. Kobirinsky NL, Letts RP, Patel RL, et al. DDAVP shortens the bleeding time and decreases blood loss in hemostatically normal subjects undergoing spinal fusion surgery. Ann Intern Med 1987; 107: 446.

10. Salzman EW, Weinstein MJ, Weintraub RM, et al. Treatment with desmopressin acetate to reduce blood loss after cardiac surgery: a double-blind randomized trial. N Engl J Med 1986; 314: 1402-6.

11.Czer LS, Bateman TM, Gray RJ, et al. Treatment of severe platelet dysfunction and hemorrhage after cardiopulmonary bypass: reduction in blood product usage with desmopressin. J Am Coll Cardiol 1987; 9: 1139-47.

12. Hackman T, Gascoyne RD, Naiman SC, et al. A trial of desmopressin to reduce blood loss in uncomplicated cardiac surgery. N Engl J Med 1989; 321: 1437-43.

13. Kohler M, Hellstern P, Reiter B, von Blohn G, Wenzel E. The subcutaneous administration of the vasopressin analogue 1-desamino-8-D-arginine vasopressin in patients with von Willebrand's disease and hemophilia. Klin Wochenschr 1984; 62: 543-8.

14. DeSio L, Mariani G, Muzzucconi MG, Chistolini A, Tirindelli MC, Mandelli F. Comparison between subcutaneous and intravenous DDAVP in mild and moderate hemophilia A. Thromb Haemost 1985; 54: 387-9.

15. Mannucci PM, Vicente V, Alberca I, et al. Intravenous and subcutaneous administration of desmopressin (DDAVP) to hemophiliac: pharmacokinetics and factor VIII responses. Thromb Haemost 1987; 58: 1037.

16. Kohler M, Hellstern P, Miyashita C, von Blohn G, Wenzel E. Comparitive study of intranasal, subcutaneous and intravenous administration of desamino-D-arginine vasopressin (DDAVP). Thromb Haemost 1986; 55: 108-11.

17. Lethagen S, Harris AS, Sjorin E, Nilsson IM. Intranasal and intravenous administration of desmopressin: effect on FVIII/vWF, pharmacokineticsd reproducibility. Thromb Haemost 1987; 58: 1033-6.

18. Rose, EH, Aledort, LM. Nasal spray desmopressin (DDAVP) for mile hemophilia A and von Willebrand Disease 1991; 114:563-568.

19. Harris AS, Ohlin M, Lethagen S, Nilsson. Effects of concentration volume on nasalbioavailability and biological response to desmopressin. J Pharm Sci 1988; 77: 337-9.

20. Lethagen , Harris AS, Nilsson IM. Intranasal desmopressin (DDAVP) by spray in mild hemophilia A and von Willebrand's disease type I. Blut. 1990;60:187-91.

21. Smith TJ, Gill JC, Ambruso DR, Hathaway WE. Hyponatremia and seizures in young children given DDAVP. Am J Hematol 1989; 31: 199-202.

22. Shepard LL, Hutchinson RJ, Worden EK, Koopman CF, Coran A. Hyponatremia and seizures after intravenous administration of desmopressin acetate for surgical hemostasis. J Pediatr 1989; 114: 470-2.

DISCUSSION

Stuart: What happens in the common cold? Is there less or more absorption?
Seremetis: We had two experiences. One person did not absorb DDAVP when she had a cold, but did so afterwards. One patient with chronic sinusitis and scarring was never able to show a response.

Nilsson: We were doubtful about nose bleeding, but it worked well in such cases.

Lusher: Dr. Seremitis, when did you start treatment for menorrhagia?
Seremetis: On the day that bleeding started.

Harris: All studies suggest that it is equivalent to a parenteral dose of 0.2 mcg. and inferior to the standard parenteral dose of 0.3 mcg. Should there not be a dose response study to determine the optimal intranasal dose?
Nilsson: We are doing such a study in Malmo.

Rao: You had two patients with vW disease with multiple hemarthroses. What were their pre- and post-drug vWf antigen levels?
Seremetis: Both were below the level of detection pre-treatment. Afterwards, the Factor VIII levels were above 40% and the vWf and ristocetin factor levels were above 30%.

Mannucci: What is the role of intranasal DDAVP? I used to use Rinile. I would not use it except in children.
Seremetis: In adults a larger dose would give a more consistent response, which would be useful for home treatment and easier to give.

Mannucci: I do not understand why intranasal DDAVP is used in surgery, in which a maximum response is needed and there is no easy access to the nostril.

Lusher: While we have never advocated its use in surgery, the highly concentrated spray form of DDAVP is quite useful in certain situations, not only children but for adolescents and for adults. In the United States the only preparation available for subcutaneous use is fairly dilute. Thus a large volume is required. Additionally, for occasional use of the drug, particularly at home, a small, intranasal spray bottle is much more convenient than having to use a needle and syringe.
Nilsson : It can also be difficult enough to persuade children to visit the dentist for extractions without having to add the fear of a subcutaneous injection.

Nilsson: In surgery I always use the intravenous route, but I recommend a spray dose before dental surgery.
Seremetis: Our surgery is outpatient, and there is a minimum of tubes, so that the intranasal route is convenient. I agree with Dr Lusher that people do not feel comfortable about bringing out needles and syringes in public.

Kobrinsky: We have had two young adults who have abused the drug by rapid intravenous bolus. This may be a cause for concern.

Rodeghiero: Is there a risk of over-treatment or over-use of the intranasal preparation? It is not completely safe.
Lusher: Patients have a limited amount at home, and are required to call in each time it is used. It is similar to the home treatment of hemophilia.
Seremetis: There may be more potential for the intranasal regimen than for the subcutaneous form.

DDAVP AND TACHYPHYLAXIS IN HEALTHY SUBJECTS

V.Vicente[1], A. Estellés[2], J. Laso[1], J. Rivera[1], J.M. Moraleda[1], J.Aznar[2]

[1]Division of Haematology. Hospital General Universitario. Murcia
[2]Centro de Investigation. Hospital La Fe. Valencia (Spain)

SUMMARY

Although the vasopressin analogue desamino-d-arginine vasopressin (DDAVP) induces a very well characterized increase in factor VIII (FVIII), von Willebrand factor (vWF), tissue plasminogen activator (t-PA) and urokinase-type plasminogen activator (u-PA), the mechanism(s) by which DDAVP enhances the plasma levels of these proteins is poorly understood. Some clinical evidence suggests that certain patients repeatedly treated with DDAVP at closely spaced intervals become progressively unresponsive (tachyphylaxis). The mechanism(s) for tachyphylaxis has not been investigated. The aims of this study are: a) to investigate the effect of repeated DDAVP infusion on the behaviour of FVIII, vWF, t-PA and u-PA, and b) to examine the role noradrenaline in these changes. After a rest period a blood sample was taken from six healthy males (19-26 years old, mean 22). Then 0.3 µg/Kg of DDAVP was infused in 50 ml of saline over a period of 30 min. Immediately after the infusion a second blood sample was collected. Two more additional infusions of DDAVP were repeated after 12 and 24 hours. Blood samples were collected immediately before and after DDAVP.

The second and third infusion of DDAVP induced a low response of FVIII and vWF. If this phenomenon of tachyphylaxis observed in healthy subjects is extended to hemophiliacs and von Willebrand's patients, the usefulness of desmopressin may be limited when these proteins must be raised therapeutically for a prolonged period of time. In contrast, t-PA and u-PA exhibited a consistent response after each DDAVP infusion. These data suggest that the mechanism(s) regulating the realise of vWF and plasminogen activators after DDAVP are independently regulated. Noradrenaline is also released consistently after each infusion of DDAVP. These changes suggest that norepinephrine may play a role in mediating endothelial cell plasminogen activator release.

INTRODUCTION

It has been demonstrated that desmopressin (DDAVP) can raise circulating levels of

Desmopressin in Bleeding Disorders, Edited by G. Mariani *et al.*
Plenum Press, New York, 1993

Factor VIII (FVIII), von Willebrand Factor (vWF), tissue plasminogen activator (t-PA) and urokinase-type plasminogen activator (u-PA)[1-3]. Consequently, DDAVP is established as a nontransfusional form of treatment for mild or moderate hemophilia and von Willebrand's disease[1,4]. It has also been claimed that DDAVP is useful for shortening the prolonged skin bleeding time accompanying uremia, cirrhosis and different platelet congenital and acquired dysfunctions[5-8]. In recent years, there has been increasing evidence that DDAVP reduces the blood loss and transfusion requirements of patients undergoing surgery[9-11].

There is some clinical evidence that patients become progressively unresponsive with DDAVP infusions at closely-spaced intervals[12,13]. This phenomenon (tachyphylaxis) may limit the usefulness of DDAVP when hemostasis must be maintained for a prolonged period of time. Information on the mechanism of tachyphylaxis is very limited.

The mechanism(s) that govern the plasma increases in FVIII, vWF and plasminogen activators induced by DDAVP are incompletely understood. It has not yet been established whether the effects of DDAVP are direct or act through a mediator or second messenger[1,4]. Many aspects of possible mechanisms of DDAVP action must be clarified.

Our interest in the study of the tachyphylaxis phenomenon of FVIII, vWF and plasminogen activators induced by repeated infusions of DDAVP, prompted us to examine the response of these proteins to three infusions of the drug within a short period of time. Another aim of this study was to examine the potential role of noradrenaline mediation in these responses. Finally we monitored the haemodynamic response to repeated infusions of desmopressin and recorded any side effects of the drug.

MATERIAL AND METHODS

Design of the study

Six healthy male subjects (age range 19-26 years old, mean 22) were fully informed of the aims and procedures involved in the study which was approved by the Human Experimental Committee of the University Hospital, and carried out according to the principles of the Declaration of Helsinki as amended in Venice (1983).

Subjects fasted overnight and abstained from smoking for 12 hours before the experiment which started at 9.00 a.m. After a rest period of 15 min., a baseline blood sample was collected (time 0), then 0.3 µg/Kg of DDAVP (Ferring AB, Malmo, Sweden) were added to 50 ml physiologic saline and infused over a period of 30 min. Immediately after the infusion a second blood sample was collected (time 30). Two more additional infusions of DDAVP were repeated after 12 and 24 hours. Blood samples were taken immediately before (time 12 h and 24 h, respectively) and after DDAVP (time 12 h 30 min and 24 h 30 min, respectively).

The haemodynamic effects of DDAVP were assessed by continuous monitoring of systolic and diastolic blood pressure and heart rate before and after samples were taken. Any side effects due to the drug were noted. At the same time plasma osmolarity, hematocrit and electrolytes were monitored.

Blood samples

Samples were collected by venipuncture through a 19-gauge needle. Blood was added to one-tenth volume of 0.129 mmol/L sodium citrate solution, centrifuge immediately at 4°C at 3000 x g for 20 min, snap frozen at -80°C in small aliquots and assayed for the different parameters within 10 days.

Assays

VIII:C was assayed with a one stage method using platelet poor plasma from a patient with severe hemophilia as substrate, as previously described[14]. vWF: Ag was determined with an electroimmunoassay using a commercial rabbit antibody (Behringwerke AG, Marburg, Germany) as described[14]. VIII:C and vWF:Ag assay were standardised against a calibrated pool of normal plasma. t-PA antigen was measured with a commercially available enzyme-linked immunosorbent assay (ELISA) (Imulyse t-PA, Biopool, Sweden)[15]. The assay detects free and complexed t-PA with similar efficiency. u-PA and activable single-chain u-PA (scu-PA) activities were determined by an immunoabsorbent activity assay (Chromolize, u-PA, Biopool, Sweden). Plasma noradrenaline levels were measured by radioenzymatic assay (CAT-A-Kit; Amersham Corp.,Amersham, England), followed by thin-layer chromatography[16].

Statistical analysis

Statistical analysis was performed using both the Mann-Whitney U-test and the paired t-test.

RESULTS

Flushing occured in all subjects after infusions of DDAVP. No clinically important alterations in either blood pressure or heart rate were observed. No evidence of hemodilution following DDAVP infusions was revealed by the unchanging concentrations of sodium and total plasma protein. One subject developed nausea and a feeling of "shakiness" after the second administration of DDAVP, but this was overcome spontanously.

The pretreatment values and the response to each infusion of DDAVP for VIII:C, vWF: Ag, t-PA and u-PA are shown in table 1. Table 2 shows the responses of these proteins, expressed as percentage increase over baseline values (100%) after DDAVP.

As expected, the first infusion of DDAVP induced a significant sharp rise in all parameters (Tables 1 and 2). There was a 2.69-fold increase in mean VIII:C (309±13, $p < 0.05$) and a 2.10-fold increase in vWF: Ag (212±21 vs. 104±12, $p < 0.05$). Similarly, a 3.09-fold increase was observed for t-PA (12.67±1.2 vs. 4.10±0.8, $p < 0.001$) and 2.36-fold increase for u-PA (0.63±0.08 vs. 0.36±0.04). Before the second (time 12 h) and third (time 24 h) infusion of DDAVP, VIII:C (235±30 and 234±36 respectively) and vWF: Ag (233±36 and 257±30 respectively) levels were significantly increased with respect to the baseline values found before beginning the study (time 0) ($p < 0.05$). In contrast, (Table 1) no differences in baseline t-PA and u-PA levels were found with respect to the values found at time 0.

After the second and third infusions of DDAVP, a modest, but significant response of VIII:C and vWF: Ag ($p < 0.05$) with respect to immediate pre-DDAVP levels was observed /Table 1). However, the response expressed in percentage increases over the immediately pre-DDAVP values were significantly decreased with respect to the levels obtained after the first DDAVP infusion ($p < 0.05$) (Table 2).

Table 1. The effect of repeated infusions of DDAVP on VIII:C, vWF:Ag, t-PA and u-PA in 6 healthy subjects (Mean ± SEM).

TIME	VIII:C (%)	vWF:Ag (%)	t-PA (ng/ml)	u-PA (ng/ml)
0	115±13	104±12	4.10±0.8	0.33±0.03
30 m	309±35*	218±21*	12.67±1.2*	0.78±0.04**
12 h.	253±30****	233±36****	3.33±0.4	0.37±0.04
12 h.30m	346±51*	260±46*	8.33±0.6*	0.69±0.10*
24 h.	234±36****	257±30	4.25±0.4	0.36±0.04
24h.30m	278±35***	289±35*	8.67±0.8**	0.63±0.08*

* $p < 0.05$ with respect to the value obtained before the immediate infusion of DDAVP
** $p < 0.001$ with respect to the value obtained before the immediate infusion of DDAVP
*** p N.S. with respect to the value obtained before the immediate infusion of DDAVP
**** $p < 0.05$ with respect to the basal value (time 0)

Table 2. Response of VIII:C, vWF:Ag, t-PA and u-PA, expressed as percentage increased over immediate baseline values after three different infusions of DDAVP. Mean±SEM).

TIME	30 min.	12h.30min.	24h.30min.
VIII:C	269±44	136±7[A]	119±10[AC]
vWF:Ag.	210±21	110±5[A]	112±4.8[AC]
t-PA.	309±47	260±21[B]	207±19[B]
u-PA.	236±19	188±29[B]	186±32[B]

[A] $p < 0.05$ with respect to the increase obtained after first infusion
[B] N.S. with respect to the increase obtained after first infusion
[C] N.S. with respect to the value obtained after second infusion

On the other hand, the plasminogen activators, t-PA and u-PA, exhibited a good and similar response after the second and third infusion of DDAVP (Table 1 and 2). t-PA increased 2.6 and 2.07-fold respectively. Similarly, a 1.90 and 1.86-fold increase in u-PA levels was observed at the same times. These responses, though slightly lower than those obtained after the first infusion of the drug, were not significantly different.

All plasma samples collected immediately before DDAVP (time 0, 12 h and 24 h) showed similar levels of noradrenaline (166±21, 227±42 and 165±32 ng/ml, respectively) (Table 3). After DDAVP infusions, a consistent (315±38; 314±53 and 269±36 ng/ml, respectively) and significant ($p < 0.01$) increase in this hormone was found.

Finally, no significant correlations between the intensity of response of the several parameters studied and noradrenaline plasma level were found.

Table 3. Plasma noradrenaline concentrations during the study (Mean±SEM).

TIME	0	30m	12h	12h 30m	24h.	24h 30m
Noradre-naline (pg/ml)	166±21	315±38*	227±42	314±53*	165±32	269±36*

*$p < 0.01$ with respect to the immediate pre-DDAVP value.

DISCUSSION

Very little information is available on the effect of repeated infusions of DDAVP on FVIII/vWF and plasminogen activator plasma levels. Our studies demonstrate that following three repeated intravenous infusions of DDAVP acetate every 12 h in healthy subjects, FVIII and vWF become unresponsive. We do not know if this phenomenon of tachyphylaxis observed in healthy subjects can be extended to hemophiliacs and von Willebrand's patients. If it can, this would limit the usefulness of desmopressin when these proteins must be maintained well above the resting level for a prolonged period of time. in fact, there is some evidence that hemophiliacs treated with DDAVP at short intervals become progressively unresponsive[1,12]. Closely spaced infusions of desmopressin may lead to a reduction in or absence of bleeding time shortening in uremics too[13].

We have previously seen that healthy subjects or patients with high vWF circulating plasma levels, as induced by a short-acting stimulus such as exercise[17] or long-acting stimuli such as hematological malignancies, cirrhosis or chronic hemolytic anemia, have lower vWF responses to DDAVP than subjects with normal vWF levels[7,14]. Furthermore, the increase in vWF following DDAVP infusion was markedly blunted in severe hemophiliacs, who had high vWF levels after treatment with vWF rich plasma concentrates[18]. A possible explanation for these findings is the existence of negative feedback by high plasma levels of vWF which would temper the release of these proteins from stores. Before the second and third infusion of DDAVP, the plasma levels of vWF and FVIII were significantly higher than basal values (time 0). This may explain the low response observed in these proteins after DDAVP by a negative feedback. Another possible mechanism explaining tachyphylaxis might be the exhaustion of vWF stores after the first stimulus or the impairment of the release mechanism, due to the development of insensitivity in the receptors following repeated challenges from the agonist.

On the other hand, in this study we have demonstrated that tachyphylaxis does not occur in the response of plasminogen activators. The response pattern of plasminogen activators to DDAVP was different from that of vWF. Both activators, t-PA and u-PA exhibited a consistent response after each stimulus. Previously, we showed that circulating levels of vWF do not affect the plasminogen activator response to DDAVP[18]. All these data suggest that the mechanisms regulating the release of vWF and plasminogen activators, t-PA and u-PA, are independently regulated. The dissociated response of these proteins to DDAVP observed by Brommer et al[19] in a number of normal volunteers or patients with prethrombic conditions is consistent with this view.

Although DDAVP has been successfully employed for nearly a decade for the diagnosis and management of congenital and acquired disorders of hemostasis, the mechanism by which DDAVP releases plasminogen activators and vWF from vascular endothelium is still poorly understood. An immediate effect of DDAVP on vessel walls seems less likely because release of plasminogen activator and von Willebrand factor could not be induced by adding DDAVP to endothelial cell cultures[20]. The hypothesis of plasminogen activator and vWF releasing hormone produced by the pituitary gland was also rejected[21].

Catecholamines are important mediators of hemostatic function. Recently,it has been demonstrated that DDAVP induces increased levels of noradrenaline[22,23]. Furthermore, the fact that plasma levels of t-PA and norepinephrine undergo a parallel increase has suggested that norepinephrine may play a role in mediating the release of plasminogen activators from endothelial cells[22]. Since noradrenaline and plasminogen activators respond consistently to all three different stimuli of DDAVP, an attractive hypothesis is that DDAVP stimulates norepinephrine release, and this hormone acts on endothelial cells and induces plasminogen activator release. These data suggest that an increase in levels of circulating noradrenaline might be an additional mechanism though which DDAVP may interact with hemostasis. The fact that DDAVP failed to shorten prolonged bleeding time in patients with platelets lacking a-adrenergic receptors[24] would support this hypothesis.

Several possibilities might explain the difference between the pattern of responses of vWF and plasminogen activators. These proteins have different half-lives (hours versus minutes)[17]. Moreover the period of synthesis in the endothelial cells is probably quite different for vWF and plasminogen activators. Finally, the existence of different receptor sites on the endothelial cells for the release of vWF and fibrinolytic activators cannot be ruled-out.

In summary,this study demonstrates that repeated infusions of DDAVP are capable of producing tachyphylaxis for FVIII and vWF. In contrast, a consistent response of plasminogen activators was observed. We do not know the mechanism by which DDAVP induces release of these proteins, but our data suggest that the mechanisms for regulating the release of vWF and plasminogen activators are independently regulated. The noradrenaline released after DDAVP may play a role in mediating the release of plasminogen activators from endothelial cells.

ACKNOWLEDGEMENTS

This work was supported by research grants from Programa de Promociòn General del Conocimiento en el àrea de Biomedicina y Ciencias de la Salud (PM 89-0070), Ministerio de Educaciòn y Ciencia, and Fundaciòn Ramòn Areces.

REFERENCES

1. Mannucci PM. Desmopressin (DDAVP) for treatment of disorders of hemostasis. In: Progress in Hemostasis and Thrombosis. Coller BS(ed). Grune & Stratton,1986;8: 19-45.
2. Levi M, ten Cate JW, Dooijewaard G, Sturk A, Brommer EJP, Agnelli G. DDAVP induces systemic release of urokinase-type plasminogen activator. 1989;62: 686-689.
3. Agnelli G, Levi M, Cosmi B, ten Cate JW, Nenci GG. Additive effect of DDAVP and standard heparin in increasing plasma t-PA. Throm Haemostas 1989;61: 507-510.
4. Mannucci PM. Desmopressin: A nontrasfusional form of treatment for congenital and acquired bleeding disorders. Blood 1988;72: 1449-1455.
5. Mannucci PM, Remuzzi G, Pusineri F, Lombardi R, Valsecchi C, Mecca G, Zimmerman TS. Deamino-8-D-arginine vasopressin shortens the bleeding time in uremia. N Engl J Med 1983;308: 8-12.
6. Mannucci PM, Vicente V, Vianello R, Cattaneo M, Alberca I, Mari D. Controlled trial of Desmopressin in liver cirrhosis and other conditions associated with prolonged bleeding time. Blood 1986;67: 1148-1153.
7. Cattaneo M, Tenconi PM, Alberca I, Vicente V, Mannucci PM. Subcutaneous desmopressin (DDAVP) shortens the prolonged bleeding time in patients with liver cirrhosis. Thromb Haemostas 1990;64: 358-360.
8. Nieuwenhuis HK, Sixma JJ. Deamino-8-D-arginine vasopressin (desmopressin) shortens the bleeding time in storage pool deficiency. Ann Intern Med 1988;108: 65-67.
9. Salzman EW, Weinstein MJ, Weintraub RM. Treatment with desmopressin acetate to reduce blood loss after cardiac surgery. N Engl J Med 1986;314: 1402-1406.
10. Czer LSC, Bateman TM, Gray RJ, Raymond MR, Stewart ME, Lee S, Golfinger D, Chaux A, Matloff JM. Treatment of severe platelet dysfunction and haemorrhage after cardiopulmonary bypass: reduction in blood product usage with desmopressin. J Am Coll Cardiol 1987;9: 1139-1147.
11. Kobrinsky NL, Letts RP, Patel RL, Israel ED, Monson RC, Schwetz N, Cheang MS. DDAVP shortens the bleeding time and decreases blood loss in haemostatically. normal subjects undergoing spinal fusion surgery. Ann Intern Med 1987; 107:446-450.
12. Mannucci PM, Ruggeri ZM, Pareti FI, Capitanio A. DDAVP: a new pharmacological approach to the management of haemophilia and von Willebrand's disease. Lancet 1977; 1:672-689.

13. Canavese C, Salomone M, Pacitti A, Mangiarotti G, Calitri V. Reduced response of uremic bleeding time to repeated doses of desmopressin. Lancet 1985; 1:867-868.
14. Vicente V, Coppola R, Mannucci PM. The role of the spleen in regulating the plasma levels of factor VIII-von Willebrand factor after DDAVP. Blood 1982; 60:1402-1406.
15. Tabernero MD, Estellés A, Vicente V, Alberca I, Aznar J. Incidence of increased plasminogen activator inhibitor in patients with deep venous thrombosis and/or pulmonary embolism. Thromb Res 1989; 56:565-570.
16. Peuler JD, Johnson GA. Simultaneous single isotope radioenzymatic assay of plasma norepinephrine and dopamine. Life Sci 1977; 21:625-636.
17. Vicente V, Alberca I, Mannucci PM. Reduced effect of exercise and DDAVP on factor VIII-von Willebrand factor and plasminogen activator after sequential application of both the stimuli. Thromb Haemostas 1984; 51:129-130.
18. Vicente V, Alberca I, Mannucci PM. High levels of circulating von Willebrand factor inhibit the release of this protein but not plasminogen activator after DDAVP. Thromb Res 1985; 38:101-105.
19. Brommer EJP, Leuven JAG, Barret-Bergshoeff MM, Schouten JA. Response of fibrinolytic activity and factor VIII-related antigen to stimulation with desmopressin in hyperlipoproteinemia. J Lab Clin Med 1982; 100:105-114.
20. Moffat EH, Giddings JC, Bloom AL. The effect of desamino-d-arginine vasopressin (DDAVP) and naloxone infusions on factor VIII and possible endothelial cell (EC) related activities. Br J Haematol 1984; 57:651-662.
21. Vicente V, Corrales J, Miralles J, Alberca I. Normal response to DDAVP in patients with pathology of the hypothalamoneurohypophyseal axis. Thromb Res 1987; 45:695-697.
22. Grant MB, Guay C, Lottenberg R. Desmopressin stimulates parallel norepinephrine and tissue plasminogen activator release in normal subjects and patients with diabetes mellitus. Thromb Haemostas 1988; 59:269-272.
23. Escolar G, Cases A, Monteagudo J, Garrido M, Lopez J, Ordinas A, Revert L, Castillo R. Uremic plasma after infusion of desmopressin (DDAVP) improves the interaction of normal platelets with vessel subendothelium. J Lab Clin Med 1989; 114:36-42.
24. Schulman S, Johnsson H, Egberg N, Blomback M. DDAVP-induced correction of prolonged bleeding time in patients with congenital platelet function defects. Thromb Res 1987; 45:165-174.

BIOLOGICAL RESPONSES TO REPEATED DOSES OF DESMOPRESSIN (DDAVP) IN PATIENTS WITH HEMOPHILIA AND VON WILLE BRAND'S DISEASE

Pier Mannuccio Mannucci, Donato Bettega and Marco Cattaneo

Angelo Bianchi Bonomi Hemophilia and Thrombosis Center
Institute of Internal Medicine
IRCCS Maggiore Hospital and University of Milan
Milano
Italy

INTRODUCTION

1-deamino-8-D-arginine vasopressin (DDAVP, desmopressin) has been used for many years to treat patients with mild hemophilia and von Willebrand disease (vWD), because it raises transiently the plasma levels of factor VIII coagulant activity (FVIII:C) and von Willebrand factor (vWF) (Mannucci, 1986;1988), probably through the release of these moieties from endothelial storage sites towards plasma and subendothelium (Takeuchi et al, 1988). In these conditions, DDAVP also shortens the prolonged bleeding time of patients with type I vWD and a few rarer subtypes of vWD, probably through the increase of plasma vWF levels (Mannucci, 1986; 1988). DDAVP is usually preferred to replacement therapy with plasma concentrates because it is less expensive and carries no risk of transmitting blood-borne viral infections.

Soon after our first report on the clinical usefulness of DDAVP (Mannucci et al, 1977a), it became apparent that a few patients repeatedly treated at intervals of 12-24 hours became less responsive or unresponsive (Lowe et al, 1977; Mannucci et al, 1977b; Theiss & Schmidt, 1978). It is thought that tachyphylaxis is due to the partial or complete depletion of FVIII:C and vWF in storage sites. Even though a full response can usually be re-established after DDAVP has been stopped for 3-4 days (Mannucci et al, 1977b; Theiss & Schmidt, 1978), a decrease in or abolishment of responsiveness would limit the clinical usefulness of DDAVP, particularly when high plasma levels of FVIII:C and vWF must be maintained for a prolonged time, such as, for instance, during the post-operative period. On the other hand, it appears that the development of tachyphylaxis is not a consistent phenomenon, since patients have been described (particularly with von Willebrand disease) in whom repeated doses of DDAVP elicit FVIII:C and vWF responses as good as those elicited by the first dose (Mannucci et al, 1977a and b; Mariani et al, 1984; de La Fuente et al, 1985).

Desmopressin in Bleeding Disorders, Edited by G. Mariani *et al.*
Plenum Press, New York, 1993

The pattern of development of tachyphylaxis after DDAVP has not been studied in controlled conditions and the information available stems from scattered clinical reports of patients given repeated infusions for the prevention or treatment of bleeding 22 patients with hemophilia and 15 patients with type I vWD ("platelet normal" subtype). In hemophilia, the goal of treatment is to increase FVIII:C to hemostatic levels; in vWD, to increase FVIII:C and shorten the bleeding time, the laboratory hallmarks of the bleeding tendency of these patients. Accordingly, we evaluated whether repeated doses of DDAVP affect FVIII:C, vWF and the bleeding time. We also evaluated the effects of DDAVP on tissue plasminogen activator (Gader et al, 1973) and cardiovascular parameters such as blood pressure and heart rate, which also change after DDAVP (Bichet et al, 1988).

RESULTS AND DISCUSSION

We found that when DDAVP is administered repeatedly to patients with hemophilia and vWD, responses are significantly lower after the second dose ($p < 0.001$), but little further reduction is seen after subsequent doses (not significant); and that this early reduction occurs for all the moieties that DDAVP usually raises in plasma (FVIII:C, vWF, tPA), but not for the bleeding time response which remains unchanged in patients with vWD.

The individual FVIII:C responses to the first dose of DDAVP varied considerably in absolute and relative terms in both hemophiliacs and vWD patients. Since the degree of the response on different occasions in rather consistent for each patient (Mannucci, 1986; Rodeghiero et al, 1989), one can predict the response to the first DDAVP dose by giving a test dose at the time of diagnosis or before the clinical utilization of DDAVP. After the second dose of DDAVP, we found an average reduction of the FVIII:C responses of approximately 30%, in both hemophilia and in vWD. Yet, a response greater than twice the baseline values could still be elicited in approximately half of the patients with hemophilia and 80% of the patients with vWD.

FVIII:C and the bleeding time, i.e., the measurements that are held to correlate better with clinical responses, were improved to values that are usually clinically useful (to 7 minutes or less for the bleeding time, to 30 U/dL or more for FVIII:C) in the majority of patients. In vWD patients the average relative increase in FVIII:C was greater that in hemophiliacs. Although it has previously been observed that patients with type I vWD, "platelet normal", respond briskly to DDAVP (Mannucci et al, 1985; Rodeghiero et al, 1988), our observations give the first direct demonstration that they respond better than patients with mild hemophilia. Why there is such a different response is not understood.

The effect of repeated infusions of DDAVP on the bleeding time had not been evaluated previously. In vWD patients, there was little reduction in bleeding time responses after repeated doses of DDAVP, despite lower vWF responses. Although there is in general a negative correlation between plasma vWF levels (measured as Ricof activity) and bleeding time in type I vWD (Weiss, 1974), the bleeding time response was not clearly affected in our patients by the lower Ricof response, perhaps because the response was still of sufficient magnitude to support the bleeding time. Moreover, DDAVP may shorten the bleeding time independently of released Ricof (Cattaneo et al, 1989).

After repeated doses of DDAVP we found a reduction in tPA:Ag response similar in magnitude and pattern to those of FVIII:C and vWF:Ag, indicating a similar mechanism of release for the three moieties. There was no significant change of the mild hemodynamic effects seen after DDAVP.

Recently, it has been shown that young children are at risk of developing severe hyponatremia and related symptoms after repeated infusions of DDAVP (Smith et al, 1989; Weinstein et al, 1989). Hence, we chose to monitor plasma sodium in the last eight patients enrolled in our study. None of them developed hyponatremia, indicating that in our patients (adolescents and adults) this risk is not high. In the original case observed by Lowe et al (1977), hyponatremia developed in an adult who was treated at more frequent intervals (every 12 hours). Therefore, it is advisable to give DDAVP at 24 hour intervals to reduce this risk.

The information gathered in our study is of practical use in planning the clinical management of patients. After repeated infusions of DDAVP at 24 hour intervals, one can expect a reduction of about 30% of the initial FVIII:C responses in hemophilia and vWD, but no important reduction of the bleeding time response in vWD. Hence, the type of bleeding episodes that might be handled with DDAVP without resorting to blood products will depend on the patients baseline FVIII:C levels, on the levels needed to stop or prevent that bleeding episode, and on the likelihood to achieve and maintain such levels as it can be predicted from our findings.

Addendum: This study will be published in full in the British Journal of Haematology (1992, volume 82).

REFERENCES

Bichet, D.C., Razi, M., Lonergan, M., Arthus, M.F., Papukna V., Kortax, C. & Barjon, J.N. (1988). Hemodynamic and coagulation responses to 1-desamino-8-D-arginine vasopressin in patients with congenital nephrogenic diabetes insipidus. New England Journal of Medicine 318: 881-884.

Cattaneo, M., Moia, M., Della Valle, P., Castellana, P. & Mannucci, P.M. (1989). DDAVP shortens the prolonged bleeding times of patients with severe von Willebrand disease treated with cryoprecipitate. Evidence for a mechanism of action independent of released von Willebrand factor. Blood 74: 1972 - 1976.

De la Fuente, B., Kasper, C.K., Rickles, F.R. & Hoyer, L.W. (1985). Response of patients with mild and moderate hemophilia A and von Willebrand disease to treatment with desmopressin. Annals of Internal Medicine 103: 6-14.

Gader, A.M.A., De costa, J. & Cash, J.D. (1973). A new vasopressin analogue and fibrinolysis. Lancet 2: 1417 - 1419.

Lowe, G., Pettigrew, A., Middleton, S., Forbes, C.D. & Prentice, C.R.M. (1977). DDAVP in hemophilia. Lancet 2: 614 - 615.

Mannucci, P.M. (1986). Desmopressin (DDAVP) for treatment of disorders of hemostasis. Progress in Hemostatis and Thrombosis 8: 19 - 45.

Mannucci, P.M. (1986). Desmopressin: a nontransfusional form of treatment for congenital and acquired bleeding disorders. Blood 72: 1449 - 1455.

Mannucci, P.M., Ruggeri, Z.M., Pareti, F.I. & Capitanio, A.M. (1977a). DDAVP: a new pharmacological approach to the management of hemophilia and von Willebrand disease. Lancet 1: 889 - 872.

Mannucci, P.M., Ruggeri, Z.M., Pareti, F.I. & Capitanio, A.M. (1977b). DDAVP in hemophilia. Lancet 2 : 1171 - 1172.

Mannucci, P.M., Lombardi, R., Bader, R., Vianello, L., Federici, A.B., Solinas, S., Mazzucconi, M.G. & Mariani, G. (1985). Heterogeneity of type I von Willebrand disease. Evidence for a subgroup with an abnormal von Willebrand factor. Blood 66: 796-802.

Mariani, G., Ciavarella, N., Mazzucconi, M.G., Antoncecchi, S., Solinas, S., Ranieri, P., Pettini, P., Agrestini, F. & Mandelli, F. (1984). Evaluation of the effectiveness of DDAVP in surgery and bleeding episodes in hemophilia and von Willebrand' disease. A study of 43 patients. Clinical and Laboratory Haematology 6: 229-238.

Rodeghiero, F., Castaman, G.O.C, Di Bona, E., Ruggeri, M., Lombardi, R. & Mannucci, P.M. (1988). Hyper-responsiveness to DDAVP for patients with type I von Willebrand's disease and normal intraplatelet von Willebrand factor. European Journal of Haematology 40: 163-167.

Rodeghiero, F., Castaman, G., Di Bona, E. & Ruggeri, M. (1989). Consistency of responses to repeated DDAVP infusions in patients with von Willebrand's disease and hemophilia A. Blood 74: 1997-2000.

Smith, T.S., Gill, J.C., Ambruso, D.R. & Hathaway, W.E. (1989). Hyponatremia and seizures in young children given DDAVP. American Journal of Hematology 31: 199-202.

Takeuchi, M., Naguza, H. & Kanedu, T. (1988). DDAVP and epinephrine induced changes in the localization of von Willebrand factor antigen in endothelial cells of human oral mucosa. Blood 72: 850-854.

Theiss, W., Schmidt, G (1978). DDAVP in von Willebrand disease: repeated administration and the behaviour of the bleeding time. Thrombosis Research 13: 1119-1123.

Weinstein, R.E., Bona, R.D., Altman, A.J., Quinn, J.J., Weisman, S.J., Bartolomeo, A. & Rickles, F. (1989). Severe Hyponatremia after repeated intravenously administration of desmopressin. American Journal of Hematology 32: 258-261.

Weiss, H.J. (1974). Relation of von Willebrand factor to bleeding time. New England Journal of Medicine 291:420.

DISCUSSION

Lusher: You showed that your patients returned to baseline Factor VIII levels at 24 hours. In repeated doses in the clinic, one would not like to have these troughs. would it be better to study its use every 12 hours?
Mannucci: This is a critical point. The choice of protocol depends on the circumstances. The baseline levels are important. I would not perform surgery with a baseline Factor VIII level of 5%, even if it rose to 50%, if it were to return to a baseline of 5%. I recognise this as a weakness of the study.

Kinter: Dr Vicente, did you see tachyphylaxis in the hemodynamic parameters?
Vicente: The blood pressure response after the second and further doses was slightly less, but not significant. electrolytes did not change. The flushing was similar after each infusion.
Mannucci: Our impression was that there was no reduction in flushing.

Mariani: Although your data are convincing, can you rule out that there are special patients who do have clear tachyphylaxis after the first dose? Say, a subset of 10% of patients?
Mannucci: It is possible, but we studied patients who were not bleeding and not being treated. In this set of patients we had none, but they may be more common in groups of patients who are bleeding, whose consumption of Factor VIII is higher.

Rao: Were the hemodynamic responses measured one hour after the dose?
Vicente: Yes.
Rao: Then perhaps you missed some blood pressure data.
Vicente: We did see the usual hemodynamic response at 60 minutes.

Brommer: Did you try to restore the response with higher subsequent doses, or give it more often than 12 hourly?
Vicente: No.

Kobrinsky: All the hemophiliac patients were male, and half the vW patients were female. As estrogens may have made a difference, did you examine the sex difference, and would it be worthwhile studying tachyphylaxis in the two sexes separately? When Danazol is given to mild hemophiliacs it does raise constitutive Factor VIII production.
Mannucci: I do not remember how many females were seen, but I think it is a good idea to look at sex differences. There is doubt that Danazol works to a significant extent, any more than estrogen. However, on theoretical grounds it is interesting.

Vicente: Do you see liver changes with Danazol?
Kobrinsky: We use it for carriers of Factor IX deficiency with menorrhagia, and it has helped. It increased Factor IX by about 40%, and in one patient with Factor VII deficiency there was also 40% increase. We have seen no liver toxicity.

Mannucci: Why not give estrogen? That would give the same results.
Kobrinsky: They were already on the birth control pill for hemostatic purposes.

Lusher: Professor Mannucci, how do you relate your old findings of a subset showing tachyphylaxis, and the new finding of everyone showing a smaller response?
Mannucci: Perhaps the patients were in a different state: the former were bleeding patients, the latter not bleeding.

Mayadas-Norton: Referring to the decreases in vWf release over successive DDAVP administrations, my in vitro studies of thrombin stimulation of human umbilical vein endothelial cells for 15 minutes or continuous stimulation for up to 48 hours did not result in an increase in vWf synthesis to replenish the depleted stores. This suggests that the replenishment of Weibel-Palade bodies with vWf occurs at the same rate as that of unstimulated cells.

Cattaneo: Knowing what goes on in the Weibel-Palade bodies does not explain everything.
Mannucci: I agree: there are things that do not fit, such as differences in time courses and relatively larger release of Factor VIII than vWf.

Kinter: Do we wish to refer to these responses as tachyphylaxis, which implies very dramatic reduction of response to zero? It is more accurately described as tolerance.

MYOCARDIAL INFARCTION AND STROKE--IS THE RISK INCREASED BY DESMOPRESSIN?

Jeanne M. Lusher

Division of Hematology-Oncology
The Children's Hospital of Michigan and
Wayne State University School of Medicine
Detroit, Michigan 48201

INTRODUCTION

Following early reports in the mid-1970's by Mannucci and colleagues[1] and Cash, et al[2] which described the effectiveness of desmopressin (1-desamino-8-D-Arginine vasopressin, DDAVP) in increasing Factor (F) VIII and von Willebrand factor (vWF) in normal individuals as well as in those with von Willebrand disease (vWD) and mild or moderate hemophilia A,[3-5] this synthetic agent has gained widespread use. Not only is DDAVP considered to be the treatment of choice for persons with vWD type I and for those with mild and moderate hemophilia A, it has been shown to be effective in preventing or treating bleeding in a wide variety of other clinical entities including many platelet function defects (both congenital and acquired),[6-13] unexplained prolonged bleeding time,[14] hepatic cirrhosis,[15] the carrier state for hemophilia A,[16,17] some persons with vWD type IIA,[13] and in persons with no underlying hemostatic defect who undergo cardiopulmonary bypass surgery[18,19] or other surgical procedures known to be associated with considerable blood loss.[13,20]

In addition to its clinical use in controlling or preventing bleeding, in Sweden DDAVP has been used to increase FVIII levels in blood donors, thereby increasing yields of FVIII in cryoprecipitate or FVIII concentrates prepared from the plasma.[21,22] This synthetic agent has also proven to be useful as a diagnostic tool, in improving carrier detection, in analyzing the relationships between responses to DDAVP and different types of vWD,[13] and in measuring the fibrinolytic potential in patients with a thrombotic tendency by measuring plasminogen activator release after DDAVP administration.[23]

Despite its increasing use in a wide variety of situations, DDAVP has been associated with relatively few undesirable side effects.

Desmopressin in Bleeding Disorders, Edited by G. Mariani *et al.*
Plenum Press, New York, 1993

The most serious potential side effect reported has been that of acute thrombosis of coronary or cerebral arteries; however, it would appear that only certain individuals are at risk.

SIDE EFFECTS ASSOCIATED WITH THE USE OF DDAVP

Common Side Effects Resulting From Vasodilation

The most common side effects following IV administration of DDAVP are facial flushing and a feeling of facial warmth, resulting from mild vasodilatation of the skin. This is thought to be related to the systemic release of prostacyclin by DDAVP.[24] Less common side effects include mild headache and slight falls in systolic and/or diastolic blood pressure. These minor side effects probably result from vasodilatation as well.

Hyponatremia and Water Intoxication

Since DDAVP is a potent antidiuretic agent, there is a risk of water retention and dilutional hyponatremia[25] which has on rare occasions resulted in generalized convulsions. The risk of water intoxication appears to be greatest in infants or very young children[26,27] and in the elderly, as well as in post-operative patients receiving large amounts of IV fluids along with DDAVP. Greater awareness of this potential complication, with fluid restriction and monitoring of electrolytes, should prevent water intoxication. The high degree of safety of DDAVP probably relates to the relatively low level of thirst in humans, which becomes symptomatic only above a plasma osmolality of about 290 m osmol/kg.

Reports of Acute Myocardial Infarction and Cerebral Arterial Thrombosis

The possibility of another more serious complication was first reported in early 1989, when O'Brien and colleagues,[28] and van Dantzig and co-workers[29] reported instances of acute myocardial infarction immediately following DDAVP infusion. These reports were soon followed by an editorial in Lancet[30] concerning the possible triggering of thrombotic events by DDAVP. Following a few more such reports,[31-33] Professor P.M. Mannucci and I sought to determine whether or not DDAVP did indeed carry a risk of arterial thrombosis. As we reported in a letter to the editor of Lancet,[34] when one compared the number of documented cases of acute myocardial infarction or other arterial thrombotic events to the estimated number of persons receiving IV DDAVP, it did *not* appear that the drug increased the incidence of such complications. In reviewing the reported cases of thrombotic events it is noteworthy that they occurred in elderly men who had other risk factors for arterial thrombosis. However, we cautioned that even though there was no clear evidence indicating such a causative association, close surveillance of DDAVP seemed warranted, especially in persons with clinical and/or laboratory evidence of coronary or cerebral atherosclerosis.[34]

In 1990, McLeod reported that a 47 year old plasma exchange program donor, who was thought to be in excellent health, developed acute myocardial infarction approximately 30 minutes following IV DDAVP, 0.3μg/kg. It is noteworthy that this man recovered uneventfully without thrombolytic therapy, and while he had 50%

narrowing in the left anterior descending and right coronary arteries on angiography 5 days later, no occlusion of even a small terminal branch could be identified.[35] While McLeod noted that paradoxical vasospasm might have accounted for this man's chest pain and electrocardiogram changes, coronary artery spasm is unlikely to be caused by DDAVP, which (unlike vasopressin) does not act on the V_1 pressor receptors.

Following this occurrence, McLeod noted that he and his colleagues had decided to restrict the use of DDAVP in plasma exchange donors to "highly motivated younger donors without risk factors for vascular disease" such as hypertension, diabetes, smoking, hyperlipidemia and family history of premature vascular disease.[35]

As noted by Lowe,[36] in most healthy persons DDAVP stimulates both fibrinolysis and coagulation, increasing plasma levels of tissue plasminogen activator (t-PA) and plasmin activity as well as plasma levels of FVIII and von Willebrand factor. However, plasma levels of t-PA inhibition are often increased in patients with coronary artery disease, and have been shown to predict recurrent myocardial infarction. In the presence of high levels of t-PA inhibition, DDAVP infusion does *not* increase t-PA activity or plasmin activity. Lowe has thus suggested that one possible mechanism for the increased risk of thrombosis in patients with underlying coronary artery disease could be high levels of t-PA inhibition, which prevent the normal fibrinolytic response to DDAVP.[36] Another possible mechanism is increased platelet adhesion at injury sites in the vessel wall, mediated via vWF release, or by a direct effect on the vascular endothelium.[37]

Nonetheless, the paucity of reported instances of myocardial infarction or cerebral thrombosis in persons receiving DDAVP makes a causal relationship uncertain.

Symptomatic Hemodynamic Changes

Alauro and Johns reported two patients, a 73 year old woman and a 63-year old man (both with unstable angina), who developed sudden unexpected decrease in arterial blood pressure shortly after receiving IV DDAVP prophylactically to prevent bleeding following cardiopulmonary bypass surgery. The authors noted that in both cases a decrease in arterial blood pressure (to 70/36 and 78/48 in the two patients) appeared within 5 minutes after DDAVP infusion was begun. While the authors admit that many confounding factors could have lowered arterial blood pressure in their patients (such as hypovolemia, myocardial depression or delayed protamine reaction), they note that a sudden unexpected decrease in arterial pressure in such patients could lead to ischemia and conclude that one should be cautious in administering DDAVP in the post-bypass period.[38]

Israels and Kobrinsky reported the sudden development of severe cyanosis and dyspnea in a 21 month old child with tetralogy of Fallot who was given a test dose of IV DDAVP, 0.3μ/kg. These authors note that while the normal cardiovascular system can compensate for a decrease in mean arterial pressure of 10-15%, in this child with cyanotic congenital heart disease the decrease in peripheral vascular resistance induced by DDAVP increased right-to-left shunting and resulted in severe cyanosis and dyspnea.[39] This experience suggests that some patients with cyanotic heart disease may be jeopardized by the vasodilatory effects of DDAVP.

SUMMARY

DDAVP has now been used for fifteen years, for an expanding list of clinical problems associated with bleeding. This synthetic agent has proven to be remarkably free of serious side effects, despite widespread usage. Nonetheless, two potentially serious side effects have been reported in very small numbers of subjects: 1) hyponatremia and water intoxication; and 2) acute myocardial infarction and cerebral arterial thrombosis. The risk of both of these potential complications can be greatly reduced by being aware of them. While a direct causative effect has not been proven for the complication of arterial thrombosis, it would seem prudent to carefully consider the risk-benefit ratio in deciding whether to use DDAVP in persons *known* to have risk factors for coronary or cerebral thrombosis. In many instances, it may be decided that the benefits outweigh this possible risk.

REFERENCES

1. P.M. Mannucci, M. Aberg, I.M. Nilsson and B. Robertson, Mechanism of plasminogen activator and factor VIII increase after vasoactive drugs. *Br J Haematol*, 30:81-93(1975).

2. J.D. Cash, A.M.A.Gader and J. DaCosta, The release of plasminogen activator and factor FVIII by LVP, AVP, DDAVP, AT III and OT in man. *Br J Haematol*, 27:363-364(1974).

3. P.M. Mannucci, F.I Pareti, L. Holmberg, I.M. Nilsson and Z.M. Ruggeri, Studies on the prolonged bleeding time in von Willebrand disease. *J Lab Clin Med*, 88:662-671(1976).

4. P.M. Mannucci, Z.M. Ruggeri, F.I. Pareti and A. Capitanio, DDAVP: A new pharmacological approach to the management of haemophilia and von Willebrand disease. *Lancet*, 1:869-872, (1977).

5. G. Mariani, N. Ciavarelli, M.G. Mazzuconi, S. Antoncecchi, S. Solinas, P. Ranieri, P. Pettini, F. Agrestini and F. Mandelli, Evaluation of the effectiveness of DDAVP in surgery and bleeding episodes in hemophilia A and von Willebrand's disease. A study of 43 patients. *Clin Lab Haematol*, 6:229-238(1984).

6. N.L. Kobrinsky, E.D. Israel, J.G. Gerrard, M.S. Cheang, C.M. Watson, A. J. Bishop, and M.L. Schroeder, Shortening of the bleeding time by 1-deamino-8-D-arginine vasopressin in various bleeding disorders. *Lancet*, 1:1145-1158(1984).

7. H.K. Nieuwenhuis and J.J. Sixma, 1-desamino-8-D-arginine vasopressin (desmopressin) shortens the bleeding time in storage pool deficiency. *Ann Intern Med*, 108:65-67(1988).

8. S. Schulman, H. Johnsson, N. Edberg and M. Blomback, DDAVP-induced correction of prolonged bleeding time in patients with congenital platelet function defects. Thromb Res, 45:165-174(1987).

9. A.J. Watson and J.A.B. Keogh, Effect of 1-deamino-8-D-arginine vasopressin on the prolonged bleeding time in chronic renal failure. *Nephron*, 32:49-52(1982).

10. A.J. Watson and J.A.B. Keogh, 1-deamino-8-D-arginine vasopressin as a therapy for the bleeding diathesis of acute renal failure. *Am J. Nephrol*, 4:49-51(1984).

11. P.M. Mannucci, G. Remuzzi, F. Pusineri, R. Lombardi, C. Valsecchi, G. Mecca and T.S. Zimmermann, Deamino-8-d-arginine vasopressin shortens the bleeding time in uremia. *N Engl J Med*, 308:8-12(1983).

12. T.B. Kentro, R. Lottenbery and C.S. Kitchens, Clinical efficacy of desmopressin acetate for hemostatic control in patients with primary platelet disorders undergoing surgery. *Am J Hematol*, 24:215-219(1987).

13. P.M. Mannucci, Desmopressin (DDAVP) for treatment of disorders of hemostasis. *Progr Hemostas Thrombos*, 8:19-45(1986).

14. H.C. Kim, K. Salva, P.L. Fallot, G.I. Karp, J. Eisele, L. Matts, I. Heller and P. Saidi, Patients with prolonged bleeding time of undefined etiology and their response to desmopressin. *Thrombos Haemostas*, 59:221-224,(1988).

15. P.M. Mannucci, V. Vicente, L. Vianello, M. Cattaneo, I. Alberca, M.P. Coccato, E. Faioni and D. Mari, Controlled trial of desmopressin in liver cirrhosis and other conditions associated with a prolonged bleeding time. *Blood*, 67:1148-1153(1986).

16. W. Theiss and E. Sauer, DDAVP: Alternative to replacement treatment in mild haemophilia A and von Willebrand-Jurgens syndrome. *Dtsch Med Wschr*, 109:1769-1772(1977).

17. J.M. Lusher, Desmopressin acetate (DDAVP): Its use in disorders of hemostasis. *Thrombos Hemostas*, No. TH 84-5(TH-35), 6:1-8(1985).

18. E.W. Salzman, M.J. Weinstein, R.M. Weintraub, J.A. Ware, R.L. Thurer, L. Robertson, A. Donovan, T. Gaffney, V. Bertele, J.T. Roll, M. Smith and L.E. Chute, Treatment with desmopressin acetate to reduce blood loss after cardiac surgery. A double-blind randomized trial. *N Engl J Med*, 314:1402-1406(1986).

19. L.S. Czer, T. M. Batemen, R.J. Gray, M. Raymond, M.E. Stewart, S. Lee, D. Goldfinger, A. Chaux, J.M. Matloff, Treatment of severe platelet dysfunction and hemorrhage after cardiopulmonary bypass: reduction in blood product usage with desmopressin. *J Am Coll Cardiol*, 9:1139-1147(1987).

20. N.L. Kobrinsky, R.M. Letts, L.R. Patel, E.D. Israels, R.C. Monson, N. Schwetz and M.S. Cheang, 1-desamino-8-D-arginine vasopressin (desmopressin) decreases operative blood loss in patients having Harrington Rod spinal fusion surgery. A randomized, double-blinded controlled trial. *Ann Intern Med*, 107:446-450(1987).

21. I.M. Nilsson, M. Mikaelsson, H. Villhardt and H. Walter, DDAVP factor VIII concentrate and its properties in vivo and in vitro. *Thromb Res*, 15:263-271(1979).

22. M. Mikaelsson, I.M. Nilsson, H. Villhardt and H. Walter, Factor VIII concentrate prepared from blood donors stimulated by intranasal administration of a vasopressin analogue. *Transfusion*, 22:229(1982).

23. E.J.P. Brommer, M.M. Barrett-Berghoeff, R.A. Allen, I. Schicht, R.M. Bertina and M.A.D.H. Schalekemp, The use of desmopressin acetate (DDAVP) as a test of the fibrinolytic capacity of patients. Analysis of responders and non-responders. *Thromb Haemost*, 48:156-161(1982).

24. C.V. Prowse, A. Farrugia, F.E. Boulton, J. Tucker, C.A. Ludlan, M. McLaren, J.J.F. Belch, C.R.M. Prentice, J. Dawes and I.R. MacGregor, A comparative study using immunological and biological assays of the hemostatic responses to DDAVP infusion, venous occlusion and exercise in normal men. *Thromb Haemost*, 51:110-114(1984).

25. G. Lowe, A. Pettigrew, S. Middleton, C.D. Forbes and C.R.M. Prentice, DDAVP in hemophilia. *Lancet*, 2:614-615,(1977).

26. L.L. Shepard, R.J. Hutchinson, E.K. Worden, C.F. Koopman and A. Coran, Hyponatremia and seizures after intravenous administration of desmopressin acetate for surgical hemostasis. *J. Pediatr*, 114:470-472(1989).

27. T.J. Smith, J.C. Gill, D.R. Ambruso and W.E. Hathaway, Hyponatremia and seizures in young children given DDAVP. *Am J Hematol*, 31:199-202(1989).

28. J.R. O'Brien, P.J. Green, G. Salmon, P. Wier, D. Colin-Jones, M. Arnold, and S. Chopra, Desmopressin and myocardial infarction. *Lancet*, 1:664 (1989).

29. J.M. vanDantzig, D.R. Duren, J.W. tenCate, Desmopressin and myocardial infarction. *Lancet*, 1:664 (1989).

30. Editorial, Desmopressin and arterial thrombosis. *Lancet*, 1:938-939 (1989).

31. L. Bond and D. Bevan, Myocardial infarction in a patient with hemophilia treated with DDAVP. *N Engl J Med*, 318:121 (1988).

32. B. Viron, C. Michel, T. Serrato and E. Verdy, Risque thrombogene du DDAVP dans l'insuffisance renal chronique. *Nephrologie*, 8:225 (1987).

33. J.J. Byrnes, A. Larcada, J.L. Moake, Thrombosis following desmopressin for uremic bleeding. *Am J. Hematol*, 28:63-64 (1988).

34. P.M. Mannucci and J.M. Lusher, Desmopressin and thrombosis. *Lancet*, 2:675-676 (1989).

35. B.C. McLeod, Myocardial infarction in a blood donor after administration of desmopressin. *Lancet*, 336:1137-1138,(1990).

36. G.D.O. Lowe, Desmopressin and myocardial infarction. *Lancet*, 1:895-896 (1989).

37. M.I. Barnhart, S. Chen and J.M. Lusher, DDAVP: Does the drug have a direct effect on the vessell wall? *Thromb Res*, 31:239-253 (1983).

38. F.S. D'Alauro and R.A. Johns, Hypertension related to desmopressin administration following cardiopulmonary bypass. *Anesthes*, 69:962-963 (1988).

39. S.J. Israels and N.L. Kobrinksy, Serious reaction to desmopressin in a child with cyanotic heart disease. *Lancet*, 320:1563-1564(1989).

DISCUSSION

Schulman: Your last recommendation about avoiding the risk factors for coronary artery thrombosis is severe. It includes smoking, for example. How strict are you?
Lusher: The risk is very small, and may not even be related to DDAVP. It is mentioned to avoid the possible association, even if it is not causative.

Mannucci: The most convincing evidence that the problem is not large is the analysis of placebo-controlled studies in patients with cardiac surgery (who are at very high risk). We could not show any excess of thrombotic complications among the DDAVP patients than in those on placebo. However, there is something there. DDAVP releases supranormal vWf multimers, which can aggregate platelets directly in conditions of high shear stress. So a word of caution is warranted.

Lusher: This clearly has medico-legal implications as well. It might be difficult to explain away giving the drug to persons who have had previous cardiac episodes.
Rao: A cautionary note is very much required, but to word it in this way may be too strong, not only for medico-legal but also for clinical practice. The drug is much used in the elderly, who often have a cardiac risk.

Sultan: Is there a lower age limit for children because of the hyponatremia?
Lusher: It must be used with great caution in small infants, but careful monitoring of fluids and sodium levels should decrease the risk.
Bichet: The key factor is the fluid intake and balance. Fluids must not be forced. If you bypass normal thirst, this will be a problem.

Schulman: A few cases of hyponatremia are not associated with fluid administration.
Lusher: Most of the time there would not be a problem, but there must be some risk.
Brommer: Most serious side effects are associated with irregular infusion, which should not be too fast. Also, you equated flushing with prostaglandins, but high doses of aspirin do not prevent it.

Cattaneo: Would you give DDAVP to patients with mild hemophilia and known coronary disease?
Lusher: I know of no case of clotting complicating DDAVP treatment in a hemophiliac.
Cattaneo: There has been one.

Harris: The pituitary renal axis, and therefore concentrating ability and response to vasopressin, is not fully developed in an 18 month-old, and this ought to be kept in mind when DDAVP is given to infants. Also I would like to encourage people to collect all individual data from cardiac studies into a central data bank, and am ready to act as co-ordinator.

Kinter: Remember that from a toxicological perspective if you push the dose high enough in animals, you get profound hypotension perhaps not associated with release of clotting factors. There may be a very narrow therapeutic window in the infants and the elderly.

Sultan: Must we take Dr Harris' suggestion of not giving DDAVP to infants under 18 months?
Lusher: Dr Harris has made a suggestion, but it still may be needed in a one year old child and careful monitoring of fluids and electrolytes should be enough to avoid harm.
Weinstein: We have used it in infants 10 days old and younger who underwent cardiac bypass and found no thrombotic complications, but no beneficial effects.

DDAVP IN THE MANAGEMENT OF CONGENITAL AND ACQUIRED BLEEDING DISORDERS: SOLVED AND UNSOLVED ISSUES

P.M. Mannucci, J. Lusher, Y. Sultan
on behalf of the workshop

MECHANISM OF ACTION

DDAVP is a V2 agonist. At low plasma concentrations DDAVP stimulates the adenylate cyclase coupled V2 receptor in the kidney. At high plasma concentrations it stimulates a V2-like receptor. Endothelial cells are the most likely target for DDAVP stimulation of release of vWf. However the cell type responsible for release of Factor VIII is unknown. Although these factors appear to be released in parallel, there is evidence that may distinguish the release of vWf from that of Factor VIII.

CELLULAR SITE(S)

Endothelial cells do not release vWF when exposed to DDAVP in vitro. However, they release vWF when incubated with whole blood from subjects treated with DDAVP, indicating that a second messenger, probably derived from mononuclear leukocytes, is involved in DDAVP stimulated release of vWF. This messenger is presently unknown; candidates include platelet activating factor (PAF), P-selectin, and cyclic GMP. Mediators that have been ruled out include catecholamines, endorphins and prostaglandins.

vWF, tPA and uPA are generally released in parallel, although there may be manipulations that will permit one or more of these factors to be selectively released.

High plasma concentrations of DDAVP cause vasodilation, flushing and mild hypotension with reflex tachycardia. These effects also appear to be mediated through a V2 like receptor mechanism. The response is largely parallel to the release of clotting factors. The relationship between these hemodynamic effects and release of clotting factors (if any) is unknown.

EFFECTS ON HEMOSTASIS

How does DDAVP affect hemostasis? The preponderance of the evidence is consistent with a relationship between DDAVP stimulation of Factors VIII and vWF release, and increase in platelet adhesion to the subendothelium and a potentiation of platelet aggregation induced by high shear. There is no direct effect of DDAVP on platelet aggregation under low shear

Desmopressin in Bleeding Disorders, Edited by G. Mariani *et al.*
Plenum Press, New York, 1993

conditions. These mechanisms outweigh the increase in fibrinolytic potential due to the concomitant DDAVP stimulated release of tPA and uPA.

There was no consensus on other effects such as general endothelial cell stimulation (PGI2, fibronectin, thrombomodulin, protein S, platelet factor 4, Factor XII).

DOSAGE

0.3 or 0.4 mcg/kg i.v. or s.c.
1 - 3 mcg/kg intranasally

ROUTE OF ADMINISTRATION

The subcutaneous and I.V. routes are clinically equivalent in onset, peak response and duration, with good reproducibility. The 0.3mcg/kg dose is sufficient, and intrapatient variability is more predictable than interpatient variability.

The response from the new highly concentrated intranasal spray formulation which concentrates in the anterior half of the nose is consistent. It is clinically equivalent to the I.V. and S.C. doses of 0.2 mcg/kg. This would appear to be the formulation of choice for home or outpatient use, (as for epistaxis and menorrhagia).

FORMULATION

The intravenous formulation is easy to use, but the subcutaneous and the older intranasal formulations contain too much fluid, making them uncomfortable for the patient and awkward to use.

Enthusiasm was voiced for trials of a more concentrated intranasal formulation, to make it therapeutically equivalent to the i.v. and s.c. dose.

CLINICAL INDICATIONS

Hemophilia

Prediction of the degree of response (both for different patients and with single patients) is reasonably reproducible. As for concomitant use of synthetic antifibrinolytic amino acids, the consensus is that if one is to be used anyway, as in bleeding within the oral cavity, or dental extractions, an antifibrinolytic can be used, irrespective of the decision to use concomitant DDAVP.

von Willebrand disease

Do both types I and II of vW disease have a Factor VIII response? Studies of bleeding time and Factor VIIIc in types I and II have shown that the failure to shorten BT is not an indicator that Factor VIII is not increased. It is not necessary to have complete correction of bleeding time before surgery: the response of Factor VIII is more important. Factor VIII does rise, practically in every case of Types I and II, but not in Type III. Why Type III patients do not respond is unknown.

Opinions on the necessity for testing Factor VIII responses before surgery in vW patients were divided. Those who favoured testing, and found patients to have a negative test would still use the drug, but would consider combining DDAVP with cryoprecipitate administration.

Opinions also differed on the advisability of giving DDAVP to Type IIB patients with low platelet counts because of the risk of worsening their thrombocytopenia.

Congenital platelet function defects

DDAVP has been used in platelet dysfunction with variable results. In storage pool defect and Bernard Joulier syndrome, few patients respond. Patients with abnormal release, but normal granules, do respond with shortened bleeding times. In thrombasthenia there is no consensus: although it is generally not thought to work. DDAVP shortens isolated idiopathic prolonged bleeding time, and can be used in minor surgery in such patients. In patients with thrombocytopenias of different origins (as in leukemia and ITP), with platelet counts of at least 50,000, there are reports of good clinical results, but more trials are needed. Meanwhile the standard primary therapies should be tried first, except in cases of known lack of platelet responsiveness after multiple transfusions.

Chronic renal failure and chronic liver disease

In uremia, DDAVP shortens bleeding time, correcting it in 70% of patients, and is clinically effective. It releases vWf mainly in large multimers, and is better than cryoprecipitate.

In chronic liver disease, DDAVP also shortens bleeding time, but evidence for its hemostatic effect is meagre. Addition of DDAVP to terlipressin gave no extra benefit in the treatment of variceal bleeding. Opinions differed on the advisability of the use of DDAVP to control bleeding in patients with liver disease.

Blood Loss after Surgery

If major blood loss is expected in surgery, then aprotinin, which is highly effective and free of side effects, must be the first choice. DDAVP may be an alternative to aprotinin where the risk of anaphylaxis is high, but more evidence is needed of its efficacy in specific types of surgery.

Children with acyanotic congenital heart disease and acquired vWf disease have long bleeding times. For them DDAVP is beneficial, and the disease is lost after corrective surgery.

Blood and Plasma Donors

Yields of Factor VIII can be greatly increased when donors are stimulated with DDAVP, but opinions differed about the ethics of doing so. Use of DDAVP to enhance the clotting factor yield in the manufacture of cryoprecipitate is thought to be of benefit in specific programmes designed to limit recipient exposure to a small number of donors.

Future growth of these procedures will most likely occur in developing countries, but it was thought that the unit cost of DDAVP would have to decrease substantially before it could be financially feasible.

ANTIHEMOSTATIC DRUGS AND DDAVP

DDAVP should not be used as a treatmentfor prolonged bleeding times in patients using antithrombotic drugs (such as aspirin, ticlopidine, heparin, streptokinase or tPA) While the risk of thrombotic complications after DDAVP is small, it must be kept in mind that these are high risk patients who are taking antithrombotic drugs to prevent or treat acute episodes of arterial thrombosis; hence, clinicians are advised to weigh the benefits against the risks for each individual.

DRUG COMBINATIONS

Initial studies have shown that ethamsylate (a Congo red derivative) added to DDAVP can enhance the bleeding time response in patients who respond poorly to DDAVP alone. This approach may be continued with other drugs, but further studies of this and of other combinations are warranted.

SIDE EFFECTS

In general, the hemodynamic effects associated with hemostatic doses of DDAVP are not clinically important. Also, water intoxication and hyponatremia are relatively rare, except in infants under 18 months old, in whom renal excretory mechanisms are immature. Monitoring of serum osmolarity or sodium levels is recommended in children up to the age of 3-4 years. Caution should always be exercised when DDAVP is given before, during or after administration of hypotonic fluids.

Thrombotic events have rarely been reported with hemostatic doses of DDAVP. However, the thrombotic risk of DDAVP is not known. At present patients with overt atherosclerotic disease should not be given DDAVP unless the benefits clearly outweigh the risks.

FUTURE RESEARCH

DDAVP is a very effective therapeutic agent, and new compounds offering only marginal improvements would seem to be unnecessary. However, an analogue completely free of antidiuretic effect would be a clear step forward.

Several species of monkey, including the marmoset, cynomolgus, and rhesus monkey, have emerged as good animal models in which to study DDAVP/clotting factor relationships. Of these the rhesus monkey is the most studied. The rat remains a controversial model.

Interest was also expressed in further elucidation of the precise mechanisms of clotting factor release and bleeding time shortening. Specific areas include:

- sites and mechanisms of Factor VIII and tPA release,
- the roles of cGMP, PAF, P-selectin, 13′ HODE, and other messengers.
- demonstration of mRNAs for different specific vascular vasopressin receptors related to the release of clotting factors into the circulation.

INDEX

The manufacturer's authorised representative in the EU is Springer Nature Customer Service Centre GmbH, Europaplatz 3, 69115 Heidelberg, Germany. If you have any concerns regarding our products, please contact ProductSafety@springernature.com

Printed and bound by CPI Group (UK) Ltd, Croydon, CR0 4YY
23/04/2026
02095607-0009